New Frontiers in Cataract Surgery Research

New Frontiers in
Cataract Surgery Research

Edited by Lorenzo Fernandez

hayle
medical

New York

Hayle Medical,
750 Third Avenue, 9th Floor,
New York, NY 10017, USA

Visit us on the World Wide Web at:
www.haylemedical.com

ISBN: 978-1-63241-707-7

Cataloging-in-Publication Data

New frontiers in cataract surgery research / edited by Lorenzo Fernandez.
    p. cm.
Includes bibliographical references and index.
ISBN 978-1-63241-707-7
1. Cataract--Surgery. 2. Cataract--Surgery--Research.
3. Cataract--Surgery--Complications. I. Fernandez, Lorenzo.
RE451 .N49 2019
617.742--dc23

Table of Contents

Preface

I am honored to present to you this unique book which encompasses the most up-to-date data in the field. I was extremely pleased to get this opportunity of editing the work of experts from across the globe. I have also written papers in this field and researched the various aspects revolving around the progress of the discipline. I have tried to unify my knowledge along with that of stalwarts from every corner of the world, to produce a text which not only benefits the readers but also facilitates the growth of the field.

Cataract surgery is the procedure done for the removal of the opacified natural lens of the eye and its replacement with an artificial intraocular lens. Unless treated, cataract leads to a loss of vision or vision impairment. During cataract surgery, the cloudy cataract lens is removed by emulsification or by cutting it out. High volume, minimally invasive, small incision phacoemulsification is the standard cataract surgery procedure. Cataract surgeries are performed under local anesthesia and usually done in an outpatient setting. After the surgery, anti-inflammatory and antibiotic eye drops are used. This book is compiled in such a manner, that it will provide in-depth knowledge about the theory and practice of cataract surgery. It presents researches and studies performed by experts across the globe. For all readers who are interested in cataract surgery, the case studies included in this book will serve as an excellent guide to develop a comprehensive understanding.

Finally, I would like to thank all the contributing authors for their valuable time and contributions. This book would not have been possible without their efforts. I would also like to thank my friends and family for their constant support.

Editor

Extensive bilateral corneal edema 6 weeks after cataract surgery: Keratopathy due to *Asclepias physocarpa*

Kazuki Matsuura[1*], Shiro Hatta[2], Yuki Terasaka[1] and Yoshitsugu Inoue[3]

Abstract

Background: Surgeons may be unaware of the ability of plant toxins to cause corneal damage. Therefore, corneal damage following intraocular surgery due to plant toxins may be misdiagnosed as postoperative infection.

Case presentation: A 74-year-old man presented with hyperemia and reduced visual acuity in both eyes 6 weeks after uneventful cataract surgery. We observed extensive hyperemia and corneal stromal edema with Descemet's folds in both eyes.
After obtaining a detailed patient history, we diagnosed plant toxin-induced corneal edema due to *Asclepias physocarpa*, which can induce corneal edema by inhibiting the Na^+/K^+ ATPase activity of the corneal endothelium. Antimicrobial and steroid eye drops and an oral steroid were prescribed accordingly. Symptons began to improve on day 3 and had almost completely resolved by day 6. At 1 month, the patient had fully recovered without any sequelae.

Conclusion: The correct diagnosis was possible in the present case as symptoms were bilateral and the patient was able to report his potential exposure to plant toxins. However, if the symptoms had been unilateral and the patient had been unaware of these toxins, he may have undergone unnecessary surgical interventions to treat non-existent postoperative endophthalmitis.

Keywords: Cataract surgery, Endophthalmitis, Asclepias physocarpa, Case report

Background

Bacterial endophthalmitis is a clinically significant condition that should be considered in patients complaining of vision loss accompanied by acute extensive inflammation in the anterior segment of the eye within a few weeks of cataract surgery. Frequent examinations are generally required in addition to antibiotic treatment, with emergency surgery often required. We experienced case of corneal edema accompanied by extensive inflammation occurring 6 weeks after uneventful bilateral cataract surgery. In the present case, we successfully diagnosed plant toxin-induced corneal edema [1–3] by obtaining a detailed patient history and thereby avoiding unnecessary surgical interventions.

Case presentation

A 74-year-old man with no history of uveitis, keratitis, or allergic eye disease underwent uneventful bilateral cataract surgery with one day interval in August 2015. His best corrected distant visual acuity (CDVA) following surgery was 1.0 and 1.2 in the right and left eyes, respectively (Fig. 1). Intraocular pressures and the number of corneal endothelial cells ($2301/mm^2$ in the right eye and $2171/mm^2$ in the left) were within the normal range. The patient reported hyperemia and reduced visual acuity in both eyes one evening at 6 weeks postoperatively and visited Maejima eye clinic the following day. On examination, extensive hyperemia and corneal stromal edema with Descemet's folds were observed in both eyes. His CDVA was 0.2 in both eyes, and central corneal thicknesses were 786 μm and 756 μm in the right and left eyes, respectively (Fig. 2). Intraocular pressure measurements and detailed observations of the anterior chamber were not possible due to the presence of corneal edema. We first suspected bacterial endophthalmitis;

* Correspondence: matsuura.kzk@gmail.com; matsu224@ncn-k.net
[1]Nojima Hospital, 2714-1, Sesaki-machi, Kurayoshi-city, Tottori 682-0863, Japan
Full list of author information is available at the end of the article

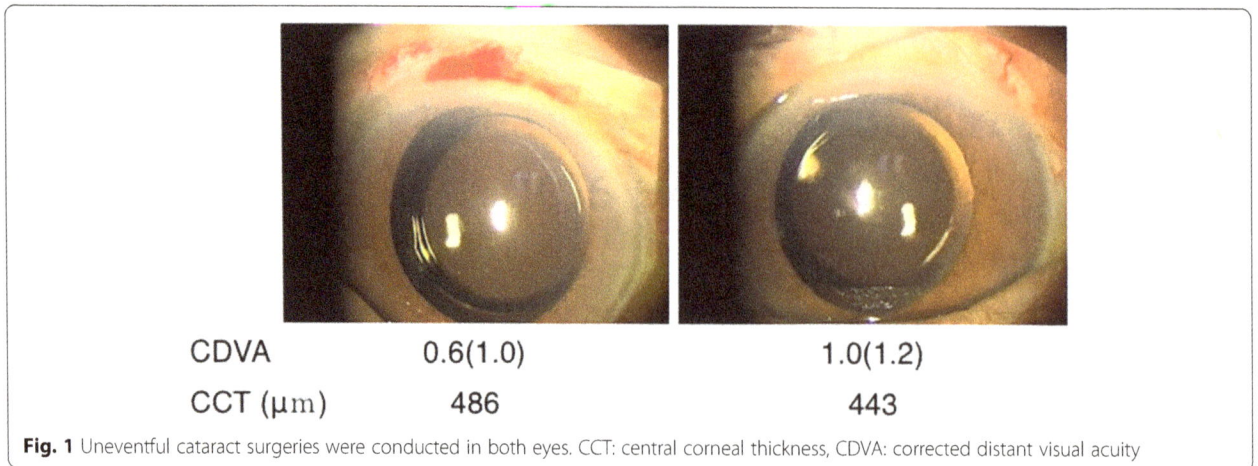

CDVA	0.6(1.0)	1.0(1.2)
CCT (μm)	486	443

Fig. 1 Uneventful cataract surgeries were conducted in both eyes. CCT: central corneal thickness, CDVA: corrected distant visual acuity

however, we considered this an atypical case due to the simultaneous development of symptoms in both eyes 6 weeks postoperatively. No apparent vitreous opacity, retinal hemorrhage, or vasculitis was evident. After obtaining a detailed patient history, it was apparent the patient had performed gardening work during the day of onset. The patient had been engaged in the cultivation and sale of ornamental plants and had heard of eye toxicity on exposure to certain plants. We requested the patient list the plants he had handled and conducted a literature search. His clinical symptoms were consistent with those reported for corneal damage due to *Asclepias physocarpa*[1]. We therefore diagnosed plant toxin-induced corneal edema accordingly. His eyes were initially thoroughly rinsed with normal saline. Topical levofloxacin 1.5% (6 times/day) and bethamethasone 0.1% (6 times/day) were administered, and he was re-evaluated daily on an outpatient basis. Small doses (10 mg) of oral steroids were added as the presence of retinal and vitreal inflammation could not be completely excluded.

The next day, conjunctival injection and corneal edema had increased, and his CDVA had decreased to 0.05 and 0.03 in the right and left eyes, respectively (Fig. 3). Corneal edema began to improve on day 3 and had almost completely resolved by day 6. The oral steroid was ceased immediately after recovery of the visibility (day5).

On day 8, his CDVA had recovered to 1.0 in both eyes (Fig. 4). No clinical signs were evident at 1 month. The intraocular pressure and number of corneal endothelial cells ($2171/mm^2$ in the right eye and $2247/mm^2$ in the left) were within the normal range.

Discussion

A. physocarpa, commonly known as tropic and subtropic milkweed, is a plant species native to tropical America and belongs to the genus *Asclepias* of the family *Apocynaceae* (Fig. 5). The plants of the *Asclepias* genus are widely distributed as horticultural or ornamental plants in Japan and other countries, and latex from their stems

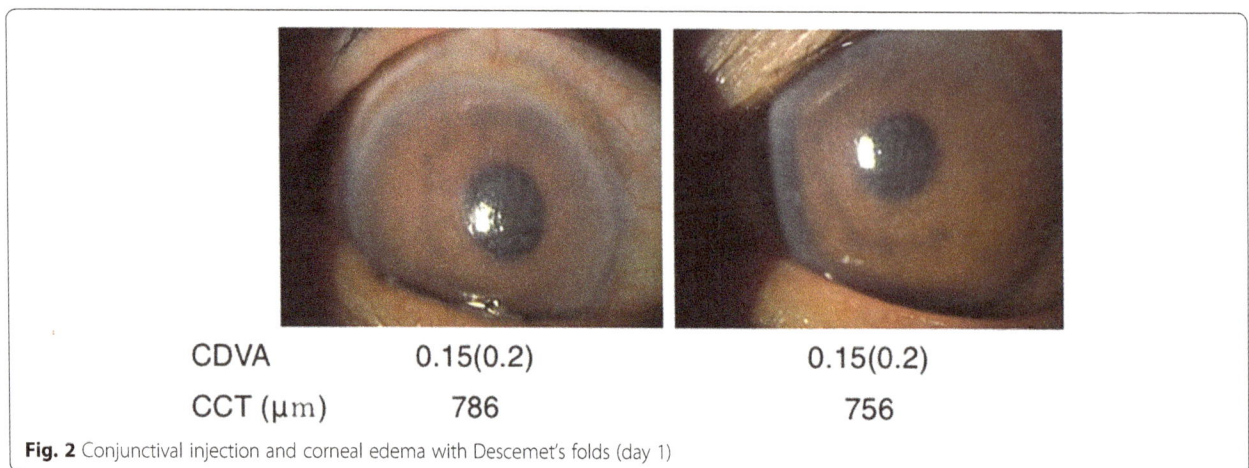

CDVA	0.15(0.2)	0.15(0.2)
CCT (μm)	786	756

Fig. 2 Conjunctival injection and corneal edema with Descemet's folds (day 1)

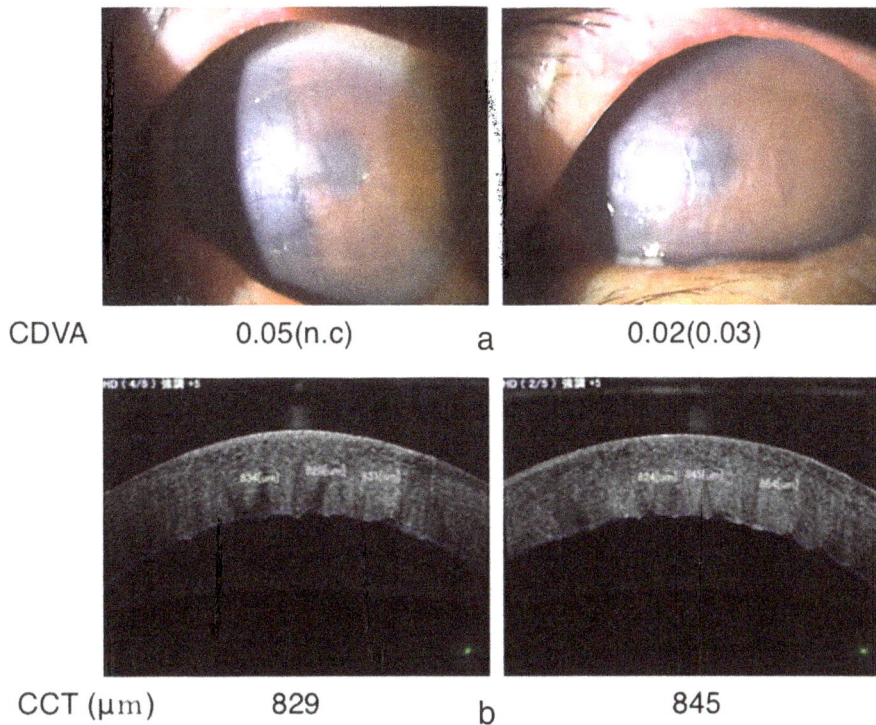

Fig. 3 a. Conjunctival injection and severe corneal edema with Descemet's folds (day 2). **b**. Anterior segment optical coherence tomography (SS-1000, TOMEY Inc, Aichi, Japan). Central corneal thickness measurements were 829 μm and 845 μm for the right and left eyes, respectively (day 2). CCT: central corneal thickness, CDVA: corrected distant visual acuity n. c: non corrigunt

has been shown to contain toxic components termed cardenolides. To our knowledge, only a few cases of cardiolides toxicity have been previously reported [1–3], and general ophthalmologists are unaware of these plants. In corneal endothelial cells, the Na^+/K^+ ATPase actively transports Na^+ from inside of the cells into the anterior chamber to create an osmotic pressure gradient; thereby resulting in the active transport of water from inside the corneal stroma to the anterior chamber. The corneal stromal edema obsereved in the present case was attributable to corneal endothelial dysfunction caused by suppression of the Na^+ active transport by cardenolides in the stem latex, thereby inhibiting the Na^+/K^+ ATPase [4].

Chakraborty et al. reported a case of *A. curassavica* exposure in which the patient rapidly attained remission with the use of artificial tear eye drops only [2]. Amiran et al. reported a case of *A. fruticosa* exposure in which the clinical signs showed marked rapid improvement after the use of 0.1% topical dexamethasone [3]. Pina et al. reported a case of *A. physocarpa* exposure in which almost complete resolution was obtained using topical dexamethasone, ofloxacin, and artificial tears. Pina et al. suggested the possibility of abnormal endothelial morphology as a sequelae at 6 months follow-up, although the cell count was within the normal range (2119 cells/mm^2).

The use of topical steroids may increase the activity of the Na^+/K^+ pump in corneal endothelial cells [5] and thus have utility in the treatment of plant-induced corneal edema. Therefore, we modelled our treatment on the approach reported by Pina et al. [1], with the patient almost completely recovering within 6 days. Our patient fully recovered without any sequelae including any damage to corneal endothelial cells.

Few plants such as those in the genus *Asclepias* have been reported to cause corneal damage. In a report of 7 cases of eye damage caused by *Euphorbia* plants, aggressive antibacterial and anti-inflammatory treatments were considered necessary as the patients presented with defects in the corneal epithelium and stromal edema, iritis, and other symptoms; with one case ultimately leading to blindness [6].

In a report on 29 cases of eye damage due to *Calotropis procera*, the patients recovered within 3–14 days with maintenance of corneal transparency. Although visual acuity also recovered satisfactorily in the majority cases, endothelial cell counts were decreased in 74% of these cases. Epithelial defects, iritis, and increased ocular pressure were observed in 10, 31, and 24% of cases, respectively [7].

In the present case, the patient did not remember any direct entry of latex into his eyes. As in the present case,

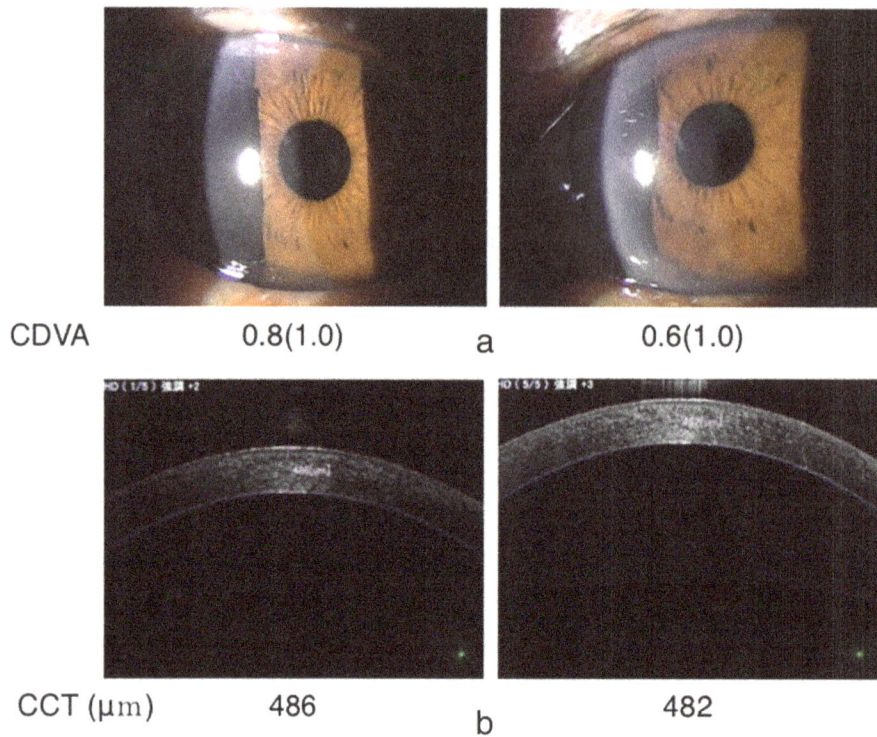

Fig. 4 a. Almost complete resolution of conjunctival injection and corneal edema (day 8). **b**. Anterior segment optical coherence tomography. Central corneal thickness measurements were normalized at 486 μm and 482 μm for the right and left eyes, respectively (day 8). CCT: central corneal thickness, CDVA: corrected distant visual acuity

corneal damage may be caused by contact between the eyes and hands that have been contaminated with latex, even without direct entry of latex droplets into the eyes. Therefore, physicians should proactively determine the involvement of plant toxins and conduct a detailed patient interview in such cases.

Conclusion

Although plants of the genus *Asclepias* are widely distributed, the number of the reports of ophthalmic disease due to plant toxins is surprisingly low. This may be attributable to the unfamiliarity of ophthalmologists to plant-based toxicity. In the present case, the correct diagnosis was possible as symptoms were bilateral and the patient could report his exposure to plant toxins. However, if the symptoms had been unilateral or developed more immediately postoperatively, or if the patient had been unaware of plant toxins, he may have undergone unnecessary surgical interventions. Although plant toxin-induced corneal damage is rarely encountered, all surgeons should be aware of this significant clinical condition.

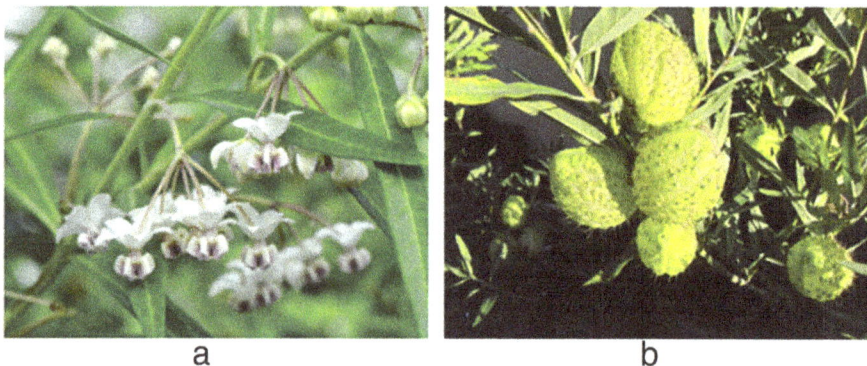

Fig. 5 a. Flower and leaves of *Asclepias physocarpa*. **b**. Follicle of *A. physocarpa*

Abbreviation
CDVA: Corrected distant visual acuity

Acknowledgements
Not applicable

Funding
There was no funding support.

Authors' contributions
KM and YI carried out the writing of the manuscript. SH and YT participated in the collection and interpretation of data. KM and YI carried out critical revision and correction of the manuscript. All authors read and approved the final manuscript.

Competing interests
The authors declare that they have no competing interests.

Consent for publication
Written informed consent was obtained from the patient for publication of this case report accompanying images. A copy of written consent is available for review by the Editor of this journal.

Author details
[1]Nojima Hospital, 2714-1, Sesaki-machi, Kurayoshi-city, Tottori 682-0863, Japan. [2]Maejima ganka, 226, Motomachi, Tottori-city, Tottori 680-0037, Japan. [3]Tottori University, 36-1, Nishi-cho, Yonago-city, Tottori 683-504, Japan.

References
1. Pina S, Pedrosa C, Santos C, Feijóo B, Pego P, Vendrell C, Santos MJ, Prieto I. Ocular toxicity secondary to asclepias physocarpa: the balloon plant. Case Rep Ophthalmol Med. 2014;2014:829469. doi:10.1155/2014/829469.
2. Chakraborty S, Siegenthaler J, Büchi ER. Corneal edema due to Asclepias curassavica. Arch Ophthalmol. 1995;113:974–5.
3. Amiran MD, Lang Y, Yeung SN. Corneal endothelial toxicity secondary to Asclepias fruticosa. Eye (Lond). 2011;25:961–3. doi:10.1038/eye.2011.59.
4. Zhang RR, Tian HY, Tan YF, Chung TY, Sun XH, Xia X, Ye WC, Middleton DA, Fedosova N, Esmann M, Tzen JT, Jiang RW. Structures, chemotaxonomic significance, cytotoxic and Na(+), K(+)-ATPase inhibitory activities of new cardenolides from Asclepias curassavica. Org Biomol Chem. 2014; 12:8919–29. doi:10.1039/c4ob01545b.
5. Hatou S, Yamada M, Mochizuki H, Shiraishi A, Joko T, Nishida T. The effects of dexamethasone on the Na, K-ATPase activity and pump function of corneal endothelial cells. Curr Eye Res. 2009;34:347–54. doi:10.1080/02713680902829624.
6. Eke T, Al-Husainy S, Raynor MK. The spectrum of ocular inflammation caused by euphorbia plant sap. Arch Ophthalmol. 2000;118:13–6.
7. Basak SK, Bhaumik A, Mohanta A, Singhal P. Ocular toxicity by latex of Calotropis procera (Sodom apple). Indian J Ophthalmol. 2009;57:232–4. doi:10.4103/0301-4738.49402.

2

Influence of corneal power on intraocular lens power of the second eye in the SRK/T formula in bilateral cataract surgery

Young Choi[1], Youngsub Eom[1,2]*(iD), Jong Suk Song[1] and Hyo Myung Kim[1]

Abstracts

Background: To evaluate the effect of different adjustments of the refractive outcome of the first eye according to corneal power (K) in order to improve the intraocular lens (IOL) power calculation of the second eye in the SRK/T formula.

Methods: One hundred thirty-four patients who underwent uncomplicated bilateral, sequential phacoemulsification with AcrySof IQ implantation were enrolled. The optimal partial adjustment of the refractive outcome of the first eye according to K was retrospectively analyzed using a regression formula.

Results: In all patients, the optimal partial adjustment of the refractive outcome of the first eye was calculated as 56%. For K values between 42.8 D and 44.6 D, the optimal partial adjustment was calculated as 30%; however, this adjustment of the first eye did not significantly improve the refractive outcome in the second eye of the subgroup with K values between 42.8 D and 44.6 D. For K values greater than 44.6 D or less than 42.8 D, the optimal partial adjustments were calculated as 69% and 81%, respectively. According to these results, the adjustment of the first eye significantly improved the refractive outcome in the second eye from 0.36 to 0.26 D ($P < 0.001$) in the entire data set. This result was significantly lower than that using a single partial adjustment (56%) (0.28 D; $P = 0.027$).

Conclusions: For K values greater than 44.6 D or less than 42.8 D, an approximately 70–80% adjustment of the first eye error should be considered. In contrast, for K values between 42.8 D and 44.6 D, a 30% or less adjustment should be considered in the SRK/T formula.

Keywords: Bilateral cataract extraction, Corneal power, Intraocular lens power, SRK/T formula

Background

Postoperative vision after cataract surgery has been greatly improved by advances in surgical techniques, precise biometry techniques, and intraocular lens (IOL) power calculation formulas [1–7]; however, the refractive error is still a major concern in cataract surgery.

A previous study demonstrated that using corneal power (K)-specific constants improved the refractive outcomes predicted by the Sanders-Retzlaff-Kraff (SRK)/T formula because it predicts a myopic refractive error for a steep cornea and a hyperopic refractive error for a flat cornea [4]. In that study, the refractive error showed a distribution between 0.25 D to −1.00 D for K values between 46.0 and 47.0 D. In cases of bilateral, sequential cataract surgery, previous studies have shown that the refractive outcome of the first eye can be used to improve the IOL calculation for the second eye due to the symmetry between the two eyes [8–10]. Thus, if the first eye shows a − 1.00 D myopic shift with a K of 47 D, the second eye is likely to show a similar myopic shift, which is different from the average refractive error. Therefore, we hypothesized that increasing the magnitude of the adjustment for the first eye error for a steep or flat cornea would improve the refractive outcome in the second eye when using the SRK/T formula. This study was designed to evaluate the effect of different adjustments of the refractive outcome of the first eye according to K for improving the IOL power calculation of the second eye in the SRK/T formula.

* Correspondence: hippotate@hanmail.net
[1]Department of Ophthalmology, Korea University College of Medicine, Seoul, South Korea
[2]Department of Ophthalmology, Ansan Hospital, Korea University College of Medicine, 123, Jeokgeum-ro, Danwon-gu, Ansan-si, Gyeonggi-do 15355, South Korea

Methods

Study population

This retrospective cross-sectional study included 268 eyes from 134 patients who underwent uncomplicated bilateral, sequential phacoemulsification with IOL implantation at Korea University Anam Hospital, Seoul, Korea between April 2008 and December 2015. An AcrySof IQ (SN60WF, Alcon, Fort Worth, TX, USA) IOL was implanted in both eyes of each patient. Patients who had best corrected visual acuities (BCVA) better than or equal to 20/40 in both eyes after cataract surgery were included. Patients with a traumatic cataract, prior ocular surgery (such as penetrating keratoplasty or refractive surgery), complicated surgery (such as posterior capsule rupture), or postoperative complications were excluded. Institutional Review Board (IRB) approval was obtained from Korea University Anam Hospital, Seoul, Korea for this study. All research and data collection methods followed the tenets of the Helsinki agreement. The data used in this study were de-identified for the sake of privacy for subjects.

Patient examination

All measurements were taken by a trained ophthalmic examiner who measured the preoperative axial length (AL) and K with optical biometry using an IOLMaster version 5.02 or higher (Carl Zeiss Meditech, Jena, Germany). IOL power was calculated using the SRK/T formula of the IOLMaster. The data-adjusted A-constant for AcrySof IQ was 119.0, calculated in our previous study using the Haigis constant optimization Excel spreadsheet (Microsoft Inc., Redmond, WA, USA) for optical biometry [4, 11].

Postoperative uncorrected visual acuity (UCVA), manifest refraction, and BCVA were measured at postoperative visits between three and 10 weeks.

Surgical technique

Phacoemulsification and IOL implantation were performed under topical anesthesia with 0.5% proparacaine hydrochloride (Alcaine; Alcon, Fort Worth, TX, USA) via a 2.2 or 2.75 mm temporal clear corneal incision by an experienced surgeon (HM.K.). The IOL was inserted into the capsular bag.

Main outcome measure(s)

The refractive error was defined as the difference between the observed refractive spherical equivalent three to 10 weeks postoperatively and the predicted refraction (spherical equivalent) by IOLMaster using the SRK/T formula (refractive error = postoperative spherical equivalent − preoperative predicted refraction). The mean absolute refractive error (MAE) was defined as the mean absolute value of the refractive error.

The optimal partial adjustment of the refractive error of the first eye according to K for improving the IOL calculation of the second eye was analyzed in retrospect using the corrective regression formula [9]: $Rx_{cor} = Rx_{exp} + \beta \times Px_{err}$, where Rx_{cor} is the observed refractive spherical equivalent of the second eye, Rx_{exp} is the expected refractive prediction of the second eye, Px_{err} is the refractive error of the first eye, and β is a correlation coefficient that is a magnitude of adjustment of first-eye error for improving the refractive outcome of the second eye.

The adjusted MAE of the second eye without considering K (MAE_{WCP}) was defined as the MAE of the second eye using a partial adjustment for the refractive error of the first eye with a calculated correlation coefficient from the entire data set by the corrective regression formula. The adjusted MAE of the second eye according to K (MAE_{ACP}) was defined as the MAE of the second eye using a partial adjustment for the refractive error of the first eye with calculated correlation coefficients for within cut-off and outside cut-off values. To decide the K cut-off value, the correlation coefficient for the partial adjustment was calculated from the cumulative subgroups based on K. Each cumulative subgroup was made according to both an increase in K from 42 to 47 D and a decrease in K from 47 to 42 D at 0.2 D intervals. After that, the lower and upper cut-off K values, which showed a deviation from the correlation coefficient increasing or decreasing trend, were decided.

Statistical analysis

Descriptive statistics were obtained using the Statistical Package for the Social Sciences (SPSS) version 21.0 (IBM Corp., Armonk, NY, USA). The Kolmogorov-Smirnov test was performed to assess data distribution normality. Paired t-tests were used for parametric continuous variables and the Wilcoxon signed rank test was used for nonparametric continuous variables according to the results of normality distribution tests. Repeated-measures analysis of variance (ANOVA) with the Bonferroni correction were performed to assess statistical differences among the unadjusted MAE, MAE_{WCP}, and MAE_{ACP}. Results were considered statistically significant if the p-value was less than 0.05. A post-hoc power analysis using the Wilcoxon signed-rank test option of G*power, version 3.1.9.2 (Franz Paul, Kiel, Germany), was conducted to determine study power.

Results

One hundred thirty-four patients were included in this study. Of the 134 patients, 50 (37.3%) were men and 84 were women. The mean age (± SD) was 68.6 ± 8.5 years (range, 43 to 90 years). The mean K, AL, calculated IOL power, preoperative predicted refraction, postoperative refraction, and refractive error are shown in Table 1.

Table 1 Clinical characteristics of patients and eyes included in the present study ($n = 134$)

Parameter	Patients	First eye	Second eye	P value[a]
Age, years (SD)	68.6 (8.5)			–
Sex (Male:Female) (%)	50 (37.3): 84 (62.7)			–
Corneal power, D (SD)		44.22 (1.43)	44.20 (1.47)	0.687
Axial length, mm (SD)		23.55 (0.95)	23.52 (0.89)	0.691[b]
IOL power, D (SD)		20.8 (2.7)	20.9 (2.4)	0.395[b]
Predicted refraction, D (SD)		−0.26 (0.24)	−0.26 (0.23)	0.847
Refraction at postop 3 to 10 weeks, D (SD)		−0.22 (0.55)	−0.21 (0.50)	0.884[b]
Refractive error, D (SD)		0.04 (0.49)	0.04 (0.45)	0.990

Data are mean (SD) except for parameter sex, which are n (%)
SD standard deviation, D diopters, OL intraocular lens
[a]Paired t-test was used for parametric continuous variables
[b]Wilcoxon signed rank test was used for nonparametric continuous variables

There was a significant correlation in K ($R^2 = 0.915$, $P < 0.001$), AL ($R^2 = 0.912$, $P < 0.001$), and IOL power ($R^2 = 0.883$, $P < 0.001$) between the first and second eyes. There was also a significant correlation between the refractive error of the first and second eyes ($R^2 = 0.366$, $P < 0.001$; Fig. 1). According to the corrective regression formula[6], the correlation coefficient (β) was 0.56 in all patients using the SRK/T formula. This means that the

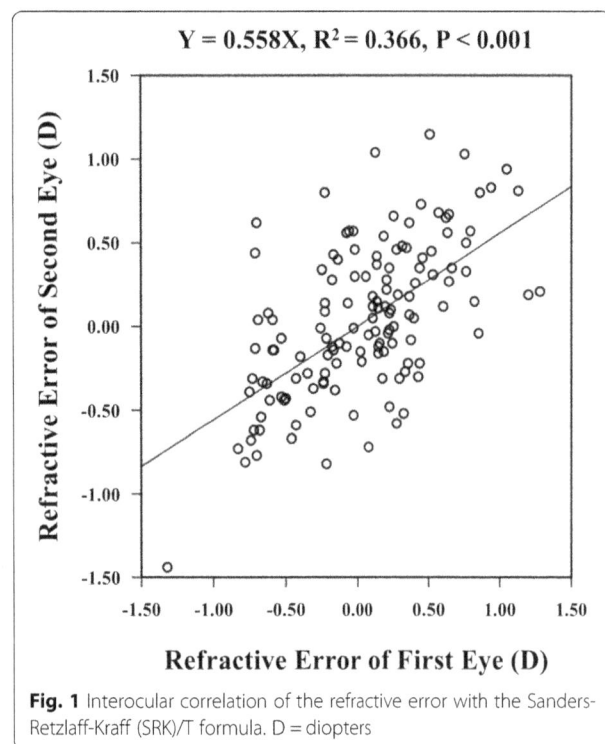

Fig. 1 Interocular correlation of the refractive error with the Sanders-Retzlaff-Kraff (SRK)/T formula. D = diopters

optimal partial adjustment of the refractive error of the first eye for IOL calculation of the second eye was determined to be 56%. According to these results, the MAE of second eyes decreased from 0.36 to 0.28 D ($P < 0.001$; Table 2).

There was a very weak positive correlation between AL and refractive error ($R^2 = 0.025$, $P = 0.010$; Fig. 2a). On the other hand, a negative correlation was observed between K and refractive error ($R^2 = 0.140$, $P < 0.001$; Fig. 2b). According to the regression equation, the refractive error could be zero when K was 44.43 D. As K increased, the refractive error showed a tendency for myopic refractive outcomes. On the contrary, as K decreased, the refractive error showed a tendency for hyperopic refractive outcomes.

Figure 3 shows the correlation coefficients of each cumulative subgroup which were calculated according to both an increase in K from 42 D (heavy line) and a decrease in K from 47 D (light line). The correlation coefficients of the cumulative subgroups tended to decrease as K increased from 42D and tended to decrease as K decreased from 47 D. The lower and upper cut-off K values were determined to be 42.8 and 44.6 D, respectively. The correlation coefficient for values less than the lower cut-off (K < 42.8 D) was calculated as 0.81 and that for values over the upper cut-off (44.6 D ≤ K) was calculated as 0.69. The lowest correlation coefficient was observed between 42.8 and 44.6 D (correlation coefficient = 0.30).

The MAE_{ACP} (± SD) (0.26 ± 0.23 D) was smaller than the MAE_{WCP} (0.28 ± 0.22 D) in the entire dataset ($P = 0.027$; Table 2 and Fig. 4). In a subgroup analysis, neither the MAE_{WCP} nor MAE_{ACP} of the subgroup within the cut-off values improved the refractive outcome in the second eye. Otherwise, both the MAE_{WCP} and MAE_{ACP} of the subgroup outside the cut-off values significantly improved the refractive outcome from 0.40 D to 0.24 D and 0.21 D, respectively ($P < 0.001$, $P < 0.001$, respectively). The MAE_{ACP} (0.21 ± 0.21 D) was significantly smaller than the MAE_{WCP} (0.24 ± 0.20 D) in the subgroup outside of the cut-off values ($P = 0.032$).

The MAE_{ACP} and MAE_{WCP} in the subgroup outside of the cut-off values were used in a post-hoc power analysis. The correlation between the MAE_{ACP} and MAE_{WCP} was 0.925 and the effect size was 0.375. The effect size of 0.375 and a two-tailed alpha of 0.05 in the subgroup analysis with 70 patients led to a power of 0.86.

Discussion

A high degree of interocular symmetry of biometry between the two eyes is helpful in IOL power calculation for the second eye in bilateral sequential cataract surgery [12]. Most patients in this study showed strong interocular correlation with K ($R^2 = 0.915$), AL ($R^2 = 0.912$), and

Table 2 Comparison of the unadjusted mean absolute refractive error (MAE$_{UNADJ}$), adjusted MAE without considering corneal power (MAE$_{WCP}$), and adjusted MAE according to corneal power (MAE$_{ACP}$) of the second eye in each subgroup (Repeated measures ANOVA with Bonferroni correction)

MAE of second eye (D)		Total (n = 134)	Within cut-off values [line break] 42.8D ≤ K < 44.6D (n = 64)	Outside cut-off values [line break] K < 42.8D or 44.6D ≤ K (n = 70)
Unadjusted MAE (MAE$_{UNADJ}$), D (SD)		0.36 (0.27)	0.33 (0.26)	0.40 (0.28)
Adjusted MAE without considering corneal power (MAE$_{WCP}$), D (SD)		0.28 (0.22)	0.33 (0.24)	0.24 (0.20)
Adjusted MAE according to corneal power (MAE$_{ACP}$), D (SD)		0.26 (0.23)	0.31 (0.24)	0.21 (0.21)
P value	MAE$_{UNADJ}$ vs. MAE$_{WCP}$	< 0.001	> 0.999	< 0.001
	MAE$_{UNADJ}$ vs. MAE$_{ACP}$	< 0.001	> 0.999	< 0.001
	MAE$_{WCP}$ vs. MAE$_{ACP}$	0.027	0.549	0.032

D diopters, MAE mean absolute refractive error, K mean corneal power, SD standard deviation

IOL power (R^2 = 0.883). Similarly, Covert et al., [8] showed strong interocular correlations with K (R^2 = 0.88) and AL measurements (R^2 = 0.96) and several other studies have shown a high degree of interocular correlation with K, anterior chamber depth, and AL measurements [10, 12, 13]. Actually, refractive outcome of the second eye was improved using the refractive error observed in the first eye [8–10].

This study evaluated the effect of different adjustments of the refractive error observed in the first eye according to K on the refractive outcome of the second eye using the SRK/T formula. The results showed that the method of different adjustments according to K value significantly improved the refractive outcome of the second eye compared to the method of fixed partial adjustments. When corneal power was not considered, the optimal partial adjustment of the refractive error of the first eye was calculated to be 56% in the entire dataset. The results of the present study using the SRK/T

formula were similar to the previous studies. Covert et al. [8] performed a study demonstrating the effectiveness of a partial adjustment (50%) to the refractive error observed in the first eye for IOL power calculation of the second eye to improve the refractive outcome of the second eye using the Holladay I and SRK II formulas. Olsen [9] demonstrated similar results using the SRK II (56%), SRK/T (38%), and more recent Olsen formulas (27%). Otherwise, there was no benefit to full adjustment of the refractive error of the first eye [8, 13].

Olsen [9] showed that the magnitude of the partial adjustment of refractive outcome of the first eye and the improvement in refractive outcome of the second eye differ depending on the IOL power calculation formula. When the formula was less accurate, more adjustments were needed, and greater benefits were shown after the correction. In the present study, the correlation coefficients of each cumulative subgroup were calculated to determine the cut-off values according to K and the cut-

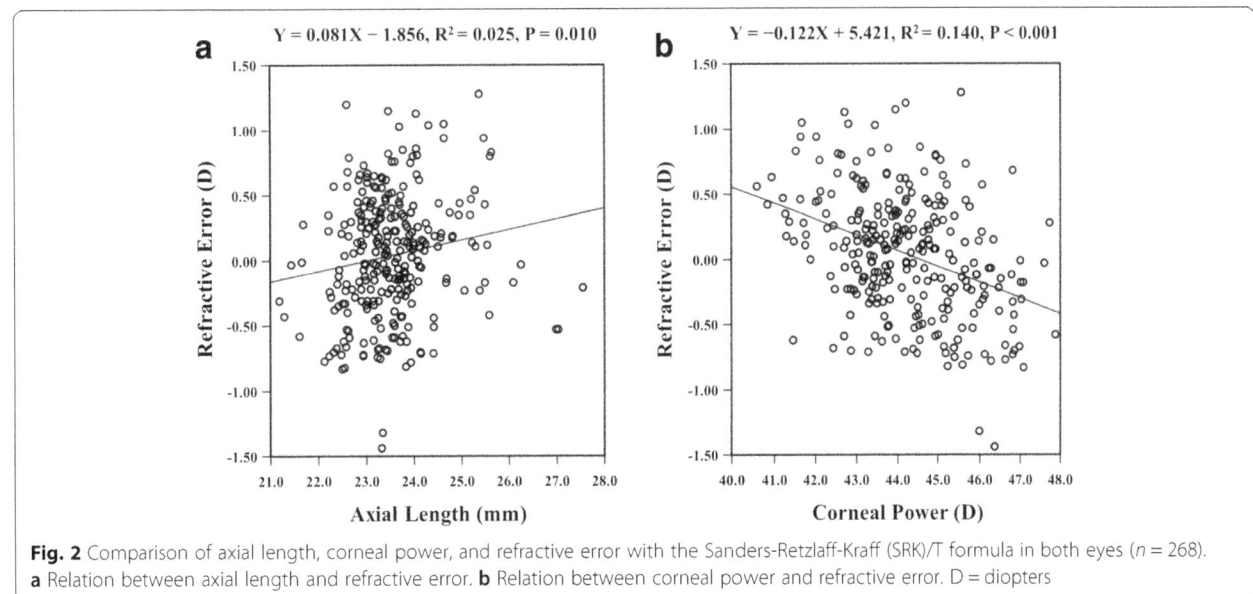

Fig. 2 Comparison of axial length, corneal power, and refractive error with the Sanders-Retzlaff-Kraff (SRK)/T formula in both eyes (n = 268). **a** Relation between axial length and refractive error. **b** Relation between corneal power and refractive error. D = diopters

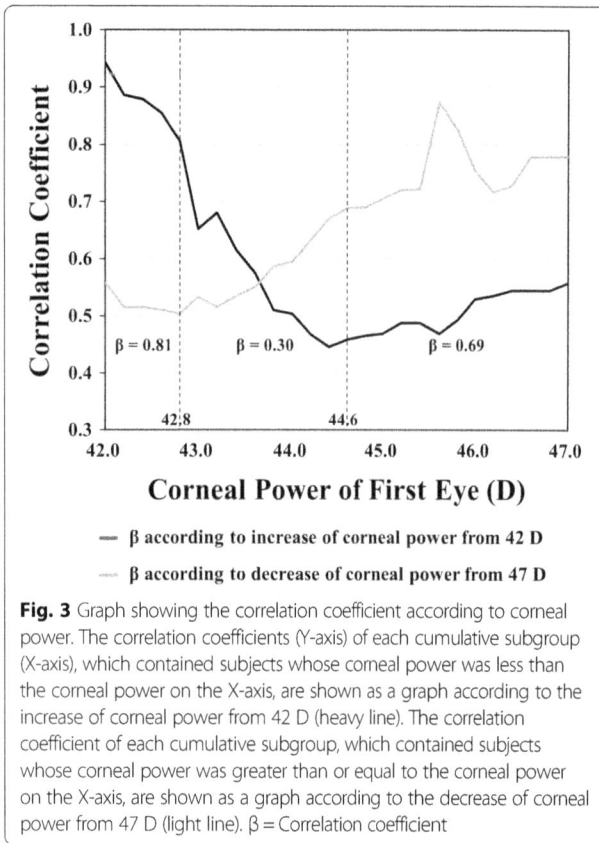

Fig. 3 Graph showing the correlation coefficient according to corneal power. The correlation coefficients (Y-axis) of each cumulative subgroup (X-axis), which contained subjects whose corneal power was less than the corneal power on the X-axis, are shown as a graph according to the increase of corneal power from 42 D (heavy line). The correlation coefficient of each cumulative subgroup, which contained subjects whose corneal power was greater than or equal to the corneal power on the X-axis, are shown as a graph according to the decrease of corneal power from 47 D (light line). β = Correlation coefficient

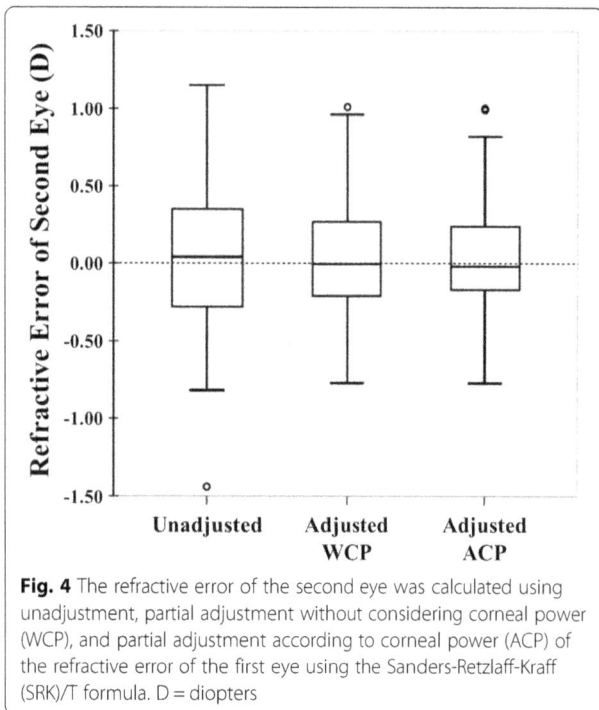

Fig. 4 The refractive error of the second eye was calculated using unadjustment, partial adjustment without considering corneal power (WCP), and partial adjustment according to corneal power (ACP) of the refractive error of the first eye using the Sanders-Retzlaff-Kraff (SRK)/T formula. D = diopters

off values were set at 42.8 D and 44.6D. When the cornea was steeper than the upper cut-off value or flatter than the lower cut-off value, the magnitude of optimal partial adjustment of the first eye refractive error (69%, 81%, respectively) were larger than that of the whole period (56%). The lowest magnitude of optimal partial adjustment (30%) was observed within the cut-off values. There was no benefit to partial adjustment for first eye error within the cut-off values. Otherwise, there was an improvement in the refractive outcome in the subgroups outside of the cut-off values. The MAE_{ACP} showed a greater effect than the MAE_{WCP} in the subgroup outside of the cut-off values. Thus, the magnitude of the partial adjustment of the first eye refractive error and the improvement in refractive outcome of the second eye could differ depending on the K in the SRK/T formula.

Sheard et al., [14] demonstrated that the SRK/T formula has non-physiologic behavior in the corrected AL and corneal height calculation. According to the non-physiologic behavior in the corneal height calculation, [14] the predicted corneal height tends to be overestimated as K increases and tends to be underestimated as K decreases in the SRK/T formula. Our previous study [4] and the present study demonstrated a negative correlation between K and the refractive error using the SRK/T formula. In the present study, the refractive error was smallest when K was 44.43 D. The refractive outcome became more myopic as K increased and became more hyperopic as K decreased. These findings were similar to those noted above [14]. These results imply that the accuracy of the SRK/T formula decreases when the cornea becomes steeper or flatter. Therefore, the magnitude of adjustment of the first eye outcome should be changed according to K in the SRK/T formula.

There are some limitations in the present study. First, the sample size was relatively small and medical records were retrospectively reviewed. Second, UCVA, manifest refraction, and BCVA were measured at postoperative visits between three and 10 weeks, due to the retrospective nature of this study [6]. However, a previous study showed that the changes in effective lens position and refractive error of the in-the-bag AcrySof IOL were insignificant from 1 week to 6 months after surgery [15]. Third, there were a few patients who had severe differences in K between both eyes, and the differences in K were not considered in the present study. Therefore, a study on the optimal partial adjustment of the refractive error of the first eye according to K with a large number of patients will be necessary.

Conclusions

Partial adjustment of the refractive error of the first eye according to the regression formula improved the refractive outcome in the second eye. When the cornea is steep or flat, an approximately 70–80% magnitude adjustment of the first eye error should be considered in the SRK/T formula. On the contrary, when K is within the range of cut-off values, a magnitude adjustment of 30% or less should be considered.

Abbreviations
AL: Axial length; BCVA: Best corrected visual acuity; IOL: Intraocular lens; K: Corneal power; MAE: Mean absolute refractive error; MAE$_{ACP}$: Adjusted MAE of the second eye according to K; MAE$_{WCP}$: Adjusted MAE of the second eye without considering K; SRK/T: Sanders-Retzlaff-Kraff /T; UCVA: Uncorrected visual acuity; β: Correlation coefficient

Acknowledgements
None

Funding
This paper was supported by Bumsuk Academic Research Fund in 2017. The funding source had no role in the design or conduct of this research.

Authors' contributions
Y.C. has made substantial contributions to acquisition of data and been involved in drafting the manuscript. Y.E. has made substantial contributions to conception and design, acquisition of data, and analysis and interpretation of data, been involved in drafting the manuscript and revising it, and given final approval of the version to be published. JS.S. and HM.K. have made substantial contributions to analysis and interpretation of data and given final approval of the version to be published. All authors have read and approved the final version of this manuscript.

Consent for publication
Not applicable (no identifying patient data).

Competing interests
The authors declare that they have no competing interests.

References
1.   Mamalis N. Intraocular lens power accuracy: how are we doing? J Cataract Refract Surg. 2003;29(1):1–3.
2.   Olsen T. Improved accuracy of intraocular lens power calculation with the Zeiss IOLMaster. Acta Ophthalmol Scand. 2007;85(1):84–7.
3.   Olsen T. Calculation of intraocular lens power: a review. Acta Ophthalmol Scand. 2007;85(5):472–85.
4.   Eom Y, Kang SY, Song JS, Kim HM. Use of corneal power-specific constants to improve the accuracy of the SRK/T formula. Ophthalmology. 2013;120(3):477–81.
5.   Eom Y, Hwang HS, Hwang JY, Song JS, Kim HM. Posterior vault distance of Ciliary Sulcus-implanted three-piece intraocular lenses according to Ciliary Sulcus diameter. Am J Ophthalmol. 2017;175:52–9.
6.   Eom Y, Song JS, Kim HM. Modified Haigis formula effective lens position equation for Ciliary Sulcus-implanted intraocular lenses. Am J Ophthalmol. 2016;161:142–9. e141-142
7.   Eom Y, Kang SY, Song JS, Kim YY, Kim HM. Comparison of Hoffer Q and Haigis formulae for intraocular lens power calculation according to the anterior chamber depth in short eyes. Am J Ophthalmol. 2014;157(4):818–24. e812
8.   Covert DJ, Henry CR, Koenig SB. Intraocular lens power selection in the second eye of patients undergoing bilateral, sequential cataract extraction. Ophthalmology. 2010;117(1):49–54.
9.   Olsen T. Use of fellow eye data in the calculation of intraocular lens power for the second eye. Ophthalmology. 2011;118(9):1710–5.
10. Jivrajka RV, Shammas MC, Shammas HJ. Improving the second-eye refractive error in patients undergoing bilateral sequential cataract surgery. Ophthalmology. 2012;119(6):1097–101.
11. Hill W: IOL power calculations physician downloads. Haigis forrmula optimization. Available at: http://doctor-hill.com/physicians/download.htm. Accessed 11 June 2015.
12. Li Y, Bao FJ. Interocular symmetry analysis of bilateral eyes. J Med Eng Technol. 2014;38(4):179–87.
13. Jabbour J, Irwig L, Macaskill P, Hennessy MP. Intraocular lens power in bilateral cataract surgery: whether adjusting for error of predicted refraction in the first eye improves prediction in the second eye. J Cataract Refract Surg. 2006;32(12):2091–7.
14. Sheard RM, Smith GT, Cooke DL. Improving the prediction accuracy of the SRK/T formula: the T2 formula. J Cataract Refract Surg. 2010;36(11):1829–34.
15. Eom Y, Kang SY, Song JS, Kim HM. Comparison of the actual amount of axial movement of 3 aspheric intraocular lenses using anterior segment optical coherence tomography. J Cataract Refract Surg. 2013;39(10):1528–33.

3

Case of asteroid hyalosis that developed severely reduced vision after cataract surgery

Ryosuke Ochi[1,2], Bumpei Sato[1,2], Seita Morishita[1,2], Yukihiro Imagawa[1,2], Masashi Mimura[2], Masanori Fukumoto[2], Takaki Sato[2], Takatoshi Kobayashi[2], Teruyo Kida[2] and Tsunehiko Ikeda[2*]

Abstract

Background: To report our findings in a patient with asteroid hyalosis (AH) who had a severe reduction of his visual acuity following cataract surgery. The vision was improved by vitreous surgery.

Case presentation: The patient was an 81-year-old man. Following cataract surgery on his left eye, his decimal best-corrected visual acuity (BCVA) was markedly reduced from 0.2 to 0.02. A large number of asteroid bodies (ABs) was observed to be concentrated on the posterior surface of the implanted intraocular lens. Ultrasound B-mode images showed turbidity of the vitreous that was denser in the anterior vitreous where the ABs were concentrated. During vitrectomy, the ABs were observed to be concentrated in the anterior vitreous cavity, and a complete posterior vitreous detachment (PVD) was present. After vitrectomy successfully removed the ABs, the visibility of the fundus improved and the BCVA recovered to 1.0.

Conclusion: We suggest that the visual impairment after the cataract surgery was due to the concentrated ABs in the anterior vitreous cavity. The clustering of the ABs in the anterior vitreous cavity was most likely caused by the PVD that developed during the cataract surgery.

Keywords: Asteroid hyalosis, Cataract surgery, Vitreous surgery, Posterior vitreous detachment

Background

Asteroid hyalosis (AH) is a degenerative vitreous disease that is common among the elderly and was first described by Benson in 1894 [1]. It is characterized by a mild liquefaction of the vitreous body and a reduced likelihood of a posterior vitreous detachment (PVD) [2, 3]. Ophthalmoscopic examinations of eyes with AH show many light-yellow plaques which give the appearance of stars or asteroid bodies (ABs) shining in the night sky. However, the ocular asteroids can be mobile. The presence of the ABs in the vitreous cavity can reduce the visibility of the fundus although they rarely cause vision reduction and myodesopsia [4]. Thus, it is rare for this disease to be treated with vitreous surgery.

We report our findings in a patient with AH whose best-corrected visual acuity (BCVA) decreased severely after cataract surgery but then markedly improved after vitreous surgery.

Case presentation

Patient

An 81-year-old man.

Chief complaint

Decreased vision in the left eye.

History of present illness

The patient underwent phacoemulsification and intraocular lens (Alcon Acosov UV posterior chamber lens; model number, MA 60) implantation for a cataract in his left eye at another hospital on August 26, 2014. Although the surgery was completed without complications, his decimal best-corrected visual acuity (BCVA) decreased from 0.2 to

* Correspondence: tikeda@osaka-med.ac.jp
[2]Department of Ophthalmology, Osaka Medical College, 2-7 Daigaku-machi, Takatsuki City, Osaka 569-8686, Japan
Full list of author information is available at the end of the article

0.02 following the surgery. He was then referred to the Department of Ophthalmology at Osaka Medical College Hospital, Takatsuki, Japan on October 15, 2014.

Past medical history
The patient was not diabetic. He did not report experiencing floaters.

Family history
No significant family history.

Findings on initial ocular examination
His initial examination of the left eye showed that his decimal BCVA was 0.02, the intraocular pressure was 14.0 mmHg, and the intraocular lens was well centered. A dense concentration of ABs was observed in the anterior vitreous cavity of the left eye, and the visibility of the fundus was very poor ophthalmoscopically (Fig. 1a). An ultrasound B-mode examination showed a shadow that appeared to be a cluster of ABs concentrated in the

anterior vitreous cavity (Fig. 1b). Spectrum domain optical coherence tomography (SD-OCT) was attempted but the resulting images were blurred and indistinct.

Follow-up course
On November 4, 2014, the patient underwent vitrectomy on his left eye using a 25-guage system. During the vitrectomy, a complete PVD was detected to be already present, and the ABs were found to be concentrated in the anterior vitreous (Fig. 2a). After injecting triamcinolone acetonide, it was noted that no vitreous gel remained on the retinal surface but cystoid macular edema (CME) was present. The vitreous body including the ABs just posterior to the intraocular lens were excised, and the peripheral vitreous and ABs were removed with compression on the sclera under microscopic coaxial illumination (Fig. 2b).

One day after the vitrectomy, the vision was markedly improved, and at 4-days the BCVA had improved to 0.7. The CME that was detected intraoperatively was still present although the degree of edema was reduced. The CME gradually disappeared, and at 5-months after the vitrectomy, the BCVA had improved to 1.0.

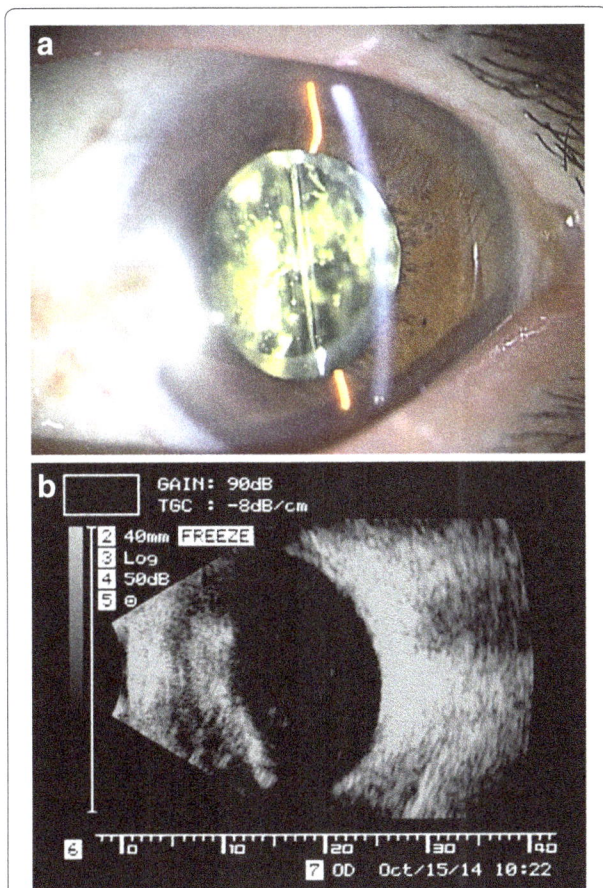

Fig. 1 Ocular findings in a patient with asteroid hyalosis (AH) after successful cataract surgery. The asteroid bodies (ABs) appear to be concentrated in the anterior vitreous cavity of the left eye (a), and an ultrasonic B-mode image shows a shadow that appears to be a cluster of asteroid bodies (ABs) in the anterior vitreous cavity (b)

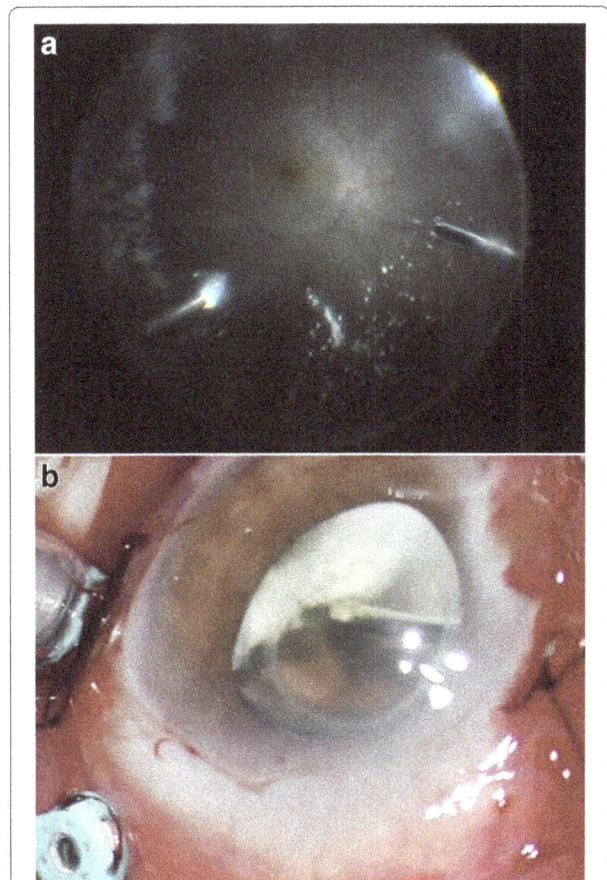

Fig. 2 Intraoperative findings. The ABs are concentrated in the anterior vitreous cavity and a complete posterior vitreous detachment is present (a, b)

Discussion

In general, the ABs have little effect on visual function, and it is rare to treat AH with vitreous surgery. The reason why the subjective symptoms such as decreased vision or floaters rarely occur in eyes with AH is that the density of ABs in the vitreous cavity is relatively low [4]. In addition, the ABs are present only in the vitreous gel and are not present in the liquid vitreous, Cloquet's canal, or posterior to a vitreous detachment [2]. In our case, it is unclear whether the PVD existed before the cataract surgery, but it is more likely that the cataract surgery caused the PVD [5]. We suggest that the visual impairment developed because the PVD forced the residual vitreous to move to the anterior vitreous cavity. This resulted in concentrating the ABs in the anterior vitreous cavity closer to the nodal point of the eye.

Even when the fundus visibility is poor in eyes with AH, it is common for the fluorescein angiographic and OCT images to be clear [6, 7]. In particular, OCT is excellent at detecting macular diseases such as age-related macular degeneration, epiretinal membrane, macular hole, and CME in eyes with AH which are all difficult to detect ophthalmoscopically. Moreover, OCT is quite useful for detecting the changes that cause the vision reduction in AH patients.

In our patient, clear SD-OCT images of the retina could not be obtained prior to the vitreous surgery. We suggest that this was because the ABs were so concentrated in the anterior vitreous cavity near the nodal point that not enough light could pass through the ABs to form a sharp tomographic image. Although the CME may have also caused some of the decreased VA in this eye, the vision did improve significantly despite the presence of the CME after the surgery. Thus, the concentrated ABs in the anterior vitreous were the more likely cause of the reduced vision. However, the true extent of the vision being affected due to asteroid hyalosis may be difficult to explain due to the inability to image the macula before the vitrectomy.

There have been several reports of AH cases in which the BCVA improved after vitreous surgery [8–10]. However, only a few of these studies reported on the exact cause of the reduced vision prior to the surgery. Jingami et al. reported on a AH patient with retinitis pigmentosa who had a decrease in the VA after cataract surgery [11]. Just as in our case, there was a significant improvement of the VA after vitreous surgery. They suggested that the cause of the decreased VA after the cataract surgery was that changes in the AB distribution caused by a change in the shape of the vitreous body due to the cataract surgery. However, it was reported that the posterior vitreous body was not detached when it was examined during vitreous surgery [12, 13]. Reviewing the published cases in which vision was improved by vitreous surgery, we were unable to find publications where the posterior vitreous was clearly detached as it was in our case.

The posterior vitreous is usually not detached in eyes with AH, and in cases of AH accompanied by advanced diabetic retinopathy in particular, there are many cases of extremely strong vitreoretinal adhesions and surgery is known to be very difficult [13]. Mochizuki et al. found that even in AH cases where it initially appeared that a PVD was present, it was common for the vitreous cortex to be found in the posterior retina and for vitreoschisis to be present [3]. However, even in AH cases, there are cases such as our case in which a complete PVD had occurred and the ABs were concentrated in the anterior vitreous. Thus, we suggest that in such cases vitreous surgery should be performed especially if the VA is reduced.

Conclusion

We suggest that the visual impairment after the cataract surgery was due to the concentrated ABs in the anterior vitreous cavity and vitreous surgery should be performed especially in such cases.

Abbreviations
ABs: Asteroid bodies; AH: Asteroid hyalosis; BCVA: Best-corrected visual acuity; CME: Cystoid macular edema; PVD: Posterior vitreous detachment; SD-OCT: Spectrum domain optical coherence tomography

Acknowledgements
The authors wish to thank Professor Emeritus Duco Hamasaki of the Bascom Palmer Eye Institution for discussions and editing the manuscript.

Funding
Not applicable.

Authors' contributions
TI and RO drafted this manuscript, collected the data, and reviewed the literature. BS, YI, SM, MM reviewed the literature. MF, TS and TK interpreted the data,and critically reviewed the manuscript. TI and TK critically reviewed the manuscript finally. All authors read and approved the final manuscript.

Competing interests
The authors declare that they have no competing interests.

Consent for publication
Informed consent was obtained from the patient for publication.

Author details
[1]Department of Ophthalmology, Osaka Kaisei Hospital, Osaka-City, Osaka, Japan. [2]Department of Ophthalmology, Osaka Medical College, 2-7 Daigaku-machi, Takatsuki City, Osaka 569-8686, Japan.

References

1. Benson AH. Disease of the vitreous: A case of monocular asteroid hyalitis. Trans Ophthalmol Soc UK. 1894;14:101–4.
2. Fawzi AA, Vo B, Kriwanek R, et al. Asteroid hyalosis in an autopsy population: The University of California at Los Angeles (UCLA) experience. Arch Ophthalmol. 2005;123(4):486–90.
3. Mochizuki Y, Hata Y, Kita T, et al. Anatomical findings of vitreoretinal interface in eyes with asteroid hyalosis. Graefes Arch Clin Exp Ophthalmol. 2009;247(9):1173–7.
4. Noda S, Hayasaka S, Setogawa T. Patients with asteroid hyalosis and visible floaters. Jpn J Ophthalmol. 1993;37(4):452–5.
5. Hilford D, Hilford M, Mathew A, Polkinghorne PJ. Posterior vitreous detachment following cataract surgery. Eye (Lond). 2009;23(6):1388–92.
6. Hampton GR, Nelsen PT, Hay PB. Viewing through the asteroids. Ophthalmology. 1981;88(7):669–72.
7. Hwang JC, Barile GR, Schiff WM, et al. Optical coherence tomography in asteroid hyalosis. Retina. 2006;26(6):661–5.
8. Parnes RE, Zakov ZN, Novak MA, Rice TA. Vitrectomy in patients with decreased visual acuity secondary to asteroid hyalosis. Am J Ophthalmol. 1998;125(5):703–4.
9. Renaldo DP. Pars plana vitrectomy for asteroid hyalosis. Retina. 1981;1(3):252–4.
10. Hanscom TA, Kreiger A. Vitrectomy for asteroid hyalosis? Ophthalmic Surg. 1984;15(6):535.
11. Jingami Y, Otani A, Kojima H, Makiyama Y, Yoshimura N. Post-cataract surgery visual disturbance in a retinitis pigmentosa patient with asteroid hyalosis. Case Rep Ophthalmol. 2011;2(2):279–82.
12. Yamaguchi T, Inoue M, Ishida S, Shinoda K. Detecting vitreomacular adhesions in eyes with asteroid hyalosis with triamcinolone acetonide. Graefes Arch Clin Exp Ophthalmol. 2007;245(2):305–8.
13. Ikeda T, Sawa H, Koizumi K, Yasuhara T, Kinoshita S, Tano Y. Vitrectomy for proliferative diabetic retinopathy with asteroid hyalosis. Retina. 1998;18(5):410–4.

4

Femtosecond laser-assisted cataract surgery in patients with phakic intraocular lenses and low endothelial cell counts

Chia-Yi Lee[1†] ⓘ, Shih-Chun Chao[1,2,3†], Chi-Chin Sun[4,5,6,10] and Hung-Yu Lin[1,7,8,9*]

Abstract

Background: Phakic intraocular lens (PIOL) implantation has been used to correct myopia and myopic astigmatism, although corneal decompensation can occur after implantation. Femtosecond laser-assisted cataract surgery (FLACS) has gained in popularity due to its lower postoperative astigmatism and endothelial loss. Herein, we report the use of FLACS in patients who previously received PIOL implantation and have a low corneal endothelial cell count.

Case presentation: Two patients with a previous iris-claw PIOL implantation were enrolled. The preoperative corrected distance visual acuity (CDVA) and diopter sphere (DS) were 20/32 and −0.25 D in patient 1 and 20/32 and −3.00 D in patient 2. Specular microscope examination revealed an endothelial cell density (ECD) of 1532/mm^2 in patient 1 and 1620/mm^2 in patient 2. Capsulotomy was performed smoothly using a femtosecond laser. Postoperative CDVA improved in both eyes, with a difference of DS less than 1 D from the preoperative estimation. Specular microscope examination revealed a decreased endothelial cell density (ECD) in patient 2, but no signs of corneal decompensation were detected.

Conclusions: The influence of using PIOL on capsulotomies performed via FLACS, in combination with preoperative refraction calculation, is minimal. A mild decrease in ECD may occur, but there is a low probability of severe corneal decompensation, even in patients with a low endothelial cell count.

Keywords: Femtosecond laser, Phakic, Intraocular lens, Endothelial cell density, Cataract

Background

Phakic intraocular lens (PIOL) implantation has been used to correct myopia and myopic astigmatism; this procedure is better than keratorefractive surgeries in patients with refractive errors of greater than 8 diopters (D) [1]. However, the implantation of iris-fixated and iris-claw PIOL rather than using the posterior chamber PIOL may lead to corneal endothelial loss or corneal decompensation, in which case the PIOL must be explanted [2–4]. Femtosecond laser-assisted cataract surgery (FLACS), introduced in 2008, has gained popularity due to its lower resulting postoperative astigmatism and endothelial loss [5, 6]. Furthermore, the capsulorhexis created by FLACS is more circular and optimally sized compared to conventional capsulorhexis [7]. To date, only two studies have evaluated the feasibility of FLACS in patients with normal corneal endothelial cell count who have received PIOL implantation [8, 9]. Herein, we report results obtained using FLACS in two patients with a low corneal endothelial cell count who had previously received PIOL implantation.

Case presentation

Case 1 is a 41-year-old Taiwanese female who presented with bilateral high myopia, measured at −13.25 D in the right eye. An iris-claw PIOL (Artisan; Ophtec BV, Groningen, The Netherlands) was implanted in May 2006; this preserved visual acuity at approximately

* Correspondence: anthonyhungyulin@hotmail.com
†Equal contributors
[1]Department of Ophthalmology, Show Chwan Memorial Hospital, No.2, Ln. 530, Sec. 1, Zhongshan Rd., Changhua City, Changhua 50093, Taiwan
[7]Institute of Medicine, Chung Shan Medical University, Taichung, Taiwan
Full list of author information is available at the end of the article

20/25. A right eye nuclear sclerosis cataract was diagnosed in this patient, who had complaints of progressively blurred vision. On examination, the corrected distance visual acuity (CDVA) was preserved at 20/32, with a diopter sphere (DS) of −0.25 D. Specular microscope examination revealed a corneal endothelial cell density (ECD) of 1532/mm^2. Considering the damage that would have been caused by a second surgery using conventional techniques, PIOL removal concurrent with FLACS was scheduled for the patient. The preoperative estimation of the remaining refractive error was −0.87D via IOLMaster (IOLMaster V.5.4, Carl Zeiss, Oberkochen, Germany). Using the normal mode of the LenSx system (Alcon Inc., Fort Worth, TX, USA) (Fig. 1a), a 4.9 mm capsulotomy (7.00 μJ) and a 2.2 mm corneal incision were made (Fig. 1b). The capsulotomy appearance was good, and cavitation bubbles were restricted below the PIOL after laser fragmentation (Fig. 1c). Nucleus materials were removed by the stop and chop technique using a phacoemulsification device (Centurion, Alcon Inc., Fort Worth, TX) (Fig. 1d). The effective phacoemulsification time was 1.45 s, with a phaco power of torsional mode of 20% to 60% and an irrigation level of 40 mmHg. The multifocal intraocular lens (IOL) (Restor, Alcon) was implanted smoothly into the capsular bag, with no intraoperative complications (Fig. 1e). The PIOL was then removed with forceps

after widening the corneal incision to 5.0 mm (Fig. 1f) and the incisional wound was sutured with two stiches. Two weeks postoperatively, the CDVA of the right eye reached 20/20, with a DS of −0.75 D. A specular microscope examination performed on the same day revealed a stable ECD of 1531/mm^2.

Case 2 is a 55-year-old Taiwanese female who received bilateral iris-claw PIOL (Artisan; Ophtec BV, Groningen, The Netherlands) implantation in 2010 due to high myopia (10 D), presenting at the time of examination with right blurred vision for more than 1 year. On examination, CDVA measured 20/32 in the right eye, and DS was −3.00. A right eye nuclear sclerosis cataract was found using a silt-lamp biomicroscope, and a specular microscope examination revealed a decreased ECD of 1620/mm^2. Since corneal decompensation may occur after two-step conventional surgery, combined surgery was recommended; the patient agreed to undergo the surgery. The estimated refractive error was −0.02 D using the EyeSuit system (EyeSuit™IOL V3.1.0, Haag-Streit Diagnostics). Using the same mode of the LenSx system (Fig. 2a), a 4.9 mm capsulotomy was made (7.00 μJ) with lens fragmentation (Fig. 2b). A laser-created corneal incision was not performed because the position of the PIOL required an adjustment of the incision site. The majority of cavitation bubbles also remained beneath the PIOL until the end of fragmentation (Fig. 2c, d). After the creation of a

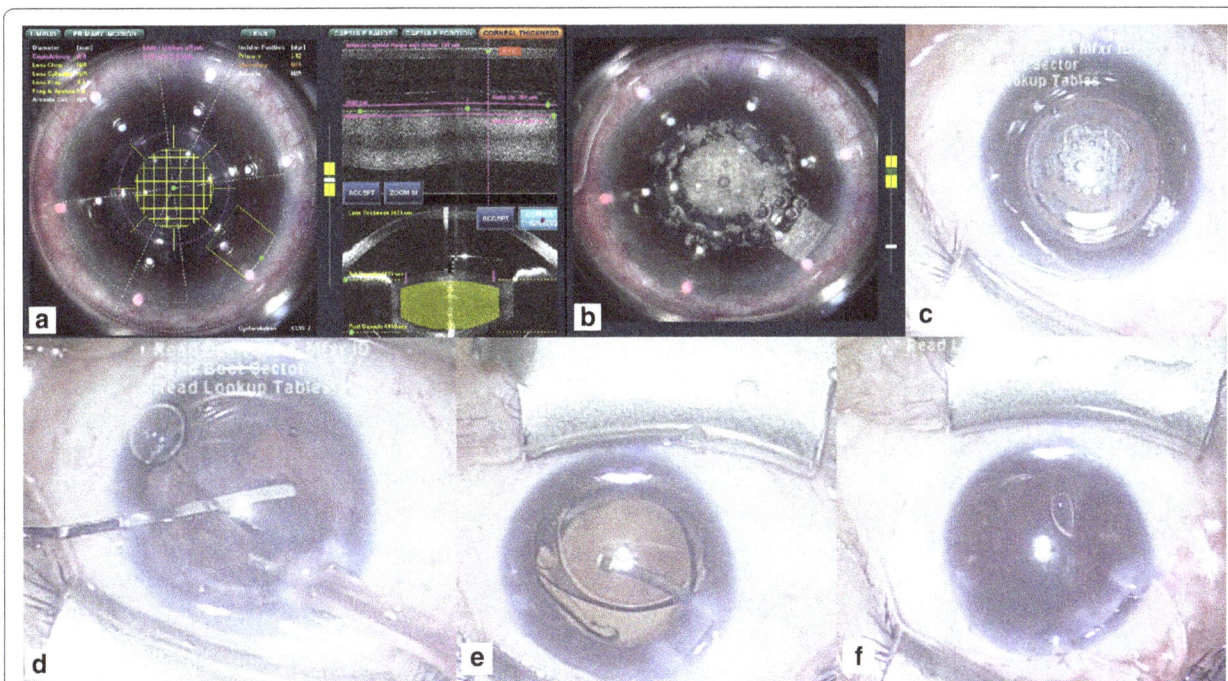

Fig. 1 Femtosecond laser-assisted cataract surgery in Patient 1 (with iris-claw phakic intraocular lens implantation). **a** Scheduling of capsulotomy, lens fragmentation and corneal incision positioning in the imaging system. **b** Completion of capsulotomy, lens fragmentation and corneal incision positioning via femtosecond laser. **c** External eye appearance prior to cataract surgery and removal of the phakic intraocular lens. **d** Phacoemulsification and aspiration under the phakic intraocular lens. **e** Implantation of a new multifocal intraocular lens. **f** Extraction of the phakic intraocular lens after widening of the corneal incision

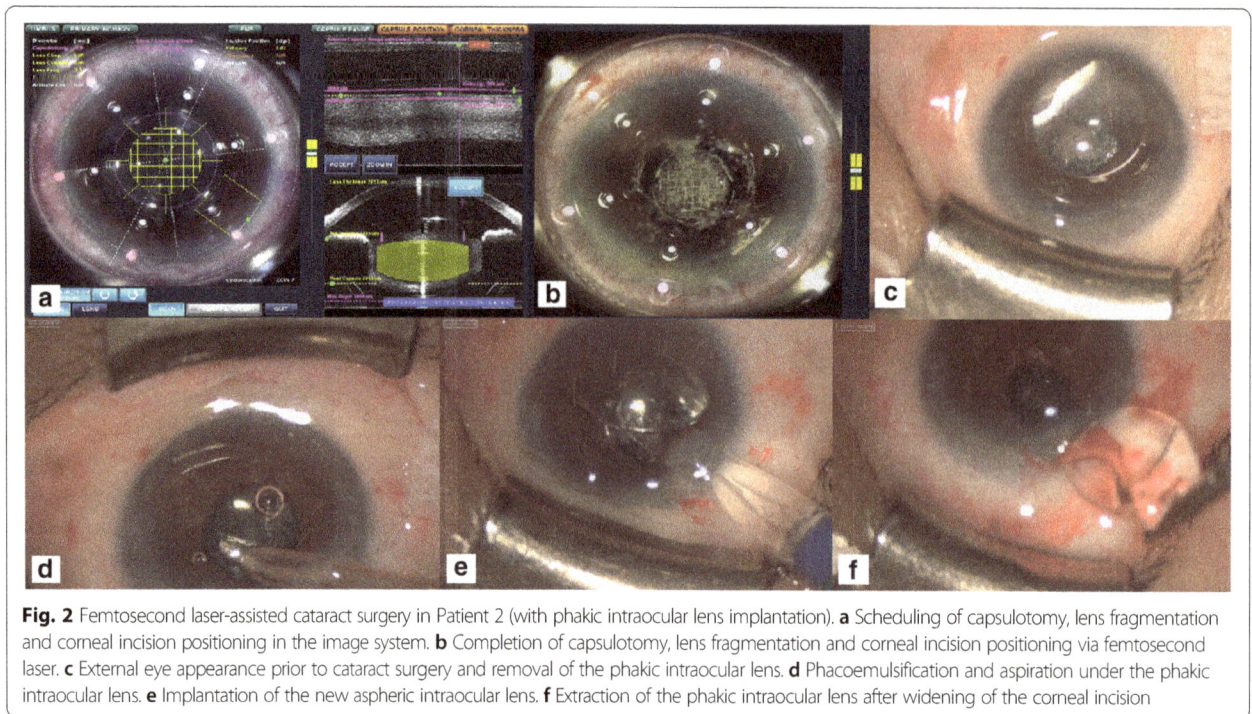

Fig. 2 Femtosecond laser-assisted cataract surgery in Patient 2 (with phakic intraocular lens implantation). **a** Scheduling of capsulotomy, lens fragmentation and corneal incision positioning in the image system. **b** Completion of capsulotomy, lens fragmentation and corneal incision positioning via femtosecond laser. **c** External eye appearance prior to cataract surgery and removal of the phakic intraocular lens. **d** Phacoemulsification and aspiration under the phakic intraocular lens. **e** Implantation of the new aspheric intraocular lens. **f** Extraction of the phakic intraocular lens after widening of the corneal incision

2.2 mm manual corneal incision, the stop and chop technique was performed to remove the nucleus using the Centurion device with the following parameters: an effective phacoemulsification time of 1.71 s, phaco power of torsional mode (20% to 60%) and an irrigation level of 40 mmHg. The IOL (Aurium, Medennium) was implanted successfully (Fig. 2e), and the corneal incision was expanded to 5.0 mm to extract the PIOL (Fig. 2f). Then, the incisional wound was closed with two stiches. The follow-up visit 1 month after surgery showed a CDVA of 20/25 and a DS of −0.25 D in the right eye. A specular microscope examination revealed a decreased ECD level of 1044/mm², but the central corneal thickness showed a value of 580 μm, which was similar to the preoperative value of 520 μm. The CDVA of the right eye had improved to 20/20 at the last visit, 10 months after surgery.

Discussion

In the current study, the feasibility of using FLACS in patients who have previously received PIOL is demonstrated. The results are similar to previous case experiences [8, 9]. In previous studies, cases with PIOL were thought to be more challenging than conventional cases needing manual adjustment [8], and incomplete fragmentation or microadhesions were not uncommon [8, 9]. However, our experience demonstrates that the technical requirements are similar in patients with PIOL because modifications were not made and no capsulotomy tags were found intraoperatively. A previous in vitro study revealed that the IOL can be transected by using

the minimum laser energy of 1 μJ [10]. This indicates that PIOL produces a small decrease in laser power.

Even with the innovation of techniques such as torsional ultrasound and viscoelastic devices, cataract surgery increases the risks of corneal decompensation in patients with a low endothelial cell count [11]. Moreover, although FLACS can effectively retard endothelial loss by reducing the effective phacoemulsification time, which correlates with the degree of endothelial damage [5, 6], laser-assisted corneal incision can also damage the endothelium [6]. In the current study, the endothelial cell counts were low for both eyes before surgery compared to an ECD of approximately 2900 cells/mm² in the normal Chinese population [12], and the ECD decreased after the surgery, but there were no signs of corneal decompensation. The combined surgery avoids endothelial damage from double surgery. Further, we removed the iris-claw IOL as the last step for several reasons. First, the PIOL can serve as a barrier to prevent damage to the corneal endothelium resulting from the ultrasound shockwave and mechanical impact. Second, both PIOLs were old products, which required a large incision to extract; late extraction can provide a more stable intraoperative corneal and anterior chamber structure. Nonetheless, synechiae between the long-term implanted PIOL and iris may lead to a hemorrhage when removing the PIOL. If PIOL extraction is done as the last step, the newly implanted IOL can block the hemorrhage, thus making the hemorrhage easier to aspirate. This is a new surgical approach, i.e., using FLACS concurrent with PIOL removal, and it may be applied in certain patients with a low endothelial cell count by using proper management. However, the prominent decline of the ECD in patient 2 makes it clear that there should be further investigation on the optimum threshold for ECD at which FLACS could be avoided.

In previous experience, the refractive outcomes when using FLACS were similar to those obtained conventional methods [5]. The refractive outcome in the current study is satisfactory, with little residual astigmatism (less than 0.75 diopters cylinder and precise DS estimation), despite the influence of the PIOL on the IOL power calculation. To prevent PIOL from interfering in the total refractive power, we used only the corneal refractive power as a reference for refractive calculation. In addition, we recommend that the refractive power of IOLs should be precisely selected in patients who have PIOL due to a high refractive error and because both aspheric and multifocal IOLs have been proven to provide acceptable outcomes in such circumstances.

Conclusion

In conclusion, the negative influence of the existing PIOL on capsulotomies performed via FLACS, in combination with preoperative refraction calculation, may be minimal. A decrease in ECD could occur in patients with a low endothelial cell count, but severe corneal decompensation does not always develop. However, further large-scale prospective studies are warranted to investigate the safety threshold of FLACS concurrent with PIOL removal in patients with a low endothelial cell count.

Abbreviation
CDVA: Corrected distance visual acuity; D: Diopter; DS: Diopter sphere; ECD: Endothelial cell density; FLACS: Femtosecond laser-assisted cataract surgery; IOL: Intraocular lens; PIOL: Phakic intraocular lens

Acknowledgements
Not applicable.

Funding
The authors have no financial sponsorship from any company or institution.

Authors' contributions
CYL and HYL contributed to the concept and study design. The patient was enrolled from HYL. CYL collected the data, made data interpretations, and drafted the manuscript. All the authors including CYL, SCC, CCS and HYL, were involved in the critical revision of the manuscript, supervision of the manuscript and final approval of the submission.

Consent for publication
Written informed consent was obtained from the patients for publication of this case report and any accompanying images. A copy of the written consent is available for review by the Editor of this journal.

Competing interests
The authors declare that they have no competing interests.

Author details
[1]Department of Ophthalmology, Show Chwan Memorial Hospital, No.2, Ln. 530, Sec. 1, Zhongshan Rd., Changhua City, Changhua 50093, Taiwan. [2]Department of Electrical and Computer Engineering, National Chiao Tung University, Hsinchu, Taiwan. [3]Department of Optometry, Central Taiwan University of Science and Technology, Taichung, Taiwan. [4]Department of Medicine, Chang Gung University, College of Medicine, Taoyuan, Taiwan. [5]Department of Ophthalmology, Chang Gung Memorial Hospital, Keelung, Taiwan. [6]Department of Chinese Medicine, Chang Gung University, College of Medicine, Taoyuan, Taiwan. [7]Institute of Medicine, Chung Shan Medical University, Taichung, Taiwan. [8]Department of Optometry, Chung Shan Medical University, Taichung, Taiwan. [9]Department of Optometry, Yuanpei University of Medical Technology, Hsinchu, Taiwan. [10]222, Mai-Chin Road, Keelung, Taiwan.

References
1. Huang D, Schallhorn SC, Sugar A, Farjo AA, Majmudar PA, Trattler WB, et al. Phakic intraocular lens implantation for the correction of myopia: a report by the American Academy of Ophthalmology. Ophthalmology. 2009;116: 2244–58.
2. de Vries NE, Tahzib NG, Budo CJ, Webers CA, de Boer R, Hendrikse F, et al. Results of cataract surgery after implantation of an iris-fixated phakic intraocular lens. J Cataract Refract Surg. 2009;35:121–6.
3. Kim M, Kim JK, Lee HK. Corneal endothelial decompensation after iris-claw phakic intraocular lens implantation. J Cataract Refract Surg. 2008;34:517–9.
4. Alfonso JF, Baamonde B, Belda-Salmerón L, Montés-Micó R, Fernández-Vega L. Collagen copolymer posterior chamber phakic intraocular lens for hyperopia correction: three-year follow-up. J Cataract Refract Surg. 2013;39: 1519–27.
5. Abouzeid H, Ferrini W. Femtosecond-laser assisted cataract surgery: a review. Acta Ophthalmol. 2014;92:597–603.
6. Abell RG, Kerr NM, Howie AR, Mustaffa Kamal MA, Allen PL, Vote BJ. Effect of femtosecond laser-assisted cataract surgery on the corneal endothelium. J Cataract Refract Surg. 2014;40:1777–83.
7. Titiyal JS, Kaur M, Singh A, Arora T, Sharma N. Comparative evaluation of femtosecond laser-assisted cataract surgery and conventional phacoemulsification in white cataract. Clin Ophthalmol. 2016;10:1357–64.
8. Li S, Chen X, Kang Y, Han N. Femtosecond Laser-Assisted Cataract Surgery in a Cataractous Eye With Implantable Collamer Lens In Situ. J Refract Surg. 2016;32:270–2.
9. Kaur M, Sahu S, Sharma N, Titiyal JS. Femtosecond Laser-Assisted Cataract Surgery in Phakic Intraocular Lens With Cataract. J Refract Surg. 2016;32:131–4.
10. Bala C, Shi J, Meades K. Intraocular Lens Fragmentation Using Femtosecond Laser: An In Vitro Study. Transl Vis Sci Technol. 2015;4:8.
11. Rosado-Adames N, Afshari NA. The changing fate of the corneal endothelium in cataract surgery. Curr Opin Ophthalmol. 2012;23:3–6.
12. Yunliang S, Yuqiang H, Ying-Peng L, Ming-Zhi Z, Lam DS, Rao SK. Corneal endothelial cell density and morphology in healthy Chinese eyes. Cornea. 2007;26:130–2.

5

Early anti-VEGF treatment for hemorrhagic occlusive retinal vasculitis as a complication of cataract surgery

Konstantinos Andreanos[1,2]* ⓘ, Petros Petrou[1], George Kymionis[1], Dimitrios Papaconstantinou[1] and Ilias Georgalas[1]

Abstract

Background: We report a case of hemorrhagic occlusive retinal vasculitis (HORV) after prophylactic intracameral vancomycin use during an uneventful cataract surgery treated with early anti-VEGF treatment.

Case presentation: A 51-year-old female underwent uneventful cataract surgery with prophylactic intracameral vancomycin during the procedure. On the seventh post-operative-day, she presented with sudden painful, visual loss. Fundus examination revealed peripheral hemorrhagic retinal vasculitis. She received anti-VEGF therapy to prevent further vision loss and retinal neovascularization due to extensive retinal ischemia. At the 6-month follow-up visit, visual acuity was 20/20 with no sign of neovascularization.

Conclusions: Postoperative HORV is a devastating condition that can occur after otherwise uncomplicated cataract surgery. The nature of this rare condition remains unknown. Early anti-VEGF administration seems to demonstrate favorable results.

Keywords: Vancomycin, Hemorrhagic occlusive retinal vasculitis, Cataract surgery, Anti-VEGF

Background

Cataract surgery is the most common operation performed in healthcare systems worldwide. Although relatively safe, intraocular infection following cataract surgery is a rare but dreaded complication that can have devastating consequences on vision. The incidence of endophthalmitis following cataract surgery is estimated between 0.04% and 0.27% [1–3]. To minimize this risk, prophylactic intracameral antibiotic use during cataract surgery has been proposed. In 2007, the European Society of Cataract and Refractive Surgeons (ESCRS) in a multinational, partially-masked placebo-controlled trial has provided strong evidence for using intracameral antibiotics in preventing postoperative endophthalmitis following cataract surgery [4]. In the wake of these results, endophthalmitis rates have dropped considerably in countries where intracameral injection was adopted as a routine method of prophylaxis at the close of cataract surgery. Therefore, in Europe, the use of intracameral antibiotics at the conclusion of the surgery represents the common practice. However, there is still debate regarding which is the optimal antibiotic to use.

Vancomycin is a branched tricyclic glycosylated non-ribosomal peptide produced by the Actinobacteria species *Amycolatopsisorientalis*. It is a broad-spectrum antibiotic that covers nearly all staphylococcal and streptococcal species, which are frequently encountered in postoperative endophthalmitis after cataract surgery [5]. Currently, it is the most commonly used prophylactic intracameral antibiotic during cataract surgery procedure in the United States [6]. Several studies have investigated its safety profile. Yoeruek et al. studied the toxic effects of cefuroxime and vancomycin on human corneal endothelial cells and found them safe in clinically used concentrations [7]. Higher concentrations could cause irreversible cell death. A recent randomized controlled trial examined the effects of intracameral vancomycin and gentamicin on macular thickness as measured by ocular coherence tomography. They found no statistically significant increase in macular thickness

* Correspondence: coandre80@icloud.com
[1]First Division of Ophthalmology, School of Medicine, National and Kapodistrian University of Athens, "G. Gennimatas" General Hospital of Athens, Athens, Greece
[2]22str Digeni E.O.K.A, Nea Penteli, 15236 Athens, Greece

in the group that received intracameral vancomycin and gentamicin [8].

However, recent reports have demonstrated the causative role of vancomycin in the pathogenesis of Hemorrhagic Occlusive Retinal Vasculitis and suggest avoiding it for chemoprophylaxis. Nicholson et al. reported severe bilateral ischemic retinal vasculitis after uncomplicated cataract surgery in 2 patients [9]. Witkin et al. presented a retrospective case series of 36 eyes with postoperative HORV development after cataract surgery in which intracameral vancomycin was used [10]. Balducci et al. recently provided strong evidence of the causative role of vancomycin in HORV [11].

This case report describes the early anti-VEGF treatment strategy in a case of unilateral hemorrhagic occlusive retinal disease after uneventful cataract surgery which to the best of our knowledge has never been reported before.

Case presentation

A 51-year-old healthy female underwent uneventful cataract surgery in her right eye. During the procedure, viscoelastic and vancomycin (1.0 mg/0.2 mL) were injected into the anterior chamber. Visual acuity on the first postoperative day was 20/20 and no other postoperative complication was detected.

On the seventh postoperative day the patient complained of acute painful visual deterioration. Visual acuity was 20/32 in her right eye with minimal anterior chamber and vitreous reaction, not suggestive of endophthalmitis. She was referred to our clinic 2 days later (post-op 9 days) for further investigation. Ophthalmic examination revealed best corrected visual acuity of 20/32 and 20/25 in the right and left eye respectively. Intraocular pressure was 15 mmHg in both eyes, pupil reaction was normal. Slit lamp examination of the right eye

revealed 1+ cell in the anterior chamber and 1+ cell in the anterior vitreous. Fundus examination of the right eye was notable for mild vitritis, vascular attenuation, and peripheral artery occlusion, as well as scattered intraretinal and perivascular hemorrhages.

Fluorescein angiography revealed delayed retinal filling, peripheral vascular occlusion, extended areas of non-perfusion, and scattered areas of perivascular staining (Fig. 1). Optical coherence tomography examination was unremarkable (Fig. 2). A 6 × 6 zone was acquired using optical coherence tomography angiography demonstrating the junction between perfusion and non-perfusion areas showing the choroidal vasculature intact.

Diagnosis of hemorrhagic occlusive retinal vasculitis was suspected based on the recent cataract surgery where intracameral vancomycin was used and characteristic clinical findings of the disease. As with previous reports of vancomycin-induced HORV, thorough systemic workup was unremarkable. Based on reports in the literature indicating the poor prognosis of the disease, the poor therapeutic effects of steroids and immunosuppressive treatment, we decided to proceed with early anti-VEGF treatment in an attempt to halt the progression of vision loss and reduce the risk of neovascular glaucoma. An intravitreal injection of bevacizumab (Avastin; Genetech, South San Francisco, CA) was administrated.

The following days the patient reported gradual pain relief and an improvement in her vision. Best corrected visual acuity was 20/25. Fundus examination showed no change, while fluorescein angiography showed reduced vascular staining. On the 25th post-operative day best corrected visual acuity was 20/20.

Despite visual acuity restoration, extended peripheral zones of non-perfusion were noted on fluorescein angiography. We discussed our concerns with the patient and we proposed continuation of anti-VEGF for at least

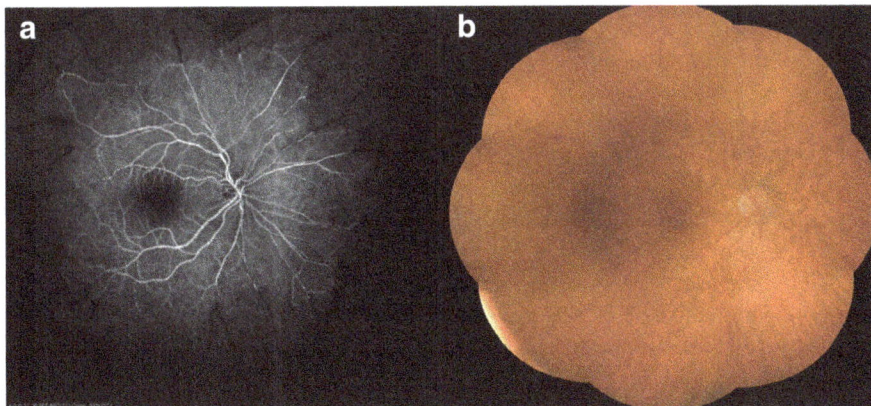

Fig. 1 a Mosaic fluorescence angiography revealing peripheral vascular occlusion, extended areas of non perfusion, and scattered areas of perivascular staining **b** Mosaic color fundus photography showing vascular attenuation, peripheral artery occlusion and few scattered intraretinal and perivascular hemorrhages

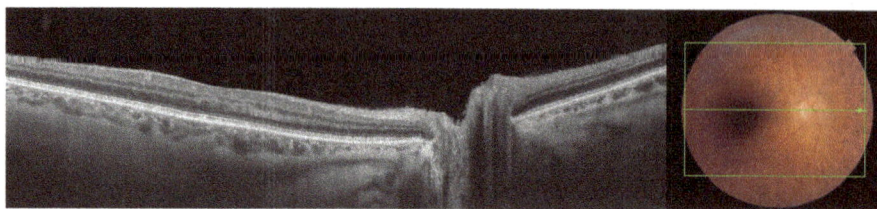

Fig. 2 Macula Optical Coherence Tomography. Fovea architecture is intact with no sign of edema

3 months to minimize the risk of neovascularization development. A total of three intravitreal injections were administrated in a 3-month period after surgery. We decided to proceed with photocoagulation treatment only in the occurrence of neovascularization.

At a 6-month follow-up examination best corrected visual acuity was 20/20 with no sign of neovascularization. Fundus examination and fluorescein angiography revealed no sign of disease activity. We decided to closely monitor the patient at regular intervals over the next 2 years in order to promptly, detect and treat a possible occurrence of neovascularization. The patient was provided a written informed consent in accordance with the tenets of the Declaration of Helsinki to having their medical data used for research purposes. Written informed consent was obtained from the patient for publication of this case report and any accompanying images.

Discussion

HORV after uneventful cataract surgery is a dreaded complication. There is an ongoing debate concerning the association of intracameral vancomycin and HORV. Nicholson et al. reported severe bilateral ischemic retinal vasculitis after uncomplicated cataract surgery in two patients. The authors associated the vasculopathy with the use of intracameral vancomycin at the close of the cataract procedure [9]. Witkin et al. discussed the findings of 36 eyes that experienced severe HORV and found that this exceedingly rare condition could represent a delayed immune reaction to intracameral vancomycin [10]. Balducci et al. presented a case where HORV developed only on the eye where vancomycin prophylaxis had been used at the end of the procedure, while the second eye of the same patient that underwent cataract surgery without vancomycin prophylaxis remained unaffected [11]. Most reported cases present poor results.

The case presented herein showed some differences from other similar reports. First, our patient complained of painful progressive loss of vision. Ophthalmodynia was not described in other cases making the diagnostic procedure difficult as endophthalmitis could not be ruled out easily. The patient described the symptom as a dull, constant ache in the affected eye, which was relieved after anti-VEGF injection. We postulate that pain

may be ischemic in origin similar to "ocular angina" presented in ocular ischemic syndrome [12]. Furthermore, fundus examination revealed few hemorrhages in contrast to the severe hemorrhagic component of previously reported cases. Moreover, OCT findings did not indicate macula pathology even though increased macula thickness and cystoid macula spaces have been described in other cases [10]. The absence of macular edema and photoreceptor disruption might explain the favorable final vision outcome.

Previous reports have presented several therapeutic approaches [9–11]. Despite intervention with high-dose topical and systemic corticosteroids, antiviral medication and early vitrectomy in many patients, visual outcomes were typically poor. Neovascular glaucoma developed in most patients and visual outcomes varied between no light perception to 20/50 [10].

In our case, we proceeded with early anti-VEGF treatment in our patient. Early outcomes were encouraging since our patient described an improvement in her symptoms. Three Intravitreal injections were performed monthly in order to halt disease progression and prevent neovascularization. At a 6-month follow-up examination the patient had 20/20 and no sign of vascularization.

This case report highlights the favorable outcome of immediate anti-VEGF therapy in cases of HORV. However, we have to take into account that the disease severity may vary and that in the presented case, HORV might have manifested with milder symptoms and a moderate visual acuity loss. Indeed, Lenci et al. reported a similar case with rapid resolution when treated with a short course of topical medications. The authors stated that the case probably represented the mild end of a spectrum of vancomycin toxicity [13]. Nevertheless, most reported cases had poor visual outcomes and further complications, thus we believe that in our patient early intervention might have modulated the course of the disease.

Conclusions

To recapitulate, HORV is a devastating condition after otherwise uneventful cataract surgery. In our case, the early intervention with anti-VEGF treatment had a favorable result in restoring vision and preventing neovascularisation. Although it is difficult to draw accurate conclusions from single cases early anti-VEGF seems to have a positive role in stopping the cascade of HORV and preventing neovascularisation which if untreated would adversely affect patients vision and quality of life. Further studies are needed to ensure such a therapeutic effect.

Abbreviations
HORV: Hemorrhagic Occlusive Retinal Vasculitis; OCT: Optical coherence tomography; VEGF: Vascular Endothelial Growth Factor

Acknowledgements
Not applicable.

Funding
No funding or sponsorship was received for this study or publication of this report.

Authors' contributions
All named authors meet the International Committee of Medical Journal Editors (ICMJE) criteria for authorship for this manuscript, take responsibility for the integrity of the work as a whole, and have given final approval to the version to be published. KA was a major contributor in writing the manuscript. PP performed the clinical examinations during the 6-month follow-up. GK performed imaging data acquisition. DP analysed and evaluated patient data. IG performed the anti-VEGF treatment and helped draft the manuscript.

Consent for publication
Written informed consent was obtained from the patient for publication of this case report and any accompanying images. A copy of the written consent is available for review by the editor of this journal.

Competing interests
The authors declare that they have no competing interests.

References
1. Taban M, Beherens A, Newcomb RL, et al. Acute endophthalmitis following cataract surgery: a systematic review of the literature. Arch Ophthalmol. 2005;123:613–20.
2. Hatch WV, Cernat G, Wong D, Devenyi R, Bell CM. Risk factors for acute endophthalmitis after cataract surgery: a population-based study. Ophthalmology. 2009;116:425–30.
3. Miller JJ, Scott IU, Flynn HW Jr, Smiddy WE, Newton J, Miller D. Acute onset endophthalmitis after cataract surgery (2000–2004): incidence, clinical settings, and visual acuity outcomes after treatment. Am J Ophthalmol. 2005;139:983–7.
4. Barry P, Seal DV, Gettinby G, Lees F, Peterson M, Revie CW. ESCRS study of prophylaxis of postoperative endophthalmitis after cataract surgery: preliminary report of principal results from a European multicenter study; the ESCRS Endophthalmitis Study Group. J Cataract Refract Surg. 2006;32:407–10.
5. Behndig A, Cochener B, Güell JL, Kodjikian L, Mencucci R, Nuijts RM, Pleyer U, Rosen P, Szaflik JP, Tassignon MJ. Endophthalmitis prophylaxis in cataract surgery: overview of current practice patterns in 9 European countries. J Cataract Refract Surg. 2013;39(9):1421–31.
6. Braga-Mele R, Chang DF, Henderson BA, et al. Intracameral antibiotics: safety, efficacy, and preparation. J Cataract Refract Surg. 2014;40:2134–42.
7. Yoeruek E, Spitzer MS, Saygili O, et al. Comparison of in vitro safety profiles of vancomycin and cefuroxime on human corneal endothelial cells for intracameral use. J Cataract Refract Surg. 2008;34:2139–45.
8. Ball JL, Barrett GD. Prospective randomized controlled trial of the effect of intracameral vancomycin and gentamicin on macular retinal thickness and visual function following cataract surgery. J Cataract Refract Surg. 2006;32(5): 789–94.
9. Nicholson LB, Kim BT, Jardón J, et al. Severe bilateral ischemic retinal vasculitis following cataract surgery. Ophthalmic Surg Lasers Imaging Retina. 2014;45:338–42.
10. Witkin AJ, Chang DF, Jumper JM, Charles S, Eliott D, Hoffman RS, Mamalis N, Miller KM, Wykoff CC. Vancomycin-associated hemorrhagic occlusive retinal vasculitis: clinical characteristics of 36 eyes. Ophthalmology. 2017;124(5): 583–95.
11. Balducci N, Savini G, Barboni P, Ducoli P, Ciardella A. Hemorrhagic occlusive retinal Vasculitis after first eye cataract surgery without subsequent second eye involvement. Ophthalmic Surg Lasers Imaging Retina. 2016;47(8):764–6.
12. Mendrinos E, Machinis TG, Pournaras CJ. Ocular ischemic syndrome. Surv Ophthalmol. 2010;55(1):2–34.
13. Lenci LT, Chin EK, Carter C, Russell SR, Almeida DR. Ischemic retinal vasculitis associated with cataract surgery and Intracameral vancomycin. Case Rep Ophthalmol Med. 2015;2015:683194.

6

Positive bacterial culture in conjunctival sac before cataract surgery with night stay is related to diabetes mellitus

Tetsuhiro Kawata[1,2] and Toshihiko Matsuo[2*]

Abstract

Background: The aim of this study is to elucidate background clinical factors in patients with positive bacterial culture for the conjunctival sac before cataract surgery in Japan.

Methods: Retrospective review was made on medical records of 576 consecutive patients who underwent conjunctival sac culture before cataract surgery with night stay at a hospital in 2 years from January 2013 to December 2014. In the patients with sequential bilateral surgeries, the data were chosen for bacterial culture in the eye which had earlier surgery. The age at surgery ranged from 33 to 100 years (mean, 76.7 years). Clinical factors, analyzed in relation with positive or negative bacterial culture, included the sex, the age, the presence of hypertension or diabetes mellitus, history of cancer, and history of hospital-based surgery at other specialties.

Results: Bacterial culture of the conjunctival sac was positive in 168 patients while negative in 408 patients. In multiple regression analysis, the positive bacterial culture was related with the older age ($P = 0.01$), the presence of diabetes mellitus ($P = 0.004$), and the history of hospital-based surgery at other specialties ($P = 0.001$).

Conclusions: Elderly patients with diabetes mellitus or previous hospital-based surgeries at other specialties have a higher rate of positive bacterial culture in the conjunctival sac before cataract surgery. This study would provide a hint for identifying patients at risk for carrying bacterial flora in the conjunctival sac.

Keywords: Conjunctival sac culture, Cataract surgery, Diabetes mellitus, History of cancer, History of hospitalization

Background

Postoperative endophthalmitis is a rare but severe complication for intraocular surgeries such as cataract and glaucoma surgeries, and vitrectomy [1, 2]. To determine a patient at risk for postoperative infection, and hence, to reduce the rate of infection related with eye surgeries, bacterial culture from swab of conjunctival sac has been commonly done in preoperative assessment for intraocular surgeries [3–5] and refractive surgery [6]. In addition, conjunctival sac culture has been used to know changing patterns in the bacterial flora in part of the body.

So far to date, only a few studies have addressed which systemic clinical factors of patients were related with positive bacterial cultures of the conjunctival sac [7, 8]. In this study, we aimed to find systemic clinical factors which

underlay culture-positive or culture-negative patients before cataract surgery in a city of Japan.

Methods

Patients

Retrospective review was made on medical records of 590 consecutive patients (248 men and 342 women) with 792 eyes who underwent conjunctival sac culture within 1 month (usually at 2 weeks) before cataract surgery at one night stay in Fukuyama City Hospital in 2 years from January 2013 to December 2014. In 202 patients with sequential bilateral surgeries, the data were chosen for bacterial culture in the eye which had earlier surgery. The second eye surgery was usually done at 1 week after the first eye surgery. The study was approved as a retrospective study by the institutional review board at Fukuyama City Hospital.

* Correspondence: matsuot@cc.okayama-u.ac.jp
[2]Department of Ophthalmology, Fukuyama City Hospital, Fukuyama City, Japan
Full list of author information is available at the end of the article

Conjunctival sac culture

To obtain conjunctival sac culture, the lower conjunctival fornix was exposed by pulling the lower lid with a finger, and swabbed with a cotton (Rayon fiber) stick, and then, the cotton stick was dipped into agar medium for transport (BBL CultureSwab Plus Amies Medium Without Charcoal, BD, Becton, Dickinson and Company, Sparks, MD, USA). At clinical laboratories of Fukuyama City Hospital, the culture on sheep blood agar medium was continued for 48 h at 37 Celsius in an incubator with 5% carbon dioxide, and a single colony was considered as positive. On the occasion that two or more bacterial strains were cultured in 13 eyes of 13 patients, one strain in a largest amount was taken as responsible in consideration of background contamination.

Inclusion and exclusion criteria

Fourteen patients were excluded from the analysis, based on the exclusion criteria: 1) eight patients with eight eyes which had preceding eye surgeries (one eye with strabismus surgery, one with pterygium resection, one with scleral buckling, one with vitrectomy, and four with intravitreous injection), 2) one patient who was involved in a clinical trial for chemotherapy, and 3) five patients with six eyes who had used antibiotic eye drops within 1 month prior to bacterial culture of the conjunctival sac due to ocular surface or eyelid infectious diseases, including keratitis, conjunctivitis, dacryocystitis, and blepharitis. After the exclusion, 576 patients remained in the analysis set.

Patients who underwent combined surgery, concurrent with cataract surgery, were not included in this study: 553 eyes of 531 patients with combined vitrectomy and 138 eyes of 123 patients with combined glaucoma surgery. Furthermore, in the 2-year period, cataract surgery was also done as day surgery in 1652 eyes of 1060 patients (551 men and 509 women with the mean age, 75.5 years, ranging from 21 to 101 years). These patients were not included in the analysis of this study because their electronic medical records had insufficient information on the history and medication. Night-stay surgery or day surgery was determined basically upon patients' wishes. The age and the sex, as background factors, were not significantly different between the patients with night-stay surgery and day surgery.

Clinical factors

Clinical factors which were collected and used for analysis in 576 patients, included the sex, the age, the presence of hypertension or diabetes mellitus, the history of cancer, the history of hospitalization for other diseases, and positive blood tests for syphilis, hepatitis B or C before cataract surgery. The presence of hypertension and diabetes mellitus was defined as taking hypotensive drugs and diabetic

medications and/or insulin injection at the time of conjunctival culture, respectively. The history of cancer, of course, did not include the history of benign tumors. The history of hospitalization was narrowly designated as hospital-based surgeries at other specialties and taken positive only when patients had experienced hospitalization for surgeries at other specialties. Hospitalization for non-surgical treatment, such as intravenous drug administration or infusion, or hospitalization for examinations was not counted as the history of hospitalization in this study. Preoperative screening blood tests included serological test for syphilis (STS) and treponema pallidum latex agglutination (TPLA), hepatitis B surface antigen (HBsAg), and hepatitis C antibody (HCV-Ab).

Cataract surgery

Cataract surgery was done from corneal incision or sclerocorneal incision on the superior side. The patients used 0.5% moxifloxacin eye drops four times daily for 3 days before the surgery, only after the results of conjunctival sac culture were obtained, irrespective of positive or negative bacterial culture. In the case that patients were using contact lenses, they were asked to stop wearing contact lenses 3 days before the surgery when prophylactic antibiotic eye drops were started. The use of eye drops for dry eye syndrome or glaucoma was not discontinued before the surgery.

At the beginning of the surgery, the ocular surface was washed with 16-time saline-diluted povidone iodine, and then, instilled with 0.3% ofloxacin gel. No intravenous antibiotics were given during the surgery. At the end of the surgery, the ocular surface was instilled with 1.5% levofloxacin eye drops, 0.3% ofloxacin and 0.1% betamethasone ointment. The patients were given cefcapene pivoxil 300 mg daily for 3 days after the surgery, and used 1.5% levofloxacin, 0.1% betamethasone, and 0.1% nepafenac eye drops four times daily for 1 month. Oral cefcapene pivoxil was not prescribed in patients with estimated glomerular filtration rate (eGFR) less than 45 mL/min/1.73 m^2. No postoperative endophthalmitis was noted in the 2-year period of the study.

Statistical analysis

The incidence of each clinical factor in two groups (culture-positive patients and culture-negative patients) were compared first by univariate analysis using chi-square test or Mann-Whitney U-test, and then compared by multivariate analysis using multiple regression analysis.

Results

The age of 576 patients (240 men and 336 women) at cataract surgery ranged from 33 to 100 years (mean, 76.7 years). Bacterial culture of the conjunctival sac was positive in 168 patients while negative in 408 patients.

Table 1 shows the list of bacteria which were cultured from the conjunctival sac. Figure 1 shows a pie chart for bacterial strains. At cataract surgery, hypertension and diabetes mellitus were noted in 228 patients and 134 patients, respectively. Positive blood tests for screening of infectious diseases (syphilis, hepatitis B, hepatitis C) were found in 51 patients. In addition, 88 patients had history of cancer and 190 patients had history of hospital-based surgeries at other specialties.

In univariate analyses (Table 2), the age (mean, 78.8 years) of patients with positive bacterial culture of the conjunctival sac was significantly older than the age (mean, 75.9 years) of patients with negative culture ($P = 0.002$, Mann-Whitney U-test).

The positive bacterial culture was also related with the presence of diabetes mellitus ($P = 0.018$, chi-square test), and the history of hospital-based surgeries at other specialties ($P = 0.001$, chi-square test). In multiple regression analysis (Table 2), the positive bacterial culture was related with the older age ($P = 0.01$), the presence of diabetes mellitus ($P = 0.004$), and the history of hospital-based surgeries at other specialties ($P = 0.001$).

Discussion

This study revealed systemic clinical factors which underlay positive bacterial culture in the conjunctival sac of patients before cataract surgery with a night stay at a major hospital in a city with the population of 471 thousands, located in the western part of Japan. Older ages of patients, current suffering of diabetes mellitus, and the history of hospital-

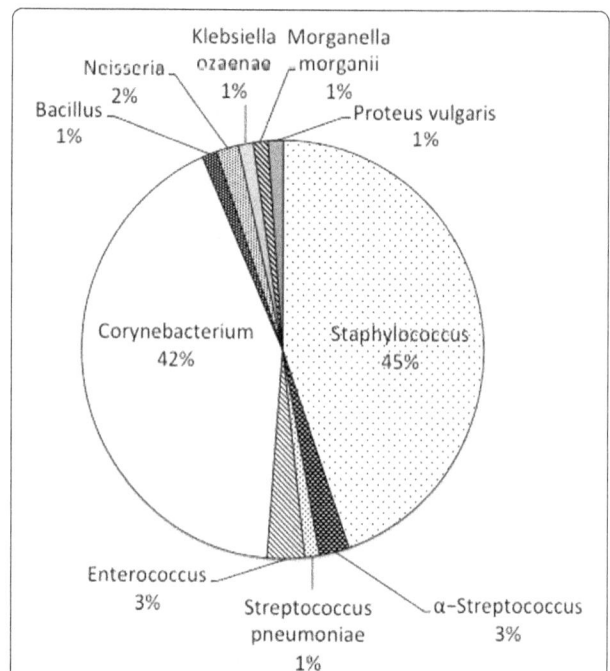

Fig. 1 Pie chart, showing bacterial strains cultured from conjunctival sac in 168 patients before cataract surgery

based surgeries at other specialties were three systemic factors which showed significant relation with the positive bacterial culture. These three factors in the patients have the common background which leads to immunologically compromised hosts. The diagnosis of diabetes mellitus in the patients of this study was strictly defined as currently having treatments as oral medication or insulin injection.

In preceding studies [7, 8], the old age of patients was found as a risk factor to have positive bacterial culture in the conjunctival sac before cataract surgeries. Furthermore, in one of the studies, patients with systemic risk factors, including diabetes mellitus, had a more chance to have positive bacterial culture of the conjunctival sac before intraocular surgeries [8]. Other series of preceding studies showed a high incidence of bacterial flora in patients with diabetes mellitus [9–11]. These preceding results, obtained in other countries, were consistent with the results in the present study which was conducted in a medium-sized city of Japan.

The bacteria which were detected in this study are considered to be part of the normal flora and rarely pathogenic. From the viewpoint of conjunctival bacterial flora, two major species, detected in the culture in this study, were Staphylococcus as a Gram-positive coccus and Corynebacterium as a Gram-positive rod (Table 1, Fig. 1). In the present study, patients with cataract surgery used moxifloxacin eye drops only for 3 days before the surgery. The prophylactic use of this antibiotic eye drop would be concluded as appropriate, based on the

Table 1 Bacteria cultured from conjunctival sac in 168 patients before cataract surgery

Classification	Bacteria	Number (%) of patients
Gram-positive cocci	Staphylococcus species	75 (44.6%)
	(Staphylococcus aureus)	(6)
	(MRSA)	(1)
	α-Streptococcus	4 (2.4%)
	Streptococcus pneumoniae	2 (1.2%)
	Enterococcus	5 (3.0%)
	(Enterococcus faecalis)	(1)
Gram-positive rods	Corynebacterium species	71 (42.3%)
	(Corynebacterium jeikeium)	(1)
	(Corynebacterium striatum)	(1)
	Bacillus	2 (1.2%)
Gram-negative cocci	Neisseria	3 (1.8%)
Gram-negative rods	Klebsiella ozaenae	2 (1.2%)
	Morganella morganii	2 (1.2%)
	Proteus vulgaris	2 (1.2%)
Total		168 (100%)

MRSA methicillin-resistant Staphylococcus aureus

Table 2 Clinical factors related with positive or negative bacterial culture in conjunctival sac of 576 patients with cataract surgery

Clinical factors	Culture-positive patients ($n = 168$)	Culture-negative patients ($n = 408$)	Univariate P value	Multivariate P value
Age (years)				
Range (median)	39–99 (79.5)	33–100 (77)		
Mean	78.8	75.9	0.002	0.010
Sex				
Male	64 (38%)	176 (43%)		
Female	104 (62%)	232 (57%)	0.265	
Hypertension				
Yes	74 (44%)	154 (38%)		
No	94 (56%)	254 (62%)	0.160	
Diabetes mellitus				
Yes	50 (30%)	84 (21%)		
No	118 (70%)	324 (79%)	0.018	0.004
History of cancer				
Yes	29 (17%)	59 (14%)		
No	139 (83%)	349 (86%)	0.396	
History of hospital-based surgeries				
Yes	80 (48%)	110 (27%)		
No	88 (52%)	298 (73%)	0.001	0.001
Screening for infectious diseases				
Yes	18 (11%)	33 (8%)		
No	150 (89%)	375 (92%)	0.313	

Univariate analysis is done with chi-square test, except for the age (Mann-Whitney U-test). Multivariate P values are calculated by multiple regression analysis

spectrum of moxifloxacin. The consecutive series of bacterial culture in the conjunctival sac in patients with cataract surgery would provide an opportunity to monitor the changing patterns of bacterial flora in the body. The monitoring would lead to an appropriate choice of antibiotics as eye drops at cataract surgery [12]. It should be noted that antibiotic-resistant bacteria, such as methicillin-resistant Staphylococcus aureus (MRSA), was detected only in one of the present series of patients. A recent regional care in a city of Japan to reduce antibiotics use might explain a low rate of MRSA detection in this study.

This study only included patients with cataract surgery at a night stay and excluded patients with day surgery. This inclusion criterion was derived from the fact that patients with hospital stay were, beforehand, screened for conjunctival flora, to avoid carrying and disseminating antibiotics-resistant bacteria in the hospital. This criterion would bring a potential selection bias in the study even though the night-stay surgery patients and day surgery patients did not show significant difference in background factors such as the age and the sex. Another potential selection bias in this study would be the exclusion of patients with combined surgeries, namely, cataract surgeries together with vitrectomy or glaucoma surgeries at one session. The patients with combined surgeries were excluded in this study simply because we aimed to focus on cataract surgeries which were a most frequent surgery in the hospital.

Another major limitation in this study is that the current use of medications was chosen as benchmarks for the presence of diabetes mellitus and hypertension in patients. These criteria would naturally miss diabetic and hypertensive patients who were not taking drugs at the time of cataract surgery. Along the same line, the use of antibiotic eye drops was used in this study to exclude patients with conjunctivitis or blepharitis which would influence the outcome of ocular surface culture. The use of medications was chosen as benchmarks to make the criteria simple and obvious in this retrospective study. Hemoglobin A1c, reliable marker for the diagnosis of diabetes mellitus, was not measured in all patients. Blood pressure at a single time point before the surgery was not reliable to make the diagnosis of hypertension. From the ophthalmic point of view, we did not pay attention to the use of eye drops for dry eye syndrome or the use of contact lenses which might also affect the ocular surface bacterial flora.

A narrow definition of previous hospital stay as hospital-based surgeries in this study is to focus on surgical intervention at other specialties. The duration of hospital stay for intravenous drug administration or examinations was usually short and sometimes difficult to differentiate from office-based or outpatient treatments or examinations. History of hospital-based surgeries at other specialties was obtained by interview with patients. The history was based on patients' memory and included the episodes long time ago. Thus, the history of hospital-based surgeries in this study has a limitation from the standpoint of its accuracy and also of undefined time span between previous surgery and current cataract surgery.

Conclusion

Elderly diabetic patients with previous history of hospital-based surgeries at other specialties would have a risk to have bacterial flora in the conjunctival sac. It is still controversial whether or not to use prophylactic antibiotic eye drops before cataract surgery. It is also controversial to screen bacterial flora in the conjunctival sac before cataract surgery. The present study would provide a hint for identifying patients at risk for carrying bacterial flora in the conjunctival sac.

Abbreviations

HBsAg: Hepatitis B surface antigen; HCV-Ab: Hepatitis C antibody; MRSA: Methicillin-resistant Staphylococcus aureus; STS: Serological test for syphilis; TPLA: Treponema pallidum latex agglutination

Acknowledgments

The authors are grateful to staff at Clinical Laboratories of Fukuyama City Hospital.

Funding

None.

Authors' contributions

TK made substantial contributions to acquisition of data, and analysis and interpretation of data, and was involved in drafting the manuscript, and gave final approval of the version for submission. TM made substantial contributions to conception and design, analysis and interpretation of data, was involved in revising it critically for important intellectual content, and gave final approval of the version for submission. Each author participated sufficiently in the work to take public responsibility for appropriate portions of the content.

Competing interests

None.

Consent for publication

Not applicable.

Author details

[1]Department Ophthalmology, Okayama University Medical School and Graduate School of Medicine, Dentistry, and Pharmaceutical Sciences, 2-5-1 Shikata-cho, Okayama City 700-8558, Japan. [2]Department of Ophthalmology, Fukuyama City Hospital, Fukuyama City, Japan.

References

1. Benz MS, Scott IU, Flynn Jr HW, Unonius N, Miller D. Endophthalmitis isolates and antibiotic sensitivities : a 6-year review of culture-proven cases. Am J Ophthalmol. 2004;137:38–42.
2. Gentile RC, Shukla S, Shah M, Ritterband DC, Engelbert M, Davis A, Hu DN. Microbiological spectrum and antibiotic sensitivity in endophthalmitis : a 25-year review. Ophthalmology. 2014;121:1634–42.
3. Mino de Kaspar H, Koss MJ, He L, Blumenkranz MS, Ta CN. Antibiotic susceptibility of preoperative normal conjunctival bacteria. Am J Ophthalmol. 2005;139:730–3.
4. Hsu HY, Lind JT, Tseng L, Miller D. Ocular flora and their antibiotic resistance patterns in the Midwest : a prospective study of patients undergoing cataract surgery. Am J Ophthalmol. 2013;155:36–44.
5. Mshangila B, Paddy M, Kajumbula H, Ateenyi-Agaba C, Kahwa B, Seni J. External ocular surface bacterial isolates and their antimicrobial susceptibility patterns among pre-operative cataract patients at Mulago National Hospital in Kampala, Uganda. BMC Ophthalmol. 2013;13:71.
6. Chung JL, Seo KY, Yong DE, Mah FS, Kim TI, Kim EK, Kim JK. Antibiotic susceptibility of conjunctival bacterial isolates from refractive surgery patients. Ophthalmology. 2009;116:1067–74.
7. Rubio EF. Influence of age on conjunctival bacteria of patients undergoing cataract surgery. Eye (Lond). 2006;20:447–54.
8. Mino de Kaspar H, Ta CN, Froehlich SJ, Schaller UC, Engelbert M, Klauss V, Kampik A. Prospective study of risk factors for conjunctival bacterial contamination in patients undergoing intraocular surgery. Eur J Ophthalmol. 2009;19:712–22.
9. Martins EN, Alvarenga LS, Hofling-Lima AL, Freitas D, Zorat-Yu MC, Farah ME, Mannis MJ. Aerobic bacterial conjunctival flora in diabetic patients. Cornea. 2004;23:136–42.
10. Fernandez-Rubio ME, Rebolledo-Lara L, Martinez-Garcia M, Alarcon-Tomas M, Cortes-Valdes C. The conjunctival bacterial pattern of diabetics undergoing cataract surgery. Eye (Lond). 2010;24:825–34.
11. Karimsab D, Razak SK. Study of aerobic bacterial conjunctival flora in patients with diabetes mellitus. Nepal J Ophthalmol. 2013;5:28–32.
12. Fintelmann RE, Naseri A. Prophylaxis of postoperative endophthalmitis following cataract surgery : current status and future directions. Drugs. 2010; 70:1395–409.

7

Real-world refractive outcomes of toric intraocular lens implantation in a United Kingdom National Health Service setting

Kanmin Xue[1,2*], Jasleen K. Jolly[1,2], Sonia P. Mall[1], Shreya Haldar[1], Paul H. Rosen[1] and Robert E. MacLaren[1,2]

Abstract

Background: With increasing availability of toric intraocular lenses (IOL) for cataract surgery, real-world refractive outcome data is needed to aid the counselling of patients regarding lens choice. We aim to assess the outcomes of toric intraocular lens use in the non-specialist environment of a typical United Kingdom NHS cataract service.

Methods: A retrospective cohort study conducted at the Oxford Eye Hospital, Oxford University Hospitals NHS Foundation Trust, UK. All patients who received a toric IOL implant over a 10 months period. Patients underwent pre-operative corneal marking, phacoemulsification and toric IOL implantation. Biometry was obtained using a Zeiss IOLMaster 500 and the toric IOLs were selected using the manufacturers' online calculators. Post-operative refractions were obtained from optometrist's manifest refraction or by autorefraction. The outcome measures were post-operative unaided visual acuity (UVA), spherical equivalent refraction, cylindrical correction and all complications.

Results: Thirty-two eyes of 24 patients aged 21–86 years (mean 66.4, SD 14.5) were included. UVA was superior to pre-operative best-corrected visual acuity (BCVA) in 81% of eyes, same in 16% and inferior in 3%, resulting in a median improvement of 0.20 LogMAR (IQR 0.10 to 0.30). 56%, 81%, 94% and 100% of eyes were within ±0.5, ±1.0, ±1.5 and ±2.0 D of predicted spherical equivalent, respectively. Three (9%) eyes required further surgery to rectify significant IOL rotation.

Conclusions: Reduced cylindrical correction and improved UVA could be expected in the majority of patients undergoing toric IOL implantation. Patients should be counselled about the risk of lens rotation.

Keywords: Toric intraocular lens, Toric IOL, Cataract surgery, Astigmatism

Background

Advances in cataract refractive surgery have enabled neutralisation of corneal astigmatism at the time of cataract surgery using toric intraocular lens (IOL) implants. Approximately 15–20% of patients presenting with cataract have > 1.5 dioptres (D) of pre-existing corneal astigmatism [1]. Before the introduction of toric IOLs (TIOL), the main method for correcting corneal astigmatism was peripheral corneal relaxing incisions (PCRI) or opposite clear corneal incisions (OCCI). However the technique is limited by variations in corneal thickness, surgical technique and scarring

response between individuals, leading to unpredictable degrees of cylindrical correction and regression of refractive correction. Creating corneal incisions of accurate depths by hand, even with a guarded diamond-tipped blade, can be operator-dependent and susceptible to patient-related variables such as intraocular pressure and eye movement under local anaesthesia. Although femtosecond laser may be able to create PCRIs with a high degree of precision thereby minimising the risk of corneal perforation, PCRIs could still be associated with the risks of wound gape, corneal infection and nerve damage leading to secondary dry eye [2–4] Alternatively, astigmatic correction through excimer laser photorefractive keratectomy could be complicated by refractive error, and all the complications associated with the technique including diffuse lamellar keratitis and corneal haze [5, 6]. It is also generally not available within

* Correspondence: kanmin.xue@ndcn.ox.ac.uk; enquiries@eye.ox.ac.uk
[1]Oxford Eye Hospital, Oxford Universities Hospitals NHS Foundation Trust, Oxford, UK
[2]Nuffield Laboratory of Ophthalmology, Nuffield Department of Clinical Neurosciences, University of Oxford, Level 6 West Wing, John Radcliffe Hospital, Headley Way, Oxford OX3 9DU, UK

the UK National Health Service (NHS) and most cataract surgery centres across Europe.

The introduction of a variety of TIOLs and manufacturer validated formulae for calculating the required lens power have enabled the correction of corneal astigmatism during cataract surgery without the need for any additional incisions. Provided the eye has regular astigmatism, the rotational alignment of the TIOL with respect to the steep meridian of the cornea is critical for achieving the desired refractive outcome. Rotation of a toric IOL from its intended orientation can degrade its cylindrical corrective power by 3.3% for every 1 degree (°) off axis. Therefore, a 30° rotation of the TIOL would completely negate the effectiveness of the astigmatic correction and a misorientation of > 30° would induce additional astigmatism. Potential risk factors for misorientation of the TIOL include erroneous measurement of the pre-operative corneal astigmatism, inaccurate marking of the cornea, incomplete viscoelastic removal, IOL dialling error (e.g. due to parallax) and postoperative rotation due to wound leak or capsule contraction. Most reports on TIOL use to date, however, are from specialist cataract surgeons who are highly experienced with high volume toric lens use and their excellent results may not necessarily be representative of the wider ophthalmology community. The purpose of this study was therefore to assess the real-world outcomes of TIOL implantation in a typical public hospital performed by a mixture of surgeons as part of routine cataract surgery in the NHS.

Methods

We conducted a retrospective analysis of all patients who received a TIOL implant at the Oxford University Hospitals NHS Foundation Trust, a tertiary referral centre in the UK, over a 10 months period. This retrospective clinical audit was conducted with local institutional review board (IRB) approval from the Clinical Effectiveness Committee, Clinical Governance and Risk Neurosciences, Orthopaedics, Trauma and Specialist Surgery (NOTSS) Division, Oxford University Hospitals NHS Foundation Trust (Datix registration no. 4916), and exempt from UK National Research Ethics Service approval (as per NHS Health Research Authority guidance). Permission was given to access patient data, which were de-identified. It adhered to the tenets of the Declaration of Helsinki. As per local policy, patients with $\Delta K > 2.00$ dioptres (D) based on biometry obtained using a Zeiss IOLMaster 500 (Carl Zeiss AG, Jena, Germany) and consistent with previous refraction, were eligible for a TIOL. Patients in whom the previous optometry report suggested inability to fully correct visual acuity (to 6/6) with glasses underwent corneal topography using Pentacam (Oculus, Wetzlar, Germany) to rule out irregular corneal astigmatism (a contraindication to TIOL implantation in this hospital). The biometry protocol followed

the recommendations within the Royal College of Ophthalmologists Cataract Surgery Guidelines 2010 (https://www.rcophth.ac.uk/standards-publications-research/clinical-guidelines). Briefly, the best of 5 repeat axial length measurements (with a minimum signal-to-noise ratio of 2.0) and the mean of 3 sets of keratometry measurements were selected for IOL power calculations. Biometry was repeated if the inter-eye axial length difference was found to be > 0.3 mm and potential causes reviewed.

All procedures were performed by surgeons ranging from specialty registrars to consultants (attending physicians) who had experience of at least 300 cataract procedures. The standard surgical approach to cataract surgery involved micro-coaxial phacoemulsification through a 2.2 mm corneal incision. Prior to surgery, the cornea was anaesthetised and marked at 90° and 270° on the slit lamp using a sterile 20 gauge needle followed by marker pen with vertical head alignment to minimise cyclotorsion. Three types of 1-piece acrylic TIOLs were available and the choice was made based on surgeons' preferences: Tecnis Toric Aspheric IOL (AMO, Illinois, USA), T-flex Aspheric Toric IOL (Rayner, Worthing, West Sussex, UK), or Acrysof IQ Toric IOL (Alcon, Fort Worth, USA). In one eye, a secondary Rayner Sulcoflex Toric (653 T) pseudophakic supplementary IOL was implanted (Table 1). TIOL power and orientation were chosen using the manufacturers' online calculators, which took into account axial length (AL), keratometry values (K-values), anterior chamber depth and surgeon-induced astigmatism. Under the operating microscope, a Mendez Degree Gauge was used to mark the steep meridian of the cornea. After cataract extraction, the TIOL was injected into the capsular bag under viscoelastic (Healon, Abbott Medical Optics, Santa Ana, USA) and dialled to align with the marked steep meridian. Healon was then removed from the bag, including from behind the IOL, and the IOL alignment rechecked before the end of surgery. Postoperatively, all patients received chloramphenicol eye drops four times per day for 2 weeks and dexamethasone 0.1% eye drops four times per day for 4 weeks, and were reviewed at 2 weeks (Fig. 1).

Outcome measures were pre- and post-operative visual acuities (unaided and best-corrected), refractions (obtained either by manifest refraction by an optometrist or by autorefraction), and all complications. The minimum follow-up of post-implantation refractive outcomes was 2 weeks. The predicted spherical equivalent (SE) following toric IOL implantation was compared with the post-operative refraction. Statistical analyses were performed using Microsoft Excel (Microsoft Corporation, Washington, USA), StatsDirect (StatsDirect Ltd., UK), and GraphPad Prism 7.0a (GraphPad Software Inc., California, USA). Paired t-tests were used when normality was noted, otherwise the Wilcoxon signed rank test was used for statistical

Table 1 A list of 32 toric intraocular lenses (TIOL) implanted over a 10 months period

ID	Age (yr)	Eye	Co-morbidity	IOL type	IOL power (D)	Pre-op BCVA	Post-op UVA
1	67	R		Tecnis ZCT 400	20.0	0.30	0.30
2	61	R		Tecnis ZCT 225	14.0	0.30	0.00
		L		Tecnis ZCT 225	14.0	0.50	0.10
3[a]	56	R		Tecnis ZCT 400	12.0	0.30	0.00
4	76	R		Tecnis ZCT 225	18.0	0.50	0.18
5	77	L[b]		Tecnis ZCT 150	20.0	0.30	0.00
		R		Tecnis ZCT 400	19.0	0.60	0.18
6	67	R		Tecnis ZCT 400	16.5	0.30	0.00
		L	ERM	Tecnis ZCT 400	13.5	0.50	0.48
7[a]	49	R	Vitrectomised	Tecnis ZCT 300	19.5	0.50	0.30
8	67	L		Tecnis ZCT 400	16.5	0.30	0.10
		R		Tecnis ZCT 225	11.0	0.20	0.00
9	78	R		Tecnis ZCT 300	20.5	0.50	0.30
10	82	L		Tecnis ZCT 225	23.5	0.00	0.00
11	82	R		Tecnis ZCT 400	24.5	0.20	0.18
12	65	L		Tecnis ZCT 400	17.5	0.30	0.00
		R		Tecnis ZCT 400	11.0	0.30	0.18
13	41	R		Tecnis ZCT 400	26.5	2.00	0.18
		L	Amblyopia	Tecnis ZCT 400	27.5	1.00	0.18
14	60	L		Tecnis ZCT 400	26.0	0.00	0.30
		R		Tecnis ZCT 400	26.5	0.30	0.30
15	80	R	Amblyopia	Tecnis ZCT 400	27.0	0.60	0.30
16	21	R		Tecnis ZCT 300	22.5	0.48	0.00
17	78	L		Tecnis ZCT 225	31.0	0.18	0.18
18	85	L		Tecnis ZCT 400	21.0	0.30	0.18
19	82	R		Tecnis ZCT 400	17.5	0.30	0.30
20	86	L		Tecnis ZCT 300	23.5	0.30	0.10
21	53	R	Previous LASIK & PCRI	AcrySof SN60 T8	23.0	0.18	0.10
		L		AcrySof SN60 T8	22.0	0.30	0.10
22	74	L		Rayner T-flex 623	18.0	0.48	0.18
23	72	L		Rayner T-flex 623	16.0	0.30	0.18
24	74	L	Corneal scar	Rayner T-flex 623	16.5	0.30	0.18

[a]Indicate cases complicated by TIOL rotation, which were corrected surgically
[b]The left eye of patient 5 received a low powered toric IOL (Tecnis ZCT 150) to correct a ΔK of 1.41 D (which is lower than the ΔK > 2.00 D inclusion criteria). This was at the clinician's discretion as the patient had already received a higher powered toric IOL in the fellow eye

comparisons. The sphero-cylindrical refractions were converted to vector notation and analysed using modified Alpins and Goggin's methodology for vector analysis [7]. For the vector analysis, the cylindrical power was resolved into its X and Y components using *sine* and *cosine* trigonometric functions. The difference in power from predicted post-operative refraction was calculated for the spherical equivalent, astigmatic refraction in both X and Y components. The surgically induced refractive correction (SIRC) was calculated. Together these allowed calculation of total error magnitude (TEM) to reflect the error in power of

the astigmatism, and angle error (orientation). Pre- and post-operative blurring strength was also calculated to evaluate the effect of the error on subjective vision [8].

Results

Thirty-two eyes of 24 patients with a mean age of 66.4 years (SD 14.5 yr., range 21–86 yr) were included in the study: 27 eyes received a Tecnis Toric Aspheric IOL, 3 eyes received a Rayner T-flex Aspheric Toric IOL, and 2 eyes received an Acrysof IQ Toric IOL (Table 1). Phacoemulsification and toric IOL implantations were

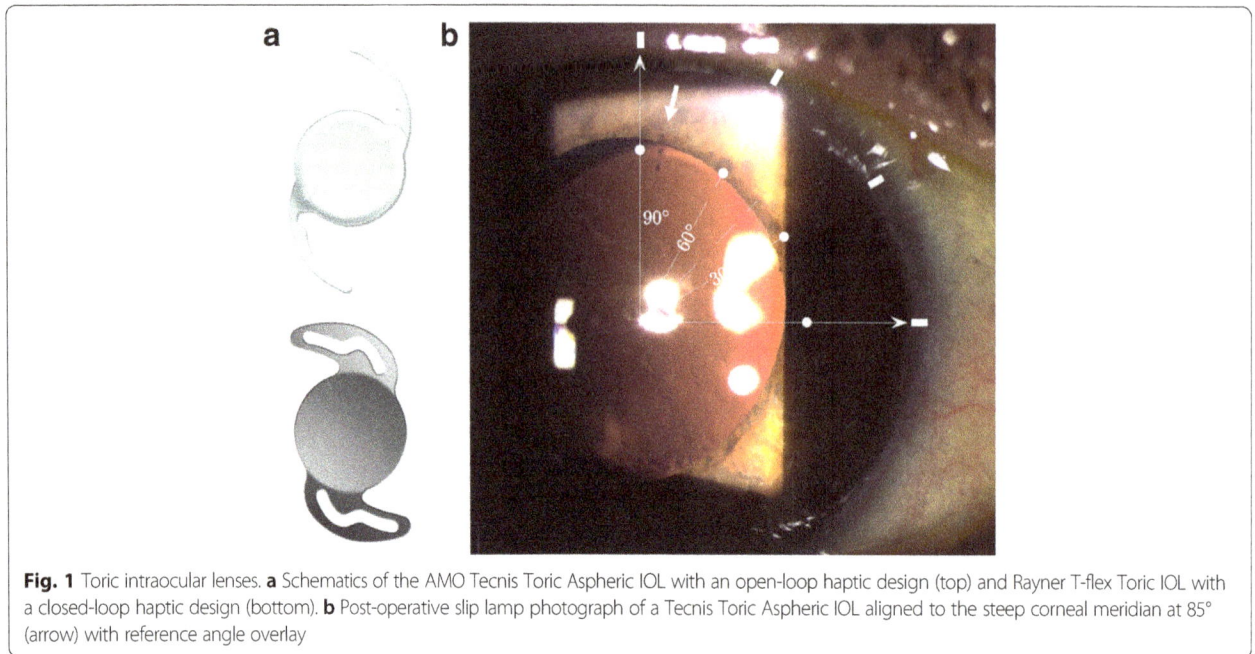

Fig. 1 Toric intraocular lenses. **a** Schematics of the AMO Tecnis Toric Aspheric IOL with an open-loop haptic design (top) and Rayner T-flex Toric IOL with a closed-loop haptic design (bottom). **b** Post-operative slip lamp photograph of a Tecnis Toric Aspheric IOL aligned to the steep corneal meridian at 85° (arrow) with reference angle overlay

performed by 15 different surgeons (3 consultants, 2 associate specialists, 4 fellows and 6 specialty registrars). One patient received a secondary Rayner Sulcoflex toric pseudophakic IOL to correct residual refractive error ($-2.75/-0.75 \times 1°$) following cataract surgery, achieving a final refraction of $0.00/-0.75 \times 10°$ with an UVA of 0.00 LogMAR. This case was however excluded from the cohort analyses as the 'piggy-back' sulcus TIOL was considered not to be comparable with other aforementioned 'in-the-bag' TIOLs.

There were no general cataract surgery related complications, such as posterior capsule rupture, zonular dialysis or endophthalmitis. However, significant TIOL rotation was found in three (9%) eyes post-operatively, which required IOL repositioning. All three eyes received a Tecnis Toric IOL. In the first case, the TIOL was found to have rotated by 10° 1 week post-operatively. IOL repositioning was performed with final unaided visual acuity (UVA) of 0.60 LogMAR and BCVA of 0.00 LogMAR, consistent with a refractive target of -2.44 D. The second case was in a vitrectomised eye following previous retinal detachment repair. The toric IOL rotated by 30° and was repositioned at 2 weeks. The IOL orientation remained stable at 3 months follow-up, achieving a final UVA of 0.30 LogMAR, consistent with a refractive target of -2.12 D. The third case was also an eye that had undergone vitrectomy for retinal detachment repair. The TIOL was found to have rotated by 25° immediately after surgery, which recurred despite IOL repositioning twice in quick succession (over 2 h). The TIOL was eventually exchanged for a single focus IOL combined with PCRIs, leading to an UVA of 0.10 LogMAR. As the TIOL was ultimately

removed in this case, it was included in the complication analysis but excluded from refractive outcomes analysis. Vector analysis was conducted using the final refractions following TIOL repositioning.

In the 32 eyes that received TIOLs, 26 (81%) eyes achieved an improvement in post-operative UVA compared with the pre-operative best-corrected VA (BCVA), 5 (16%) eyes showed no change, and 1 (3%) eye showed a reduction. The median improvement in post-operative UVA over pre-operative BCVA was 0.20 LogMAR (IQR 0.10 to 0.30), equivalent to 2 Snellen lines. The mean post-operative LogMAR UVA ranged from 0.00 to 0.48. In the one eye that showed a poorer post-op UVA than pre-op BCVA, 2.00 D of residual cylinder was found and the UVA (0.30 LogMAR) improved to 0.20 with pinhole.

In terms of final refractive outcome, 18 eyes (56%) reached within ±0.50 D of the predicted SE, 26 eyes (81%) reached within ±1.00 D, 30 eyes (94%) reached within ±1.50 D, and 32 eyes (100%) reached within ±2.00 D (Fig. 2). The range of deviation of the post-operative SE from the predicted SE (based on manufacturers' IOL calculators) was -1.66 to $+1.38$ D with a median of -0.37 D (Fig. 3).

The pre-operative median ΔK was 2.94 D (interquartile range 2.41 to 3.24). The pre-operative median refractive cylinder was 2.63 DC (IQR 1.50 to 3.50) whilst the post-operative median refractive cylinder was 0.75 DC (IQR 0.50 to 1.44), representing a statistically significant reduction (Wilcoxon signed rank test: $p < 0.0001$) (Fig. 4a). Twenty-seven (84%) eyes obtained a reduction in refractive cylindrical correction. However, two (6%) eyes showed no change in refractive cylinder, whilst three (9%) eyes showed an increase in refractive cylinder: from -1.25 to -4.00 DC,

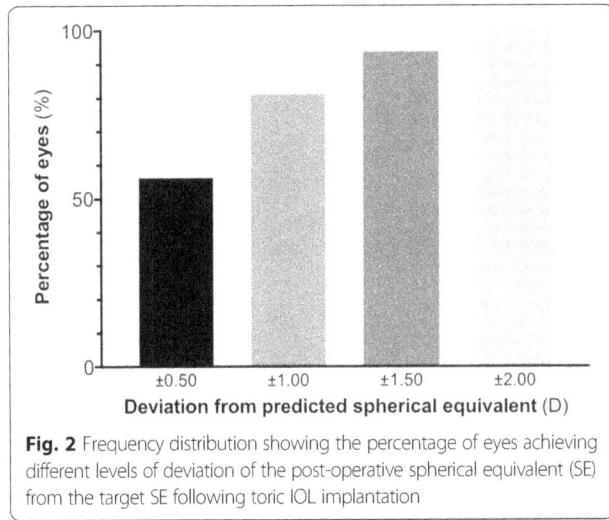

Fig. 2 Frequency distribution showing the percentage of eyes achieving different levels of deviation of the post-operative spherical equivalent (SE) from the target SE following toric IOL implantation

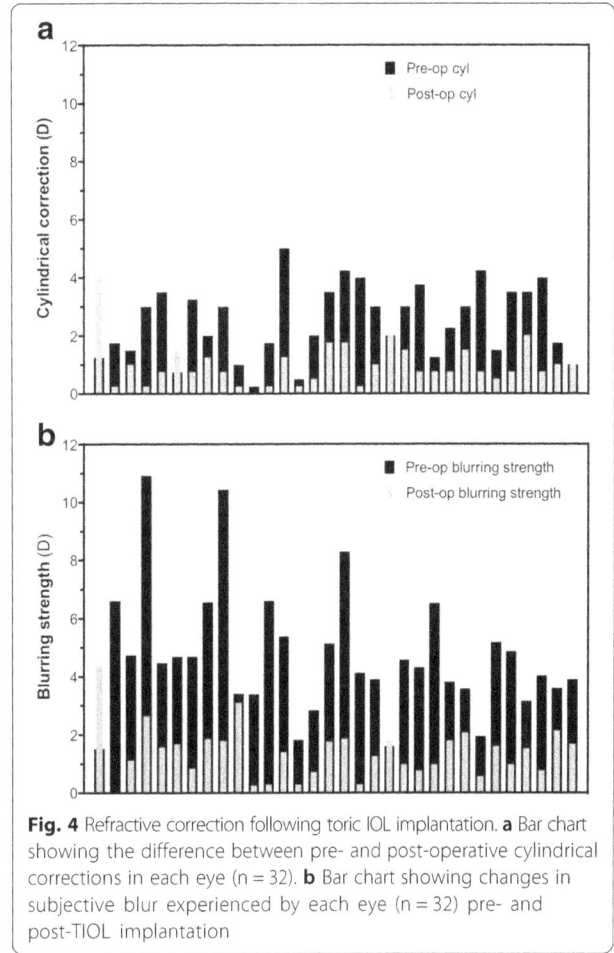

Fig. 4 Refractive correction following toric IOL implantation. **a** Bar chart showing the difference between pre- and post-operative cylindrical corrections in each eye (n = 32). **b** Bar chart showing changes in subjective blur experienced by each eye (n = 32) pre- and post-TIOL implantation

− 0.75 to − 1.50 DC, and − 1.00 to − 2.25 DC, respectively. The first of these three eyes obtained the same post-operative UVA as pre-operative BCVA (0.50 LogMAR), and was not associated with significant IOL rotation - measured to be 6°. The other two eyes both demonstrated improvement of post-op UVA compared with pre-op BCVA despite the increases in refractive cylinder, which was likely due to removal of lens opacity from cataract extraction.

Blurring strength was calculated as the geometrical representation of the sphero-cylindrical refractive errors and represented the subjective blur experienced by the patient as a result of their refractive error. A significant reduction in median blurring strength from 4.39 D (IQR 3.49 to 5.28) pre-operatively to 1.46 D (IQR 0.76 to 1.80) post-operatively was seen in this cohort of eyes following TIOL implantation (95% CI for change in blurring strength = 2.55 to 3.99 D, $p < 0.0001$) (Fig. 4b).

The discrepancy between achieved astigmatism and pre-operative astigmatism for each individual could be

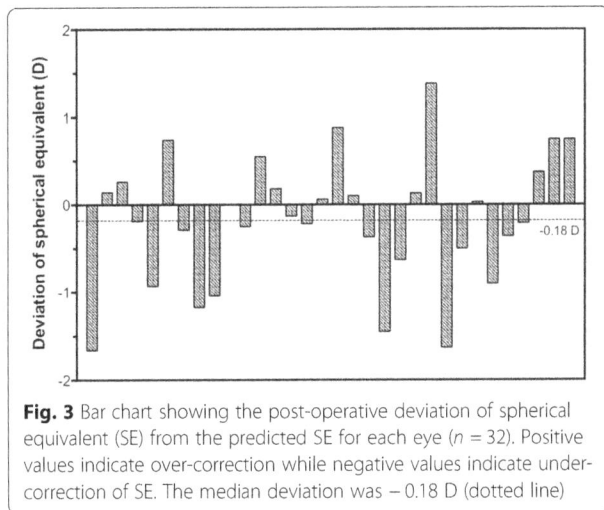

Fig. 3 Bar chart showing the post-operative deviation of spherical equivalent (SE) from the predicted SE for each eye (n = 32). Positive values indicate over-correction while negative values indicate under-correction of SE. The median deviation was − 0.18 D (dotted line)

expressed as an error vector and subjected to vector analysis in which polar coordinates (of cylinder power and axis) were converted to Cartesian values (Fig. 5) [7]. The combined error vector of the cohort had a magnitude of − 0.42 D and angle of 4.63°, indicating a tendency for slight under-correction of astigmatism.

Discussion

This study has shown that TIOLs could provide predictable correction of the sphero-cylindrical error in cases of low to moderate corneal astigmatism. It represents one of the largest cohorts assessing the refractive outcomes and rotational stability of toric IOLs within a real-world mixed surgeon public health service (NHS) setting.

The post-operative unaided distance visual acuity and refractive cylindrical corrections of this cohort were comparable to other published studies of 1-piece acrylic toric IOLs (Table 2). For instance, Hirnschall et al. [9] evaluated the outcomes of 30 eyes that received the Tecnis Toric IOL and found a post-op UVA of − 0.05 logMAR at 3 months and mean IOL rotation of 2.7° (SD 3.0). Tsinpoulos et al. [10] demonstrated that 90% of a cohort of 29 eyes that received the Alcon Acrysof toric IOL achieved UVA ≥0.30

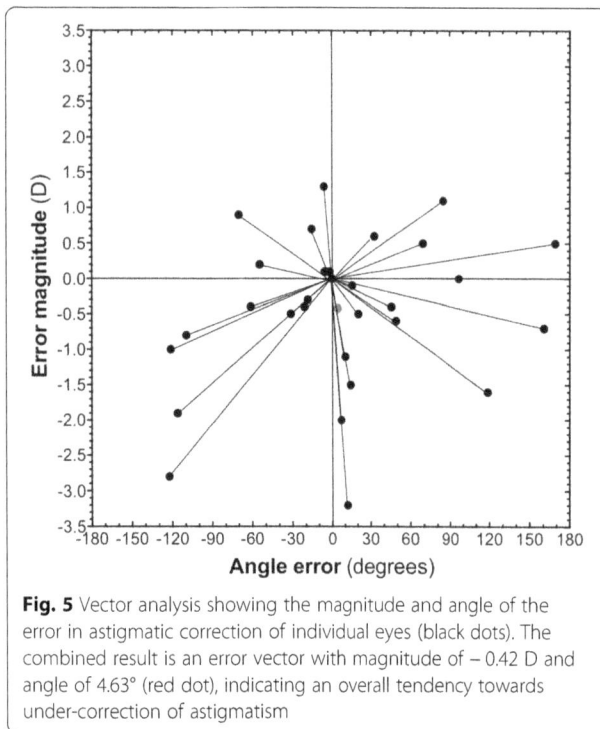

Fig. 5 Vector analysis showing the magnitude and angle of the error in astigmatic correction of individual eyes (black dots). The combined result is an error vector with magnitude of − 0.42 D and angle of 4.63° (red dot), indicating an overall tendency towards under-correction of astigmatism

logMAR and mean post-operative astigmatism of 0.64 D (SD 0.61, range 0 to 2.5). Entabi et al. [11] showed that 33 eyes that received the Rayner T-flex toric IOL achieved mean post-operative UVA of 0.28 logMAR (SD 0.23) and mean astigmatism of 0.95 (SD 0.66). They also found a mean difference between targeted and actual IOL cylinder axis of 3.44° (range 0 to 12). The apparent increase (n = 3) or lack of reduction (n = 2) in refractive cylinder observed in some individuals in this study were most likely the result of large degrees of corneal astigmatism, which were previously neutralised by the lens astigmatism, but were unmasked by cataract extraction and only partially neutralised by the TIOL (Fig. 4). The specific reasons for this may include (i) selection of a slightly underpowered TIOL, (iii) small degrees of TIOL rotation or decentration (which can be difficult to detect), (iv) surgically-induced astigmatism, or (iv) uncorrected posterior corneal astigmatism or

corneal ectasia. Despite apparently similar overall post-operative refractive cylindrical corrections obtained by this and other studies, the differences in UVA achieved may be partly related to differences in patient age, ocular co-morbidities (e.g. two eyes had mild amblyopia, 1 eye had ERM and 1 eye had a corneal scar in this cohort – Table 1), and differences in the stringency by which eyes with irregular corneal astigmatism were excluded. Only three patients in this study underwent Pentacam corneal topography to definitively rule out irregular astigmatism, but since then it has been incorporated as our standard protocol for patients undergoing toric IOL implantation in order to optimise refractive outcomes.

TIOL rotation following implantation is a well-known phenomenon and modern lens designs have sought to reduce this risk [12]. The Tecnis Toric and Alcon Acrysof IQ TIOLs used in this study both have an open-loop haptic design, whereas the Rayner T-flex TIOL has a closed-loop haptic design. However, there does not appear to be any strong linkage between these two types of haptic design and rotational stability of the IOLs [9, 11, 13]. Long-term stabilisation of the toric IOL is thought to result of fusion between the anterior and posterior capsules, which trap it in a permanent orientation, however factors that could influence this fusion include capsulorhexis size, residual viscoelastic in the bag, IOL design and material [13]. Older TIOLs were often made of silicone and were associated with poor capsular adhesion and high post-operative misalignment rates, whereas the modern TIOLs (as used in this study) are made of acrylic, which appears to induce stronger capsular adhesions [14]. The three cases of significant TIOL rotation encountered in this cohort appear to indicate previous vitrectomy as a risk factor. One possible explanation is that post-vitrectomy eyes may be associated with zonular weakness, e.g. secondary to zonular stretching by expansile gas, zonular stress from indentation, or zonular damage during vitreous base shaving [15]. If a sector of zonular weakness lies close to the desired TIOL meridian, the resulting uneven tension around the capsular bag could provide the torque for IOL rotation. It may explain why IOL misalignment recurred

Table 2 Comparison of toric IOL implantation studies

Study	Eyes	Age (years ±SD or range)	Toric IOL	Post-op UVA (logMAR) ± SD	Pre-op cyl (D) ± SD	Post-op cyl (D) ± SD	Max IOL rotation (°)
This study	32	66.6 ± 14.5	Tecnis Toric (n = 27), Rayner T-flex (n = 2), Alcon Acrysof toric (n = 3)	0.16 ± 0.12	2.45 ± 1.2	1.04 ± 0.79	30
Tsinpoulos et al. [10]	29	63 ± 5.4	Alcon Acrysof toric	≥0.30 (90%) ≥0.10 (66%)	2.38 ± 0.91	0.64 ± 0.61	8.4
Hirnschall et al [9]	30	67 (36–85)	Tecnis Toric	−0.05	1.80 ± 0.50	0.90 ± 0.40	13.7
Entabi et al. [11]	33	81 ± 8.9	Rayner T-flex	0.28 ± 0.23	3.35 ± 1.20	0.95 ± 0.66	17

almost immediately after IOL repositioning in one of our cases. This raises the question whether previous vitrectomy might be a relative contraindication to TIOL implantation but a capsule tension ring may be used to prevent TIOL rotation secondary to zonular weakness in those eyes. Interestingly, a recent close observational study of 72 eyes following Tecnis Toric IOL implantation revealed that most (around 60%) of the IOL rotation occurred within 1 h after surgery and further rotation was minimal after 1 week [16]. While TIOL rotation may be detected early, it remains unclear whether immediate repositioning would carry a significant risk of recurrence whereas allowing some capsule-IOL adhesion to develop over a short time period may help to stop the IOL from rotating again.

Vector analysis of the difference between calculated and actual refractive outcomes showed a combined error vector of -0.42 D in magnitude with an angle of $4.63°$, which would suggest a tendency towards under-correction of astigmatism and slight clockwise rotation of the IOL. There could be a range of explanations for the under-correction of astigmatism. For instance, small IOL misalignments could result from inaccurate corneal markings, ocular cyclotorsion on the slit lamp, or decentration of the IOL with regard to angle kappa. Other potential sources of error in toric IOL calculations could arise from incorrect calculation of the cylinder power using standard biometry formulae in cases where the effective lens position or the relationship between anterior and posterior corneal curvature was not as predicted. Newer techniques have now emerged to ensure accurate intraoperative alignment of toric IOLs, such as iris fingerprinting in which high-resolution iris photograph obtained pre-operatively can assist with corneal marking, and intra-operative wavefront aberrometry (IWA).

In summary, the use of the toric IOLs within routine NHS setting consistently improved UVA and reduced blurring strength in patients with significant corneal astigmatism, thereby facilitating spectacle-independence. The median refractive cylinder was reduced from 2.63 D pre-operatively to 0.75 D post-operatively. Three out of 32 (9%) eyes required IOL repositioning to correct lens rotation with previous vitrectomy being a common risk factor in two-thirds of the cases. Cost-benefit analysis of the widespread use of TIOL within a public healthcare setting would need to balance the quality of life improvements associated with spectacle-free vision with the additional costs associated with pre-operative corneal topography and toric IOL implantation, as well as the potential costs associated with lens repositioning/explantation in a proportion of cases.

Conclusions

The post-operative unaided visual acuities (UVA) and refractive outcomes of toric intraocular lens implantation were analysed in a high-volume public health service setting. Three different toric IOLs were implanted: Tecnis Toric, Alcon Acrysof Toric and Rayner T-flex. Post-operative UVA was superior to pre-operative best-corrected VA in 26 of 32 (81%) eyes. Significant IOL rotation occurred in 9% of cases with previous vitrectomy being a common risk factor in two thirds of the cases.

Abbreviations
BCVA: Best Corrected Visual Acuity; IOL: Intraocular lenses; NHS: National Health Service; OCCI: Opposite clear corneal incisions; PCRI: Peripheral corneal relaxing incisions; TIOL: Toric IOLs; UVA: Unaided visual acuity

Acknowledgements
Not Applicable

Funding
Supported by the National Institute for Health Research (NIHR) Biomedical Research Centre (BRC) Oxford, based at the Oxford University Hospitals NHS Foundation Trust and in partnership with the University of Oxford, UK. The views expressed are those of the authors and not necessarily those of the NHS, the NIHR or the Department of Health. The sponsor and funding organization had no role in the design or conduct of this research.

Authors' contributions
KX: Conception and design of study, acquisition of data, analysis and interpretation of data. Manuscript drafting and revision. JKJ: Acquisition of data, analysis and interpretation of data, and revision of manuscript. SPM: Conception and design of study, acquisition of data, analysis and interpretation of data. SH: Analysis, drafting and revision of manuscript. PHR: Conception and design of study, acquisition of data, analysis and interpretation of data. Manuscript revision. REM: Conception and design of study, acquisition of data, analysis and interpretation of data. Manuscript revision. All authors have read and approved the final manuscript.

Consent for publication
Not Applicable

Competing interests
The authors declare that they have no competing interests.

References
1. Hoffer KJ. Biometry of 7500 cataractous eyes. Am J Ophthalmol. 1980;90:360–8.
2. Wang L, Misra M, Koch DD. Peripheral corneal relaxing incisions combined with cataract surgery. J Cataract Refract Surg. 2003;29:712–22.
3. Budak K, Friedman NJ, Koch DD. Limbal relaxing incisions with cataract surgery. J Cataract Refract Surg. 1998;24:503–8.
4. Muller-Jensen K, Fischer P, Slepe U. Limbal relaxing incisions to correct astigmatism in clear corneal cataract surgery. J Refract Surg. 1999;15:586–9.

5. Netto MV, Mohan RR, Ambrosio R Jr, Hutcheon AE, Zieske JD, Wilson SE. Wound healing in the cornea: a review of refractive surgery complications and new prospects for therapy. Cornea. 2005;24:509–22.

6. Dayanir V, Azar DT. LASIK complications. In: Yanoff M, Duker J, editors. Ophthalmology. 2nd ed. St. Louis: Mosby; 2004. p. 179–85.

7. Alpins NA, M Goggin M. Practical astigmatism analysis for refractive outcomes in cataract and refractive surgery. Surv Ophthalmol. 2014;49:109–22.

8. Eydelman MB, Drum B, Holladay J, Hilmantel G, et al. Standardized analyses of correction of astigmatism by laser systems that reshape the cornea. J Refract Surg. 2006;22(1):81–95.

9. Hirnschall N, Maedel S, Weber M, Findl O. Rotational stability of a single-piece toric acrylic intraocular lens: a pilot study. Am J Ophthalmol. 2014;157(2):405–11.

10. Tsinopoulos IT, Tasaosis TD, Ziakas NG, Dimitrakos SA. Acrylic toric intraocular lens implantation: a single center experience concerning clinical outcomes and postoperative rotation. Clin Ophthalmol. 2010;4:137–42.

11. Entabi M, Harman F, Lee N, Bloom PA. Injectable 1-piece hydrophilic acrylic toric intraocular lens for cataract surgery: efficacy and stability. J Cataract Refract Surg. 2011;37:235–40.

12. Ahmed II, Rocha G, Slomovic AR, et al. Visual function and patient experience after bilateral implantation of toric intraocular lenses. J Cataract Refract Surg. 2010;36:609–16.

13. Koshy JJ, Nishi Y, Hirnschall N, et al. Rotational stability of a single-piece toric acrylic intraocular lens. J Cataract Refract Surg. 2010;36(10):1665–70.

14. Oshika T, Nagata T, Ishii Y. Adhesion of lens capsule to intraocular lenses of polymethylmethacrylate, silicone, and acrylic foldable materials: an experimental study. Br J Ophthalmol. 1998;82:549–53.

15. Cole CJ, Charteris DG. Cataract extraction after retinal detachment repair by vitrectomy: visual outcome and complications. Eye (Lond). 2009;23(6):1377–81.

16. Inoue Y, Takehara H, Oshika T. Axis misalignment of toric intraocular lens: placement error and postoperative rotation. Ophthalmology. 2017;124(6): 1424–5.

8

Complete occlusion of anterior capsulorhexis after uneventful cataract surgery, treated with YAG laser capsulotomy

Hoon Dong Kim[1], Jae Min Kim[2] and Jong Jin Jung[2*]

Abstract

Background: Capsular contraction syndrome (CCS) has been reported as an uncommon complication after an cataract extraction surgery with intact anterior capsulorhexis. This report is written to present a case of complete occlusion of the anterior capsulorhexis opening after an uneventful cataract surgery, which was treated with non-invasive treatment.

Case presentation: A 69-year-old woman complained of decreased visual acuity in her right eye, which had started 2 months ago. She underwent phacoemulsification with an uneventful anterior capsulorhexis before 3 months. A total occlusion of the anterior capsulorhexis opening with capsular phimosis was identified on slit-lamp biomicroscopy, and a circular anterior capsulotomy using neodymium-doped yttrium aluminum garnet (Nd:YAG) laser was performed immediately. The capsulotomy site remained clear after a couple of years.

Conclusions: It is supposed that proliferation of fibrotic tissue was relatively prominent in this case, rather than the appearance of capsular phimosis. This case can be an uncommon showing a total occlusion of the anterior capsulorhexis opening with prominent fibrotic proliferation pattern after an uneventful cataract surgery. Additionally, the occlusion could be removed with a non-invasive procedure, and was maintained clearly for several years.

Keywords: Anterior capsulorhexis, Capsular contraction syndrome, Fibrotic proliferation, Phacoemulsification, Total occlusion

Background

Capsular contraction syndrome (CCS) has been reported as an uncommon complication after an cataract extraction surgery with intact anterior capsulorhexis [1–3]. It is treated by surgical removal or application of laser to the thickened and opaque anterior capsulorhexis site. It is considered that most cases of CCS are associated with an underlying disease showing zonular weakness and chronic inflammation [2, 3]. However, several patients of CCS without any clinical signs of obvious zonular weakness or inflammatory reaction were presented in previous reports [1–4]. Therefore, we would like to report a

case of complete occlusion of the anterior capsulorhexis opening after an uneventful cataract surgery, that was treated with neodymium-doped yttrium aluminum garnet (Nd:YAG) laser.

Case presentation

A 69-year-old woman visited our clinic, complaining of decreased visual acuity in her right eye, which had started 2 months ago. There was no documented history of any systemic disease or drug intake. Three years ago, she had undergone laser iridotomy in the right eye following an angle-closure attack. Phacoemulsification with an uneventful anterior capsulorhexis was performed. Intraoperatively, the anterior capsulorhexis opening was noted to approximately 5.5 mm in diameter, and clinical features of prominent zonular weakness were not

* Correspondence: jiny0122@kimeye.com
[2]Myung-Gok Eye Research Institute, Department of Ophthalmology, Kim's Eye Hospital, Konyang University College of Medicine, 136, Yeongsin-ro, Yeongdeungpo-gu, Seoul 07301, Korea
Full list of author information is available at the end of the article

evident. A one-piece aspheric hydrophobic acrylic intraocular lens with an overall diameter of 13.0 mm, optic diameter of 6.0 mm and power of +22.0 diopters was implanted in the bag without any decenteration. The best corrected visual acuity (BCVA) was 20/20 in both eyes postoperatively, and there were no remarkable findings. Four months later, however, her visual acuity was found to have decreased to 20/60 in the right eye. Slit-lamp biomicroscopy revealed a total occlusion of the anterior capsulorhexis opening with capsular phimosis (Fig. 1). Immediately, a circular anterior capsulotomy using Nd:YAG laser was performed. After 1 month, the capsular phimosis had not recurred, and additional findings about zonular weakness were not apparent. The BCVA in the right eye had recovered to 20/20 with no other remarkable findings under slit-lamp biomicroscopy (Fig. 1). The capsulotomy site

remained clear after 2 years, and the visual acuity was also unchanged (Fig. 1).

Discussion and conclusions

CCS is one of the well-known complications of continuous curvilinear capsulorrhexis. It has been described as an exaggerated fibrotic response that can lead to a reduction in the size of the anterior capsulotomy [1, 2]. Thereafter, CCS results in impaired visual function secondary to the opacity in pupillary area. It has been associated with uveitis, pseudoexfoliation, myotonic dystrophy, and retinitis pigmentosa [3]. CCS has also occurred with small capsulorrhexis openings of less than 6 mm diameter, and Acrylic IOL revealed lowest rates [4]. The present case was an unusual, compared with previously reported CCS cases that were treated with Nd:YAG laser radial capsulotomy, because an uneventful

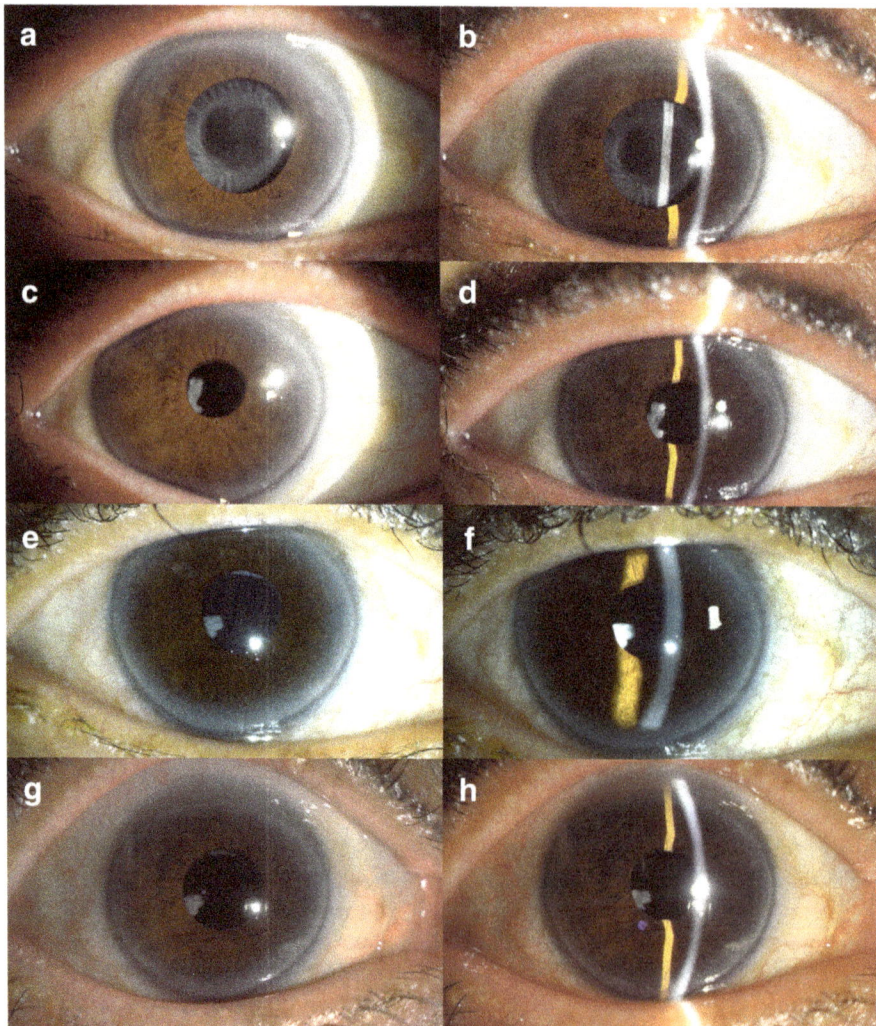

Fig. 1 Consecutive findings of silt-lamp biomicroscopy on the right eye. Total occlusion of anterior capsulorhexis opening was identified (**a**, **b**). Cleared anterior capsulorrhexis site followed by anterior capsulotomy using Nd:YAG laser (**c**, **d**). Capsulotomy site remained clearly after 6 months (**e**, **f**) and there was no remarkable change on capsulotomy site after 2 years (**g**, **h**)

surgery without zonular weakness was performed, the patient had no underlying disease except for a history of an angle-closure attack; furthermore, anterior capsulorhexis opening was completely occluded. In addition, proliferation of fibrotic tissue was relatively prominent in this case, rather than the appearance of capsular phimosis. In previous studies, CCS was thought to have been caused by two underlying mechanisms; shrinkage of the capsulorhexis leading to the formation of smaller diameter capsular opening, and the development of a fibrocellular membrane caused by lens epithelial cells closing remaining central opening [5]. Spang et al. noted that complete occluded anterior capsulorhexis opening was filled with proliferated lens epithelial cells under light microscopy, and the cellular elements revealed a positive reaction for actin filament upon immunohisto-chemical analysis [5]. In our opinion, this is an uncommon case showing a total occlusion of the anterior capsulorhexis opening with prominent fibrotic proliferation pattern after an uneventful cataract surgery. Additionally, the occlusion could be removed with a non-invasive procedure, and was maintained clearly for a couple of years.

Abbreviations
BCVA: Best corrected visual acuity; CCS: Capsular contraction syndrome; Nd:YAG: Neodymium-doped yttrium aluminum garnet

Acknowledgements
Not applicable

Funding
This work was supported by the Soonchunhyang University Research Fund.

Author's contributions
JMK, JJJ participated in the design of the study, and conceived the study. HDK, JMK were major contributors in writing the manuscript. HDK, JJJ helped to draft the manuscript. All authors read and approved the final manuscript.

Consent for publication
Written informed consent to publish this case report was obtained from the patient.

Competing interests
The authors declare that they have no competing interests.

Author details
[1]Department of Ophthalmology, College of Medicine, Soonchunhyang University, Cheonan, Korea. [2]Myung-Gok Eye Research Institute, Department of Ophthalmology, Kim's Eye Hospital, Konyang University College of Medicine, 136, Yeongsin-ro, Yeongdeungpo-gu, Seoul 07301, Korea.

References
1. Davison JA. Capsule contraction syndrome. J Cataract Refract Surg. 1993;19:582–9.
2. Werner L, et al. Anterior capsule opacification; a histopathological study comparing different IOL styles. Ophthalmology. 2000;107:463–71.
3. Hayashi H, Hayashi K, Nakao F, Hayashi F. Area reduction in the anterior capsule opening in eyes of diabetes mellitus patients. J Cataract Refract Surg. 1998;24:1105–10.
4. Joo CK, Shin JA, Kim JH. Capsular opening contraction after continuous curvilinear capsulorhexis and intraocular lens implantation. J Cataract Refract Surg. 1996;22:585–90.
5. Spang KM, Rohrbach JM, Weidle EG. Complete occlusion of the anterior capsular opening after intact capsulorhexis: Clinicopathologic correlation. Am J Ophthalmol. 1999;127:343–5.

Femtosecond laser-assisted cataract surgery in a public teaching hospital setting

Alfonso Vasquez-Perez[1], Andrew Simpson[1] and Mayank A. Nanavaty[1,2]* (iD)

Abstract

Background: To evaluate the efficiency and practicality of femtosecond laser assisted cataract surgery (FLACS) in a public teaching hospital setting using a mobile FLACS system compared to conventional phacoemulsification cataract surgery (CPCS).

Methods: Ninety eyes from 90 patients underwent either FLACS or CPCS (45 in each group). Cataracts were graded using the Lens Opacities Classification System III system. Outcome measures included total surgery duration, femtosecond laser treatment time, vacuum time (VT), total phacoemulsification time (TPT) and total phacoemulsification power (TPP).

Results: No differences were observed in the preoperative mean cataract grades and co-morbidities. FLACS took longer than CPCS with a mean difference of 5.2 ± 4.5 min (range: 0–18.8 min). The average femtosecond laser treatment time was 4.3 ± 3.4 min (range: 1–15.5 min). The VT was 2.51 ± 0.45 min (range: 1.59–4.10 min). Although not significant, TPT in FLACS showed a trend towards improvement (mean 1.0 ± 0.6 s; range: 0.1–2.4 s) compared to CPCS (mean 1.2 ± 0.6 min; range: 0.5–2.5 min). Whereas, TPP was significantly less in FLACS (mean 17.9 ± 5.0%; range: 5–27%) compared to CPCS (mean 20.3 ± 4.1%; range: 12.0–28.7%)($p = 0.031$).

Conclusions: The mobile FLACS system housed in the same operating room increased the surgical duration by 5.2 min. The average VT was 2.51 min, which was lower in comparison to published experience using non-mobile FLACS systems.

Keywords: FLACS, Femtosecond laser cataract surgery, Phacoemulsification, Teaching hospital, Conventional cataract surgery

Background

As cataract removal and its treatment options continue to evolve, the necessity of new innovations to circumvent standard phacoemulsification continues to be questioned. Femtosecond laser assisted cataract surgery (FLACS) has been shown to offer numerous potential advantages including a customized size and centration of capsulorhexis, astigmatic incisions and lens fragmentation of white and brunescent cataracts [1–6]. It also requires less phacoemulsification power and time thereby diminishing corneal endothelial injury; however its superiority over conventional phacoemulsification cataract surgery (CPCS) is still under scientific scrutiny [7–9]. Besides its cost, logistical challenges which include longer operating times and additional operating area represent major drawbacks that make cataract surgeons reluctant to adopt FLACS [4, 10–12].

In a public teaching hospital where cost and efficiency remain at the forefront of funding decisions, FLACS has generally been considered untenable due to the significant time and logistical burdens. For instance, due to the substantial clinical footprint of a femtosecond laser, almost all available platforms require their own dedicated room which is expensive, particularly in city hospitals where space comes at a premium. Additionally, unlike other theatre equipment, most FLACS lasers are completely immobile which means patients must be shuttled between rooms to complete surgery which not only adds time and increases risk of

* Correspondence: mayank.nanavaty@bsuh.nhs.uk

The results of this study were presented in parts at the European Society of Cataract & Refractive Surgery conference 2016, Copenhagen and at the American Society of Cataract & Refractive Surgery Conference 2016, New Orleans.

[1]Sussex Eye Hospital, Brighton & Sussex University Hospitals NHS Trust, Eastern Road, Brighton BN2 5BF, UK

[2]Brighton & Sussex Medical School, University of Sussex, Falmer, Brighton BN1 9PX, UK

infection but also creates an additional liability burden for a hospital in the event that a patient sustains an injury during the transfer [13].

The LDV Z8 femtosecond laser system is the only completely mobile system with a small clinical footprint that can be shuttled in and out of rooms eliminating the need to move the surgeon and patient [14]. As space, time and general efficiency are core components of successful workflow in the public hospital setting, we decided to investigate how the LDV Z8 laser would perform in the public care setting compared to traditional phacoemulsification cataract surgery (CPSC) in terms of surgical time and patient exposure to phaco energy. Publications on femtosecond lasers, which explore operating times of FLACS versus CPSC, have examined stationary platforms, which require more theatre space [15–18].

In this study we evaluate how the use of a mobile femtosecond laser platform shuttled to the required operating room changes the operating times compared with CPCS with surgeons with varying surgical experience. This study was not aimed at identifying inter-surgeon differences but rather exploring the impact of having mobile FLACS system on the surgical duration in real time during theatre lists in a public teaching hospital.

Methods

This prospective study included 90 eyes from 90 patients; 45 eyes underwent mobile FLACS and 45 eyes underwent CPCS at the Sussex Eye Hospital, Brighton & Sussex University Hospitals NHS Trust, Brighton, United Kingdom. This study was approved by the Audit and Research department at the Sussex Eye Hospital, Brighton & Sussex University Hospitals NHS Trust and followed the tenets of the Declaration of Helsinki.

Patients needing only routine cataract surgery were included in this study. No exclusions were made on the basis of cataract density, age and the depth of the eye socket. Patients with subluxated and traumatic cataracts were excluded.

The mobile laser was acquired through a local company (Instinctive UK Ltd., United Kingdom), which brought the device to the facility on scheduled surgery days and removed it the same day. Participants were recruited for the study on the day they were scheduled to undergo surgery whereby on days when the mobile Ziemer Z8 LDV was present, all patients were invited to participate in the study and offered an option for FLACS or CPCS. Patients whose surgery date did not coincide with the day the laser was present were informed, about the study and invited to participate in the CPCS arm. Patients who declined to take part in the study were offered cataract surgery as per usual United Kingdom National Health Service (NHS) protocols.

Prior to the recruitment of patients in this study, each surgeon (a senior, mid and trainee level surgeon) was assessed on 10 consecutive FLACS cases and certified. Following this, 90 patients were consecutively recruited into the FLACS and CPCS groups between October 2015 and March 2016. All surgeries were completed without moving the patient and in the same operating room that contained a mobile femtosecond laser (Z8 LDV, Ziemer, Port, Switzerland) and the Centurion phacoemulsification platform (Alcon Surgical, Fort Worth, USA). The size of the operating theatre was 10 ft × 10 ft. The arrangement of the FLACS laser, phacoemulsification machine, scrub trolley and the microscope is shown in Fig. 1.

On the day of the surgery, patients were dilated with G. Tropicamide 1% (Minims, Bausch & Lomb UK limited, UK) and G. Phenylephrine 2.5% (Minims, Bausch & Lomb UK limited, UK). Cataract density was graded using LOCS III grading [19]. At the time of the surgery, an independent theatre practitioner recorded the 'total surgery duration' or time from betadine 5% (Minims, Bausch & Lomb UK limited, UK) application to speculum removal at surgery completion.. Additionally for FLACS cases, time was recorded starting when the suction ring touched the eyeball before the suction was applied and the ring was removed to after the suction was released. This time was labeled as 'Femtosecond laser treatment time' and included anything that happened between the above two time points such as time lost due to docking issues, laser planning delays, re-checking the laser parameters whilst the ring still touching the eye but prior to vacuum application, re-dockings due to failed suction, etc. The duration of applied vacuum via the suction ring for the treatment

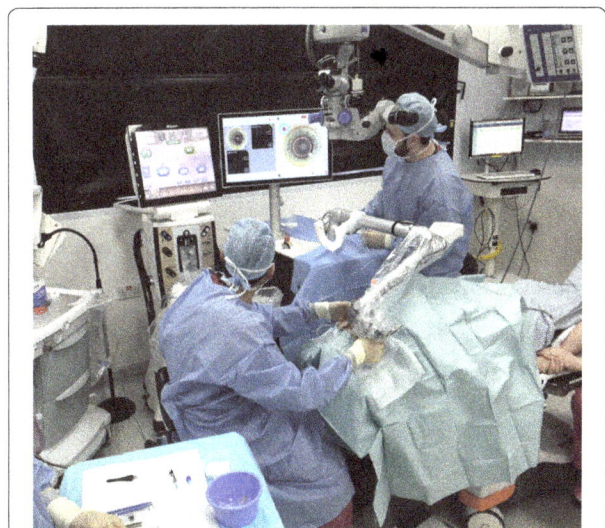

Fig. 1 The arrangement of the mobile femtosecond laser, phacoemulsification machine, scrub trolley and the microscope. This shows the mobile femtosecond laser housed in the same theatre with the phacomachine next to the patient's bed

was recorded as 'vacuum time' (VT). Any intraoperative complication or event was also noted at the end of the procedure. Total phacoemulsification time (TPT) and total phacoemulsification power (TPP) was recorded from the phacoemulsification machine.

The primary outcome measure was total surgical duration. Secondary outcome measures included femtosecond laser treatment time, VT, TPT and TPP.

Surgical technique

All surgeries were performed under topical anaesthesia (G. Proxymethacaine Minims, Bausch & Lomb UK limited, UK)). In FLACS cases, a disposable suction ring was applied to the eye and was filled with balance salt solution creating a fluid-filled interface. The mobile arm of the laser system was then docked over the cornea. Once the integrated OCT imaged the ocular structures and the surgeon confirmed the parameters, the laser was applied starting with lens fragmentation in four quadrants and then capsulotomy with a predetermined diameter. Laser power was graded as per the density of the cataract based on LOCS III cataract grading in that the energy was titrated based on the surgeons experience of the laser with the grade of the cataract. If the docking was not successful in the first attempt, subsequent attempts were made until a successful docking was achieved. The time of when the suction ring was removed was noted. All patients, irrespective of FLACS or CPCS, received manual superior corneal incisions and 2 paracentesis at 0 and 180 degrees. In the FLACS cases, the free-floating anterior capsulorhexis flap was removed with capsulorhexis forceps after viscoelastic injection followed by hydrodisection. As the nucleus was already fragmented the nucleus was split using primary chop technique. Following the removal of nucleus, a bimanual irrigation and aspiration was performed and a single piece hydrophilic acrylic intraocular lens was implanted into the capsular bag. Intracameral Cefuroxime (Aprokam, Thea Pharmaceuticals, France) was injected after thorough irrigation and aspiration to remove the residual viscoelastic. The paracentesis wound were hydrated and the speculum was removed. The time of the speculum removal was noted in all cases.

Statistical analysis

All data was recorded on Microsoft Office Excel® 2010 (Microsoft® Corporation, USA). Normality of all the data was tested by Kolmogorov-Smirnov test. The SPSS statistics version 22.0 (International Business Machines® Corporation) was used for all statistical analysis. TDS, TPT and TPP between two groups were compared using a 2 sample unpaired 2-tailed t test with pooled variance. Differences with a P value less than 0.05 were considered statistically significant.

Results

There were no significant differences in age and sex between the two groups. The mean age of the patients was 72 ± 10.4 (range: 61–83 years). In the FLACS group there were 20 females and 25 males whereas in the CPCS group there were 27 females and 18 males. In the FLACS group, 23 patients were Caucasians and 2 were Afro-Caribbean. Whereas, in the CPCS group, 44 patients were Caucasians and 1 was Afro-Caribbean and 1 was Chinese. There was no significant difference in the LOCS III grading of the cataracts between the FLACS and CPCS groups. No intraoperative complications were reported in either of the groups.

As shown in Fig. 2, FLACS (mean: 18.5 ± 5.1 min; range: 12–32.4 min) took significantly longer compared to CPCS (mean 12.8 ± 3.7 min; range: 4.5–23.2 min) ($p < 0.0001$). The mean of the difference in the total surgical duration between FLACS and CPCS was 5.2 ± 4.5 min (range: 0–18.8 min). The average femtosecond laser treatment time was 4.3 ± 3.4 min (range: 1–15.5 min). The VT was 2.51 ± 0.45 min (range: 1.59–4.10 min). As shown in Fig. 3, although TPT was less in FLACS (mean 1.0 ± 0.6 s; range: 0.1–2.4 s) compared to CPCS (mean 1.2 ± 0.6 min; range: 0.5–2.5 min) it was not statistically significant ($p = 0.348$). Whereas, TPP was significantly less in FLACS (mean $17.9 \pm 5.0\%$; range: 5–27%) compared to CPCS (mean $20.3 \pm 4.1\%$; range: 12.0–28.7%)($p = 0.031$) (Fig. 4). Although not objectively assessed but the learning curve of FLACS docking skills were similar amongst all grades of the surgeons. For the less experienced surgeons acquiring Femtosecond laser cataract surgery skills improved their overall confidence. Total surgery time for less experienced surgeons was longer for both CPCS and FLACS and shorter for more experienced surgeons.

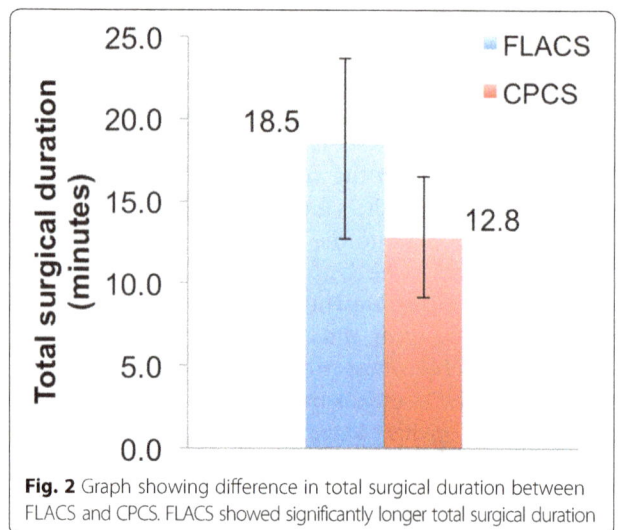

Fig. 2 Graph showing difference in total surgical duration between FLACS and CPCS. FLACS showed significantly longer total surgical duration

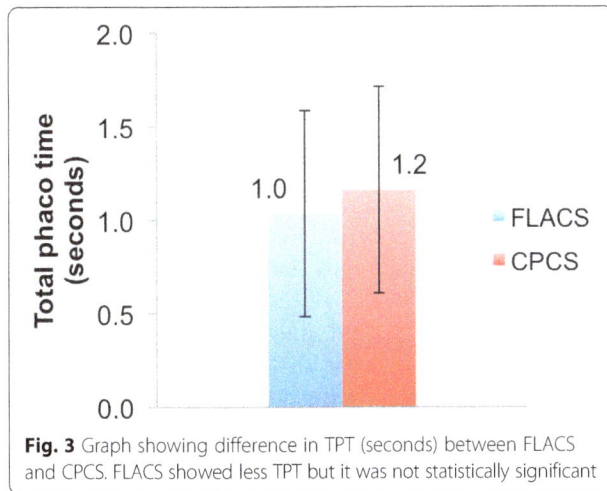

Fig. 3 Graph showing difference in TPT (seconds) between FLACS and CPCS. FLACS showed less TPT but it was not statistically significant

Discussion

FLACS has proven to be an effective and safe technique [1, 7–9, 11, 12, 14] but comparing it with conventional phacoemulsification cataract surgery, FLACS demands logistical considerations which can be challenging to overcome in the public teaching hospital setting where maintaining efficiency is critical. Additional operating times, extra operating space and the consideration for the patients/surgeon to transfer from one room to another to complete the procedure have all been associated with FLACS [4, 10–12, 15]. Information can be found in peer reviewed literature about the potential advantages and outcomes of FLACS [4, 15–18, 20], however, little has been published on how the use of mobile FLACS system affects the amount of operating time in real life in comparison to CPCS.

From the time of betadine application to the point of removal of the speculum, we found that cases undergoing FLACS spent an average of five minutes more compared with CPSC. This difference did not dissipate with surgical experience. In a non-comparative study by a

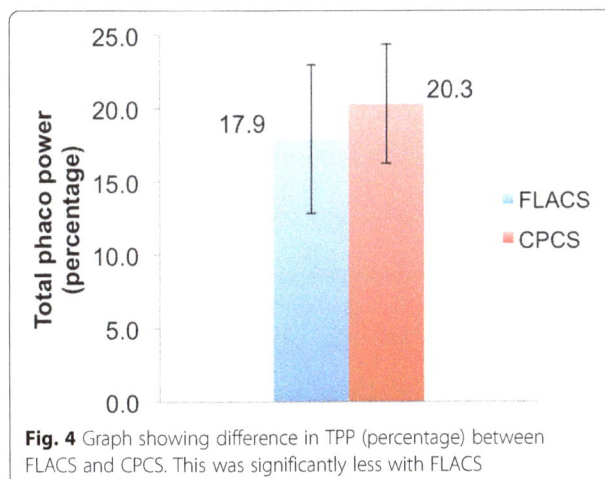

Fig. 4 Graph showing difference in TPP (percentage) between FLACS and CPCS. This was significantly less with FLACS

single surgeon using mobile Ziemer LDV Z8, the TDS was reported to be 16.3 ± 4.5 min going down to 12.5 ± 1.1 min once the learning curve had been reached by an experienced surgeon [21]. Two retrospective studies on static FLACS platforms housed in the same operating room (Catalys Precision Laser System, Abbot medical optics, Santa Ana, CA), evaluated surgical times in FLACS compared to CPCS. Lubahn et al. [17] in 162 cases, considered "total operative time", as the time the patient entered the operating room to the patient leaving the room. Grewal et al. [16] in their study in 166 cases, among different parameters, recorded "procedure time" as the time from the suction ring application in FLACS or corneal incisions in CPCS to the speculum removal. This last parameter in Grewal's study [16] was similar to our primary outcome measure (total surgical duration). Lubahn [17] reported a mean difference of 14 min longer for FLACS whilst Grewal [16] reported only 9 min. In another study but Bali et al. [15] comparing FLACS with CPCS, a non-mobile FLACS system was housed outside the operating room and the mean operating theatre time was 15.7 min for CPCS and 19.8 min for FLACS.

Because different studies have reported FLACS times differently, we decided to report the actual VT and femtosecond laser treatment time. Femtosecond laser treatment time would include VT and any additional time taken before and after suction was switched on and off. This included time to position the suction ring on the cornea, rechecking the laser parameters for the final time with the suction ring in place but before application of suction, any loss of suction and re-docking attempts, etc. A few results of VT have been published with various non-mobile platforms. Grewal et al. [16] in their study using Catalys platform, analyzing the impact of learning curve on the time durations in FLACS, noted a VT of 3.35 min after the surgeon gained experience on few cases. Whereas, Chang et al. [20], using LensAR® platform, reported the VT of 6.72 ± 4.57 min (range: 2–28 min). Using Victus® platform, Baig et al. [21] reported VT of 3.6 ± 0.25 min. Rivera et al. [22] in their study reported VT of 3.75 min (range: 2.5–9.38 min) with Catalys® and 2.88 min (range: 1.13–4.31 min) with LenSx®. Kerr et al. [23] reports the shortest time 3.05 min using the Catalys® system. In comparison to above studies, we found a lower VT of 2.51 ± 0.45 min (range: 1.59–4.10 min) with the mobile Femto LDV Z8.

Although the findings of Grewal et al. [16] and Lubahn et al. [17] cannot be compared directly due to differences in the study outcome measures, our results showed lower total surgical duration with a mobile FLACS system. But like their studies [16, 17], we also found a significantly longer total time for FLACS compared to CPCS which was consistent across surgeons' grades. As femtosecond laser treatment time reports have been similar across different laser platforms; [16–18, 20, 21, 23] the longer operating times of both studies [16, 17] compared to our results undoubtedly may be due to logistical and workflow differences. With non-mobile platforms, even if the femtosecond laser is housed in the same operating room the patients need to be transferred from the laser bed to the microscope, painted and draped before continuing with phacoemulsification under a different operating microscope. Unique to our study is that using a mobile laser platform with varying grades of the surgeon, neither the patient nor the surgeon needed to move irrespective of the patient undergoing FLACS or CPCS. We did not analyze the inter surgeon difference as the aim of our study was only to evaluate the real time difference between the procedures in a teaching environment.

We found statistically significant less TPT and TPP used in the FLACS group but these findings are well known advantages of femtosecond laser reported in vast number of publications [1, 2, 4, 7–12].

Using the only available mobile laser platform (Ziemer LDV, Z8) we found the shorter difference in operating times among published comparative studies of FLACS. This laser uses a fluid-filled patient interface and has an optical coherence tomography (OCT) integrated directly into the hand piece that uses the same optics as the laser beam [18]. In our experience, we found that the most important aspects of the Z8 system were its mobility, which simplifies patient flow, and its size, requiring only a small extra space in the operating room. In a public healthcare setting, both of these aspects are beneficial as caseload and room space are often limiting. Although we did not test other modules on the Z8, it can also be used for refractive surgery and keratoplasty which could be beneficial when sharing the device among other departments in a comprehensive ophthalmic teaching center. Moreover, studies have shown pupil miosis after femtosecond laser application during FLACS [24, 25]. However, in our study, we did not use any preoperative non-steroidal anti-inflammatory eye drops and still did not find significant pupil miosis. We believe this is because previous studies report pupil miosis after femtosecond laser application were performed using non-mobile laser systems housed in a different room and there was a small time delay between laser application and phacoemulsification. Whereas in our study, the mobile Z8 FLACS system was housed in the same operating room and the femtosecond laser application was commenced after painting and draping the patient for the cataract surgery (effectively causing now delay between femtosecond laser application and phacoemulsification).

In terms of safety and efficiency of FLACS in the public hospital setting, intra operative patient transfer has not been addressed appropriately in any study evaluating FLACS; despite requiring additional transport time and staff, it could potentially introduce risks of infections and secondary injuries when patients are moved to a different room. There are hygienic and ethical issues with patient's shuttle between non-mobile laser not housed in the same room and the operating room [23]. And if the patient requires hook or iris expanders before the use of non-mobile femtosecond laser in a clean room outside the operating room then this could be an issue from the point of view of hygiene and infection.

Limitations of our study include the relatively low number of cases and that all three surgeons despite vast experience in CPSC had only limited experience in FLACS. We could assume that with additional experience there might be a reduction in operating times as already shown by a previous study [16]. However we believe that FLACS is a safe and a well-developed technique and has a fast learning curve compared with CPSC. This study also did not focus on the astigmatic correction with femtosecond laser based incision and all surgeries where planned with superior corneal incisions.

Conclusions

Public hospitals must consider the cost/benefit and understand in which patient cases FLACS can become truly beneficial [26–29]. as well as how to share a device across multiple sub-specialties within the ophthalmology department. Centers willing to offer patients the advantages of this new technology in addition to the direct cost related with the laser, must budget the running cost of an operating room and make an effective strategy to reduce operating times and not significantly decrease their caseload. Mobile FLACS system apart from the proven advantages of FLACS requires less space and also appears to perform better in operating times than stationary platforms, however further evaluation of these parameters with direct clinical comparison of mobile and non-mobile FLACS systems are needed.

Abbreviations
CPCS: Conventional phacoemulsification cataract surgery; FLACS: Femtosecond laser assisted cataract surgery; TPP: Total phacoemulsification power; TPT: Total phacoemulsification time; VT: Vacuum time

Acknowledgements
None.

Funding
The authors did not receive any funding or fees for preparation of this report. Ziemer has agreed to cover the journal's publication cost.

Authors' contributions
AV-P: Data collection, analysis and manuscript drafting. AS: Data collection and manuscript drafting. MAN: Data collection, analysis, manuscript drafting and supervision. All authors read and approved the final manuscript.

Consent for publication

Not applicable as this study does not contain any individual patient's data in any form.

Competing interests

MAN is a consultant to Alcon, Rayner and Ziemer. one of the other authors have any financial or proprietary interests in any products or procedures mentioned. Ziemer Ophthalmic Systems, Switzerland funding the publication costs of this manuscript.

References

1. Abell RG, Darian-Smith E, Kan JB, et al. Femtosecond laser-assisted cataract surgery versus standard phacoemulsification cataract surgery: outcomes and safety in more than 4000 cases at a single center. J Cataract Refract Surg. 2015;41(1):47–52.
2. Abell RG, Kerr NM, Howie AR, et al. Effect of femtosecond laser-assisted cataract surgery on the corneal endothelium. J Cataract Refract Surg. 2014; 40(11):1777–83.
3. Hatch KM, Schultz T, Talamo JH, Dick HB. Femtosecond laser-assisted compared with standard cataract surgery for removal of advanced cataracts. J Cataract Refract Surg. 2015;41(9):1833–8.
4. Grewal DS, Schultz T, Basti S, Dick HB. Femtosecond laser-assisted cataract surgery–current status and future directions. Surv Ophthalmol. 2016;61(2): 103–31.
5. Nagy ZZ, Kranitz K, Takacs AI, et al. Comparison of intraocular lens decentration parameters after femtosecond and manual capsulotomies. J Refract Surg. 2011;27(8):564–9.
6. Sutton G, Bali SJ, Hodge C. Femtosecond cataract surgery: transitioning to laser cataract. Curr Opin Ophthalmol. 2013;24(1):3–8.
7. Day AC, Gore DM, Bunce C, Evans JR. Laser-assisted cataract surgery versus standard ultrasound phacoemulsification cataract surgery. Cochrane Database Syst Rev. 2016;7:CD010735.
8. Popovic M, Campos-Moller X, Schlenker MB, Ahmed II. Efficacy and safety of Femtosecond laser-assisted cataract surgery compared with manual cataract surgery: a meta-analysis of 14 567 eyes. Ophthalmology. 2016;123(10):2113–26.
9. Manning S, Barry P, Henry Y, et al. Femtosecond laser-assisted cataract surgery versus standard phacoemulsification cataract surgery: study from the European registry of quality outcomes for cataract and refractive surgery. J Cataract Refract Surg. 2016;42(12):1779–90.
10. Bartlett JD, Miller KM. The economics of femtosecond laser-assisted cataract surgery. Curr Opin Ophthalmol. 2016;27(1):76–81.
11. Hatch KM, Talamo JH. Laser-assisted cataract surgery: benefits and barriers. Curr Opin Ophthalmol. 2014;25(1):54–61.
12. Wu BM, Williams GP, Tan A, Mehta JS. A comparison of different operating Systems for Femtosecond Lasers in cataract surgery. J Ophthalmol. 2015; 2015:616478.
13. Dick HB, Gerste RD. Plea for femtosecond laser pre-treatment and cataract surgery in the same room. J Cataract Refract Surg. 2014;40(3):499–500.
14. Nagy ZZ, Takacs AI, Filkorn T, et al. Complications of femtosecond laser-assisted cataract surgery. J Cataract Refract Surg. 2014;40(1):20–8.
15. Bali SJ, Hodge C, Lawless M, et al. Early experience with the femtosecond laser for cataract surgery. Ophthalmology. 2012;119(5):891–9.
16. Grewal DS, Dalal RR, Jun S, et al. Impact of the learning curve on Intraoperative surgical time in Femtosecond laser-assisted cataract surgery. J Refract Surg. 2016;32(5):311–7.
17. Lubahn JG, Donaldson KE, Culbertson WW, Yoo SH. Operating times of experienced cataract surgeons beginning femtosecond laser-assisted cataract surgery. J Cataract Refract Surg. 2014;40(11):1773–6.
18. Pajic B, Vastardis I, Gatzioufas Z, Pajic-Eggspuehler B. First experience with the new high-frequency femtosecond laser system (LDV Z8) for cataract surgery. Clin Ophthalmol. 2014;8:2485–9.
19. Chylack LT Jr, Wolfe JK, Singer DM, et al. The lens opacities classification system III. The longitudinal study of cataract study group. Arch Ophthalmol. 1993;111(6):831–6.
20. Chang JS, Chen IN, Chan WM, et al. Initial evaluation of a femtosecond laser system in cataract surgery. J Cataract Refract Surg. 2014;40(1):29–36.
21. Baig NB, Cheng GP, Lam JK, et al. Intraocular pressure profiles during femtosecond laser-assisted cataract surgery. J Cataract Refract Surg. 2014; 40(11):1784–9.
22. Rivera RP, Hoopes PC Jr, Linn SH, Hoopes PC. Comparative analysis of the performance of two different platforms for femtosecond laser-assisted cataract surgery. Clin Ophthalmol. 2016;10:2069–78.
23. Kerr NM, Abell RG, Vote BJ, Toh T. Intraocular pressure during femtosecond laser pretreatment of cataract. J Cataract Refract Surg. 2013;39(3):339–42.
24. Diakonis VF, Yesilirmak N, Sayed-Ahmed IO, et al. Effects of Femtosecond laser-assisted cataract pretreatment on pupil diameter: a comparison between three laser platforms. J Refract Surg. 2016;32(2):84–8.
25. Diakonis VF, Kontadakis GA, Anagnostopoulos AG, et al. Effects of short-term preoperative topical Ketorolac on pupil diameter in eyes undergoing Femtosecond laser-assisted Capsulotomy. J Refract Surg. 2017;33(4):230–4.
26. Abell RG, Vote BJ. Cost-effectiveness of femtosecond laser-assisted cataract surgery versus phacoemulsification cataract surgery. Ophthalmology. 2014; 121(1):10–6.
27. Crema AS, Walsh A, Yamane IS, Ventura BV, Santhiago MR. Femtosecond laser-assisted cataract surgery in patients with Marfan syndrome and Subluxated lens. J Refract Surg. 2015;31(5):338–41.
28. Kranitz K, Mihaltz K, Sandor GL, et al. Intraocular lens tilt and decentration measured by Scheimpflug camera following manual or femtosecond laser-created continuous circular capsulotomy. J Refract Surg. 2012;28(4):259–63.
29. Martin AI, Hodge C, Lawless M, et al. Femtosecond laser cataract surgery: challenging cases. Curr Opin Ophthalmol. 2014;25(1):71–80.

10

Femtosecond laser-assisted cataract surgery after penetrating keratoplasty

Danmin Cao[1,2], Shiming Wang[2,3] and Yong Wang[1,2*]

Abstract

Background: Cataract surgery after penetratingkeratoplasty (PKP) is often challenging due to changes in the integrity of the cornea caused by PKP. For example, corneal endothelial cell (CEC) loss and corneal edema commonly occur after traditional phacoemulsification cataract surgery in patients that previously had successful PKP. Recent studies have reported that femtosecond laser-assisted cataract surgery (FLACS) significantly reduces the need for ultrasound energy minimizing mechanical damage to the cornea and results in a reduction of CEC loss and corneal edema.

Case presentation: We report a case in which FLACS was used in a patient with previous PKP.

Conclusion: This case supports the suggestion that the use of the femtosecond laser improves the surgical outcome of cataract surgery after PKP. This improvement may be result of the precise incision, controlled capsulorhexis, and reduced lens fragmentation experienced with the femtosecond laser which helps to reduce potential complications of cataract surgery after PKP.

Keywords: Femtosecond, Cataract, Corneal, Transplantation

Background

Previous studies report that 44–64% of patients develop cataracts within five years of PKP. Cataract surgery after PKP is often challenging due to changes in corneal integrity induced by PKP. CEC loss and corneal edema often occur after traditional phacoemulsification cataract surgery in patients that had previous successful PKP [1]. The mean annual rate of endothelial cell loss from 10 to 15 years after surgery was 0.2 +/− 5.7% [2].

Corneal distortion, irrigation solution turbulence, instrument-related mechanical trauma, nuclear fragments, IOL contact, and free oxygen radicals can cause corneal damage during cataract surgery. Several preoperative and intraoperative parameters (high nucleus grade, advanced age, long phaco time, high ultrasound energy, short axial length, and surgical skill) are associated with an increased risk of endothelial cell damage after phacoemulsification [3]. Recent studies had shown that the use of FLACS significantly reduces the need for ultrasound energy minimizing mechanical damage to the cornea and results in a reduction of CEC loss and corneal edema [4].

Case presentation

A male patient of 61-years that had 7.0 mm diameter PKP performed in his left eye two years ago. His best corrected visual acuity (BCVA) at distance in the left was light perception. Slit lamp examination showed a corneal graft transparency and a hard cataract with a 3 mm centered white anterior lens capsule calcification (Fig. 1). Due to the hardness of cataract in this case, the IOL-Master could not assess the axial length (AL) and an A-Scan (TOMEY, AL2000, Japan) was used to assess AL. Keratometry was assessed using the auto-refractometer (Topcon, KR8800, Japan).IOL power was calculated using the SRK/T formulas, using the A-Scan software. The LenSx laser system (Alcon Laboratories, Inc.) was used to perform this surgery. Based on this examination, a 5.0 mm capsulotomy diameter was selected. Anterior segment optical coherence tomography (AS-OCT) showed a bulge in the anterior lens capsule calcification of the central area. An AS-OCT-guided 2.2 mm corneal incision was created (Fig. 2a). Cylinder and chop pattern was used for lens fragmentation (Fig. 2b). After completion of the laser

* Correspondence: wangyongeye@163.com
[1]Wuhan Aier Eye Hospital, Aier Eye Hospital Group, Wuhan, China
[2]Aier School of Ophthalmology, Central South University, Changsha, China
Full list of author information is available at the end of the article

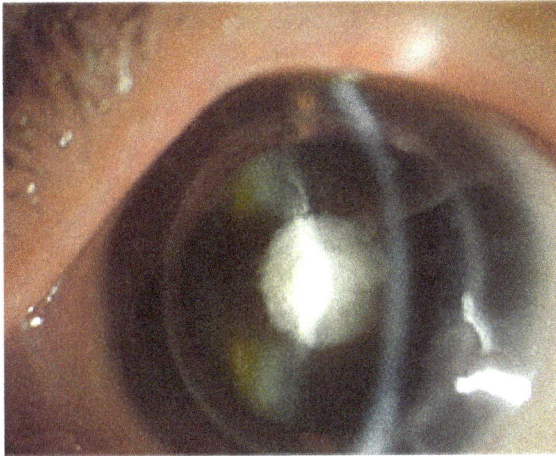

Fig. 1 A preoperative slitlamp image showing a corneal graft transparency and a hard cataract with a 3 mm centered *white* anterior lens capsule calcification

procedure, the patient was moved to the operating room. The surgery was completed with a standard phacoemulsification procedure using the Infiniti Vision System. The Cumulative Dissipated Energy (CDE) was used to assess phacoemulsification time and phacoemulsification power. The CDE was 8.69, the total surgical time was 16 mins., (from femtosecond laser to watertight), and the volume of irrigating solution used was 92 ml. A 23D Acrysof SN60WF intraocular lens(IOL) (Alcon Laboratories, Inc.) was implanted.

On postoperative day 1, the uncorrected visual acuity (UCVA) was 20/40 with a transparent cornea and a well-centered IOL with a 360-degree capsule overlap (Fig. 3). The postoperative UCVA improved to 20/25 after one month. Subjective refraction was stable at 0.75 D sphere and 2.00 D cylinder at the three month follow up. The specular microscope (Topcon, SP2000P,Japan) was used to measure CEC numbers. Preoperative CEC

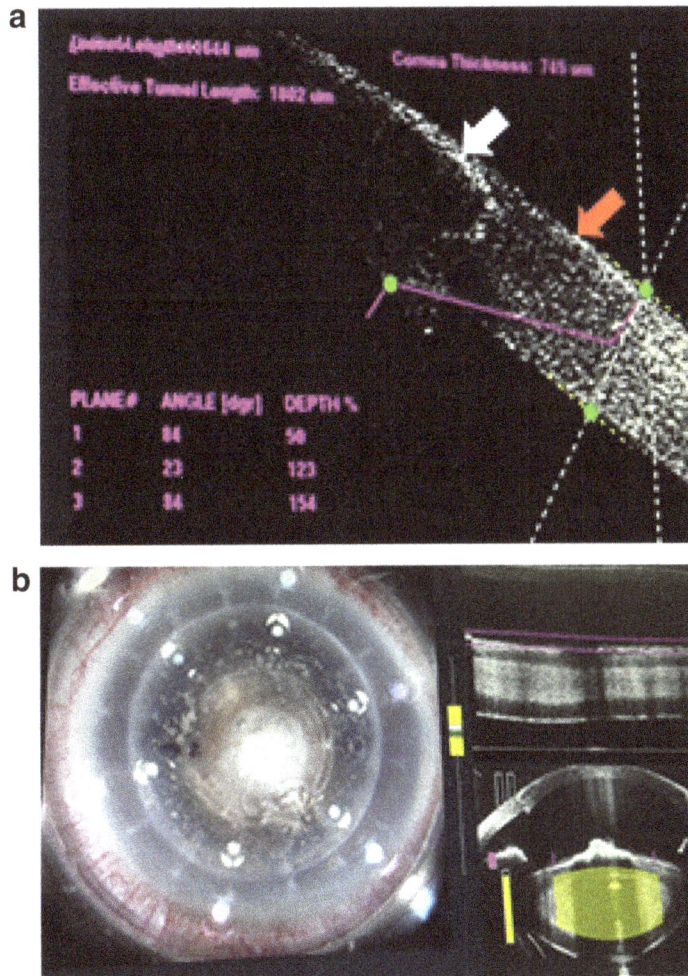

Fig. 2 a AS-OCT image depicts the architecture of clear corneal incision. The *white arrow* indicates the corneal graft. The *red arrow* indicates corneal bed. **b** A 5.0 mm capsulotomy diameter was selected. The AS-OCT indicated that the anterior lens capsule calcification of the central areas had a bulge

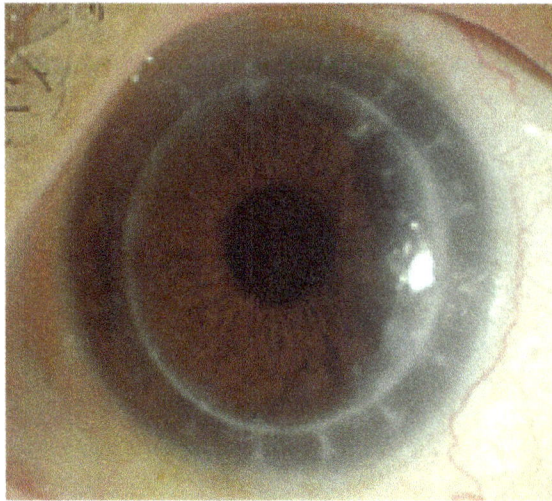

Fig. 3 A postoperative slitlamp image showing a transparent cornea and a well-centered IOL

numbers were 1947 cells/mm^2, 1792 cells/mm^2 immediately after surgery, 1628 cells/mm^2 at one month and 1517 cells/mm^2 at three months.

Discussion and conclusions

The three critical steps for successful cataract surgery after PKP areobtaining a central continuous capsular capsulotomy, minimizing ultrasound energy and ensuring a closed incision. Manual capsulorhexis is a significant challenge, such as in this case, when an intumescent cataract is present with a 3 mm centered white anterior capsule. Many studies report a decreased rate of anterior capsule tears in FLACS compared to manual phacoemulsification cataract surgery [5–7]. Additionally, the creation of a precise, safe, and reproducible capsulotomy is a prerequisite for successful cataract surgery and IOL implantation. Compared to manual capsulorhexis [8], the femtosecond laser has been shown to create a particularly well-shaped and reproducible capsulotomy geometry and circularity [9]. In this case, intraoperative AS-OCT of LenSx was able to image through white opacities of the lens anterior capsule calcifications in advanced cataracts [10]. The femtosecond laser capsulotomy diameter is highly controlled. In this case, the diameter was set to 5 mm, larger than the 3 mm central area of the anterior lens capsule calcification. Capsulotomies performed by the femtosecond laser ensures the safety of intraoperative nucleus chopping and provides accurate location of the IOL [11]. Dick, et al. compared the surgical outcome of patients who underwent the standard manual phacoemulsification versus FLACS. They report that the FLACS group had significantly less capsular bag shrinkage than the standard group at one, two, and three months, with a mean difference of 0.33 ± 0.25 mm at three months [12]. Early stabilization of

the capsular bag diameter leads to more predictable effective lens position, IOL power calculations, and refractive outcomes.

Normal function of corneal endothelial cells is essential for maintaining corneal transparency [13, 14]. Cataract surgery after corneal transplant must minimize endothelial cell damage as the transplant has fewer endothelial cells compared to normal corneas. In our case, the preoperative of CEC numbers were 1947 cells/mm^2 and a decrease in endothelial cell numbers occurred after phacoemulsification [15]. Several studies [16–18] report a direct relationship between endothelial cell loss and ultrasound power and time. Endothelial cell loss related to ultrasound use is markedly higher in cornea graft than in normal corneas [19]. Furthermore, the cataract nucleus hardness in this case was a grade IV .To perform this procedure with traditional phacoemulsification would require more energy and significantly decrease postoperative CEC numbers. Using extra capsular cataract extraction (ECCE) causes less endothelial cell loss compared to phacoemulsification [17], but often induces an astigmatism which leads to poor vision. Femtosecond laser uses ultra short pulses of near infrared light to disrupt tissue with micron precision, this minimizing tissue damage [20]. Lens fragmentation, induced by the femtosecond laser, significantly reduces endothelial cell damage by minimizing the amount of potentially injurious ultrasound energy required to emulsify the lens. Furthermore, laser energy is focused on the capsular bag and limits exposure to the endothelium [21]. Here, we report that our patient had postoperative CEC numbers of 1517 cells/mm^2 at the three-month follow up.

The thickness of the corneal graft and corneal bed are often not the same which leading to poor incision architecture during traditional phacoemulsification. Femtosecond laser improves incision architecture by increasing the precision and reducing mechanical and thermal stress at the incision site [22]. In our case, the corneal incision was made by femtosecond laser and guided by AS-OCT.

In conclusion, the use of femtosecond laser allows precise incisions, controlled capsulorhexis and reduces the amount of ultrasound energy required for lens removal. This technique reduces potential complications in cataract surgery after PKP and improves visual recovery and refractive results.

Abbreviations
AC-OCT: Anterior segment optical coherence tomography; BCVA: best corrected visual acuity; CEC: corneal endothelial cell; FLACS: femtosecond laser-assisted cataract surgery; IOL: intraocular lens; PKP: penetratingkeratoplasty; UCVA: uncorrected visual acuity

Acknowledgements
Not applicable.

Funding

This study was funded by Science Research Foundation of Aier Eye Hospital Group (AM142D17, AF1602D1, AF1602D2), Health and Family Planning Commission of Hubei Municipality(WJ2017M205).

Authors' contributions

All authors conceived of and designed the experimental protocol. DC and SW collected the data. All authors were involved in the analysis. DC wrote the first draft of the manuscript. DC and YW reviewed and revised the manuscript and produced the final version. All authors read and approved the final manuscript.

Competing interests

The authors declare that they have no competing interests.

Consent for publication

Written informed consent was obtained from the patient for publication of this case report accompanying images. A copy of written consent is available for review by the Editor of this journal.

Author details

[1]Wuhan Aier Eye Hospital, Aier Eye Hospital Group, Wuhan, China. [2]Aier School of Ophthalmology, Central South University, Changsha, China. [3]Ningbo Aier Guangming Eye Hospital, Aier Eye Hospital Group, Ningbo, China.

References

1. Acar BT, Utine CA, Acar S, Ciftci F. Endothelial cell loss after phacoemulsification in eyes with previous penetrating keratoplasty, previous deep anterior lamellar keratoplasty, or no previous surgery. J Cataract Refract Surg. 2011;37:2013–7.
2. Bertelmann E, Pleyer U, Rieck P. Risk factors for endothelial cell loss post-keratoplasty. Acta Ophthalmol Scand. 2006;84:766–70.
3. Cho YK, Chang HS, Kim MS. Risk factors for endothelial cell loss after phacoemulsification: comparison in different anterior chamber depth groups. Korean J Ophthalmol. 2010;24:10–5.
4. He L, Sheehy K, Culbertson W. Femtosecond laser-assisted cataract surgery. Curr Opin Ophthalmol. 2011;22:43–52.
5. Roberts TV, Lawless M, Sutton G, Hodge C. Anterior capsule integrity after femtosecond laser-assisted cataract surgery. J Cataract Refract Surg. 2015;41:1109–10.
6. Scott WJ. Re: Abell et al.: anterior capsulotomy integrity after femtosecond laser-assisted cataract surgery (ophthalmology 2014;121:17–24). Ophthalmology. 2014 121:e35–6.
7. Abell RG, Davies PE, Phelan D, Goemann K, McPherson ZE, Vote BJ. Anterior capsulotomy integrity after femtosecond laser-assisted cataract surgery. Ophthalmology. 2014;121:17–24.
8. Dick HB, Gerste RD, Schultz T, Waring GO. Capsulotomy or capsulorhexis in femtosecond laser-assisted cataract surgery. J Cataract Refract Surg. 2013;39:1442.
9. Mastropasqua L, Toto L, Calienno R, et al. Scanning electron microscopy evaluation of capsulorhexis in femtosecond laser-assisted cataract surgery. J Cataract Refract Surg. 2013;39:1581–6.
10. Nagy Z, Takacs A, Filkorn T, Sarayba M. Initial clinical evaluation of an intraocular femtosecond laser in cataract surgery. J Refract Surg. 2009;25:1053–60.
11. Grewal DS, Schultz T, Basti S, Dick HB. Femtosecond laser-assisted cataract surgery–current status and future directions. Surv Ophthalmol. 2016;61:103–31.
12. Dick HB, Conrad-Hengerer I, Schultz T. Intraindividual capsular bag shrinkage comparing standard and laser-assisted cataract surgery. J Refract Surg. 2014;30:228–33.
13. Dikstein S, Maurice DM. The metabolic basis to the fluid pump in the cornea. J Physiol. 1972;221:29–41.
14. MAURICE DM. The structure and transparency of the cornea. J Physiol. 1957;136:263–86.
15. Bourne RR, Minassian DC, Dart JK, Rosen P, Kaushal S, Wingate N. Effect of cataract surgery on the corneal endothelium: modern phacoemulsification compared with extracapsular cataract surgery. Ophthalmology. 2004;111:679–85.
16. Dick HB, Kohnen T, Jacobi FK, Jacobi KW. Long-term endothelial cell loss following phacoemulsification through a temporal clear corneal incision. J Cataract Refract Surg. 1996;22:63–71.
17. Zhou HW, Xie LX. Effects of Cataract Surgery on Endothelium in Transplanted Corneal Grafts: Comparison of Extracapsular Cataract Extraction and Phacoemulsification for Complicated Cataract after Penetrating Keratoplasty. Chin Med J (Engl). 2016 **129**:2096–101.
18. Walkow T, Anders N, Klebe S. Endothelial cell loss after phacoemulsification: relation to preoperative and intraoperative parameters. J Cataract Refract Surg. 2000;26:727–32.
19. Kim EC, Kim MS. A comparison of endothelial cell loss after phacoemulsification in penetrating keratoplasty patients and normal patients. Cornea. 2010;29:510–5.
20. Sugar A. Ultrafast (femtosecond) laser refractive surgery. Curr Opin Ophthalmol. 2002;13:246–9.
21. Abell RG, Kerr NM, Howie AR, Mustaffa KMA, Allen PL, Vote BJ. Effect of femtosecond laser-assisted cataract surgery on the corneal endothelium. J Cataract Refract Surg. 2014;40:1777–83.
22. Mastropasqua L, Toto L, Mastropasqua A, et al. Femtosecond laser versus manual clear corneal incision in cataract surgery. J Refract Surg. 2014;30:27–33.

11

Bacteriology of the conjunctiva in pre-cataract surgery patients with occluded nasolacrimal ducts and the operation outcomes in Japanese patients

Yuko Hayashi[1], Takeshi Miyamoto[2*] (ID), Shuko Fujita[1], Katsuo Tomoyose[1], Nobuyuki Ishikawa[1], Masahide Kokado[1], Takayoshi Sumioka[1], Yuka Okada[1] and Shizuya Saika[1]

Abstract

Background: Contamination of the conjunctiva in association with nasolacrimal duct obstruction is by all accounts a risk factor for infectious endophthalmitis post-cataract surgery.

Methods: All patients who underwent cataract day surgery routinely received nasolacrimal duct syringing with normal saline at the Wakayama Medical University Hospital, Japan, from 2011 to 2013. The microorganisms isolated from conjunctival swab samples of patients with occluded nasolacrimal ducts and their susceptibility to antibiotics, as well as the operation outcomes in all the patients were retrospectively investigated.

Results: Nasolacrimal duct obstruction was observed in 125 eyes of 90 patients (3.3%; 42 eyes of 30 male individuals, and 83 eyes of 60 female individuals) from a total of 3754 eyes of 2384 patients by using irrigation samples of nasolacrimal ducts. The mean age of the subjects with duct obstruction was 79 ± 8.5 years.. In bacterial cultures of swabs from these 125 individuals, microbial growth was detected in 56 samples (i.e. 44.8%). Coagulase-negative *Staphylococcus* was detected in 28 eyes, and *Corynebacterium* species was detected in 17 eyes. *Staphylococcus aureus*, excluding methicillin-resistant *S. aureus* was detected in seven eyes with nasolacrimal duct obstruction. Methicillin-resistant *S. aureus* was isolated in two eyes with nasolacrimal duct obstruction. Each case was treated with topical antibiotics based on the results of antibiotic sensitivity tests. After culturing of cotton swab samples from the conjunctiva, and using direct micrography of bacteria every 2 or 3 days after starting treatment, and once the results were negative (consecutively tested three times), the patients received cataract surgery. In the current case series, bacteria were not detected in conjunctival swabs obtained consecutively three times for 3 weeks after starting topical antibiotics in 118 eyes from 125 eyes (94.4%), and later in the remaining patients. No patient required dacryocystorhinostomy to eliminate bacterial contamination in the conjunctiva following topical antibiotic therapy. No patient developed infectious endophthalmitis at least 1-year post-cataract surgery.

Conclusions: All the patients receiving cataract day surgery underwent the operation after the elimination of conjunctival microorganism contamination in association with nasolacrimal duct obstruction by using appropriate topical antibiotics.

Keywords: Nasolacrimal duct obstruction, Conjunctiva, Bacterium, Cataract surgery

* Correspondence: tmiyam@wakayama-med.ac.jp
[2]Department of Ophthalmology, Wakayama Medical University Kihoku Hospital, 219 Myoji, Katsuragi-cho, Itogun, Wakayama 649-7113, Japan
Full list of author information is available at the end of the article

Background

Infectious endophthalmitis occurs in 0.04–0.075% of patients following cataract surgery [1–3]. Colonies of endogenous normal bacterial flora are the main source of bacterial contamination in the anterior chamber of the eye. *Staphylococci*, *Enterococci*, or Gram-negative bacilli could cause poor visual prognoses postinfection, although the incidence is reportedly low [4–7]. Gram negative bacteria reportedly constitute an increasing proportion of the bacteria found in chronic dacryocystitis and they may be a reservoir for postoperative intraocular infection [8]. It was suggested that these bacteria account for higher rates of nasolacrimal duct obstruction among patients who developed infectious endophthalmitis after cataract surgery [9–11]. Furthermore, these studies indicated that nasolacrimal duct obstruction might cause lacrimal sac and conjunctival bacterial contamination even in the absence of dacryocystitis. Such an occurrence could also be a intraocular infection risk factor subsequent to either trauma or surgery.

It is beneficial, therefore, to test for the presence of nasolacrimal duct obstruction prior to cataract surgery to prevent postoperative bacterial infection in the eye. We routinely perform syringing of the nasolacrimal duct in pre-cataract surgery patients. Furthermore, in all the patients having nasolacrimal duct obstruction regardless of the presence or absence of dacryocystitis we examine both their washings and conjunctival swab samples for bacteriological growth. The susceptibilities of the bacteria isolated from the conjunctival swab samples of patients with occluded nasolacrimal duct, to antibiotics, were determined to eliminate conjunctival bacterial contamination. In the current retrospective study, none of the patients received surgical treatment i.e. tubing or dacryocystorhinostomy, for nasolacrimal duct obstruction at our institution to eliminate bacterial contamination in conjunctiva. The present study retrospectively summarizes our results and the outcomes of cataract surgery during 3 years (2011–2013) along with those abovementioned cases receiving pre-surgical antibiotic treatment. As a result of being given suitable topical antibiotics prior to nasolacrimal duct obstruction surgery, even though those individuals had positive bacterial cultures, there were no cases of postoperative endophthalmitis.

Methods

Patients

This retrospective study was approved by the institutional committee for clinical research All the patients undergoing day surgery for cataract (3754 eyes of 2384 patients) received syringing (irrigation) of the nasolacrimal duct with normal saline at Wakayama Medical University Hospital, Wakayama, Japan, 3 weeks prior to the operation due date, for a 3-year period from 2011 to 2013. Bacteriological examinations and/or antibiotic susceptibility testing of samples isolated from conjunctival swabs were performed in patients with obstruction of the duct prior to surgery. Bacteria-positive patients received further examination of conjunctival swab samples at every 2 or 3 days, along with topical administration of antibiotics that were effective for the detected microorganism (Fig. 1). The patients underwent cataract surgery after obtaining negative results for bacterial infection consecutively for three times. Phacoemulsification and aspiration of the crystallin lens with implantation of an intraocular lens (IOL) was performed in 3707 eyes (98.7%) and planned extracapsular cataract extraction with IOL implantation was performed in 47 eyes (1.3%). No patient developed infectious endophthalmitis post-cataract surgery.

Bacteriological examinations

Conjunctival swab samples were obtained from patients with nasolacrimal duct obstruction by using cotton swabs under local anesthesia with topical lidocaine. On the same day, bacteriological culturing (blood agar medium, chocolate agar medium, MacConkey's medium, Colombian nutrient medium, and *Candida* medium) was conducted. Each culture was incubated in 35 °C for 16–20 h. Anaerobic culturing was not performed. The minimum inhibitory concentration was classified as "S" (susceptible) or "R" (resistant) by employing the criteria developed by the Clinical and Laboratory Institute.

All patients with nasolacrimal duct obstruction had received topical gatifloxacin 0.3%(GFLX) before receiving bacteriological examinations as described above. Patients with positive bacterial cultures received further administration of topical cefmenoxime hydrochloride0.5% (CMX) when the detected bacteria were susceptible to these antibiotics. All patients with detected microorganisms by

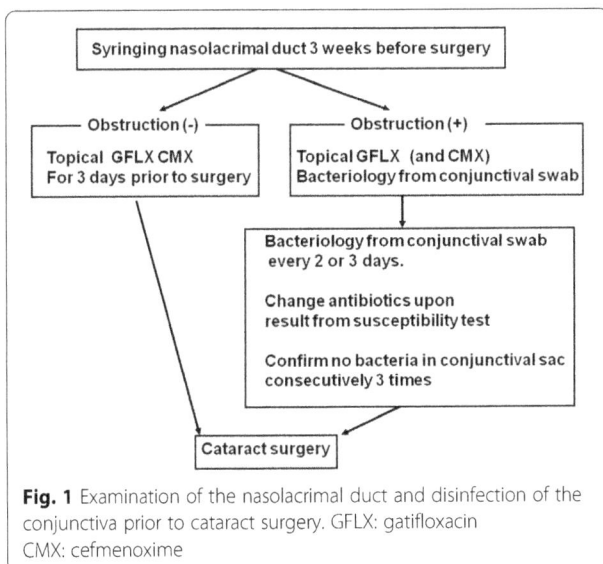

Fig. 1 Examination of the nasolacrimal duct and disinfection of the conjunctiva prior to cataract surgery. GFLX: gatifloxacin
CMX: cefmenoxime

culture examination after detecting nasolacrimal duct obstruction received further conjunctival swab examinations every 2 or 3 days along with topical antibiotics as necessary. Cataract surgery was performed after obtaining no bacterial positive results from the conjunctival swab cultures consecutively for three times.

Prior to the surgery, the eyelid skin and conjunctival sac were disinfected with povidone-iodine. The patients received intravenous sodium piperacillin during or immediately after the surgery. The affected eye received levofloxacin (LVFX) ointment after the operation. From the next day, the patients received topical GFLX for 1–3 months and oral cefcapene pivoxil hydrochloride for 4 days.

Results

The incidence of nasolacrimal duct obstruction

Nasolacrimal duct obstruction was observed in 125 eyes of 90 patients (3.3%; 42 eyes of 30 male individuals, and 83 eyes of 30 female individuals) in a total of 3754 eyes of 2384 patients. The mean age of the subjects with duct obstruction was 79 ± 8.5 years.

Bacteriological examinations of conjunctiva with nasolacrimal duct obstruction

Bacteriological cultures detected microbial growth from the swab samples of 56 of 125 subjects from 90 patients at the initial bacterial culturing (44.8%). Percentages for Gram-positive cocci, Gram-positive rods, Gram-negative bacilli, and fungi were 64, 24, 11, and 1%, respectively (Table 1). Among 125 eyes with positive results for bacteria or fungi, coagulase-negative *Staphylococcus* (CNS), *Corynebacterium* species, or *S. aureus* were detected in 28, 17, and seven eyes, respectively. Methicillin-resistant *S. aureus* (MRSA) was observed in two of seven eyes with *S. aureus*.

Table 1 Bacteria and fungus detected at the first conjunctival swab culture in patients with nasolacrimal duct obstruction

Gram-positive cocci	Coagulase-negative Staphylococci	28
	Staphylococcus aureus (including MRSA in 2 eyes)	7
	Enterococcus facalis	3
	Streptococcus speices	6
Gram-positive bacilli	Corynebacterium species	17
Gram-negative bacilli	Enterobacter	3
	Moruganella	2
	Klebsiella	2
	Proteus	1
Fungus	Candida albicans	1

MRSA methicillin-resistant Staphylococcus aureus

Bacterial results following antibiotic treatment prior to surgery

As shown in Table 2, detected microorganisms exhibited resistance to antibiotics. The majority of the bacteria detected were found to be resistant to LVFX, cefazolin (CEZ), and/or gentamycin.

Table 3 includes all the cases in the current series that required additional topical administration of antibiotic eye drops besides the new quinolone drugs and cephem antibiotics. Conjunctival bacterial contamination was successfully eliminated by administration of topical dibekacin0.3%(DKB)or arbekacin0.5%(ABK)sulfate in case 1 or in cases 2 and 3, respectively. In three eyes of two patients, MRSA was detected at the second or later examination, but not at the first examination. MRSA detected in this case series exhibited resistance to LVFX and CEZ, but was sensitive to vancomycin(VCM). In case 7, *Corynebacterium* appeared after Gram-negative bacilli were eliminated with topical GFLX0.3%. Because this occurred during topical quinolone drug administration, the *Corynebacterium* was eliminated with topical tobramycin0.3%(TOB). In the current case series, no microorganisms were detected in conjunctival swabs consecutively for three times at 3 weeks after starting topical antibiotics in 118 eyes of 125 eyes (94.4%). Durations of more than 3 weeks were required before no bacteria were detected in swab cultures from conjunctiva taken consecutively for three times in cases 4–7 (Table 3).

Table 2 Sensitivity of detected microorganisms and their resistance to each antibiotic

Bacterium species	Antibiotic	Resistant	Sensitive
Coagulase-negative Staphylococci	LVFX	5	17
	CEZ	5	15
	GM	4	15
MSSA	LVFX	1	5
	CEZ	0	6
	GM	1	5
MRSA	LVFX	3	0
	CEZ	3	0
	GM	2	1
Streptococcus species	LVFX	1	2
	CEZ	1	1
Corynebacterium species	LVFX	3	2
	CEZ	0	4
Gram-negative bacilli	LVFX	1	7
	CEZ	3	5
	GM	1	7

MSSA methicillin-susceptible Staphylococcus aureus
MRSA methicillin-resistant Staphylococcus aureus
The majority of the bacteria were found to be resistant to levofloxacin (LVFX), cefazolin (CEZ), or gentamycin (GM)

Table 3 Cases that required administration of additional topical antibiotic eye drops in addition to quinolone and cephem drugs to achieve a negative result for bacterial infection

Case #	Bacterium species	Sensitivity	Additional antibiotic
1	CNS	LVFX (R) CEZ (R) GM (R) ABK (S)	DKB
2	CNS	LVFX (R) CEZ (R) GM (R) ABK (S)	ABK
3	CNS	LVFX (R) CEZ (R) GM (R) ABK (S)	ABK
4	MRSA	LVFX (R) CEZ (R) GM (R) VCM (S)	VCM
5	MRSA	LVFX (R) CEZ (R) GM (R) VCM (S)	VCM
6	MRSA Gram-negative bacilli	LVFX (R) CEZ (R) GM (R) VCM (S)	VCM
		LVFX (S) CEZ (S) GM (S)	
7	Corynebacterium Spp. Gram- negative bacilli	LVFX (S) CEZ (S) GM (S)	TOB

CNS coagulase-negative Staphylococci
MSSA methicillin-susceptible Staphylococcus aureus
MRSA methicillin-resistant Staphylococcus aureus
DKB: dibekacin0.3%; ABK; arbekacin0.5%; VCM; vancomycin; TOB: tobramycin

Discussion

Obstruction of the nasolacrimal duct causes retention of tears in the lacrimal and conjunctival sac, leading to the acceleration of growth of the microorganisms in the accumulated tears. The likelihood of post-cataract surgery infectious endophthalmitis is much higher in patients whose nasolacrimal ducts are obstructed [9, 10]. This association suggests that this condition could be a risk factor for intraocular infection subsequent to either trauma or surgery. In addition, 82% of the bacteria detected from eyes with postoperative infectious endophthalmitis were reportedly genetically identical to those in the normal conjunctival flora [11]. There is no published guideline available in Japan describing a recommended strategy for treating patients with nasolacrimal duct obstruction and have contaminated conjunctivae prior to intraocular surgery. Therefore, examination of the nasolacrimal duct by syringing and bacteriological examinations in eyes with obstruction of the duct should be performed prior to intraocular surgeries according to our protocol.

A previous study found the incidence of adult nasolacrimal duct obstruction to be 3.1%. Anatomical differences may account for the difference in the incidence of obstruction between male and female individuals [12]. Microorganisms were detected in 44.8% of the eyes with nasolacrimal duct obstruction. We did not perform anaerobic culturing, and this could account for the difference in the detection rate (30–80%) between our study and the previous studies [13–16].

CNS was the most prevalent finding, and therefore in the current case series, *Corynebacterium* and *S. aureus*

were detected. This result is similar to that of a previous study, although we did not perform anaerobic culturing and could not detect *Propionibacterium acnes* [8]. CNS is the bacterial type most frequently observed in post-cataract surgery infectious endophthalmitis [4]. Obstruction of the nasolacrimal duct reportedly increases the percentage of Gram-negative bacilli in the conjunctiva in non-Japanese subjects [8, 16]. Bacteriology of conjunctiva in healthy Japanese subjects without nasolacrimal duct obstruction was also reported [17, 18]. Suto et al. described bacterial presence without screening for nasolacrimal duct obstruction in pre-cataract surgery patients [14]. Thus this data is not applicable to this study. Hoshi et al. reported an increased incidence of Gram-negative bacilli in Japanese subjects as compared with healthy subjects [17]. Moreover, Omatsu et al. reported that the incidence of Gram-negative bacilli was 3.2% [18]. In the current study, 6.4% of the bacilli were Gram-negative in the conjunctiva among all subjects, which is indicative of a higher incidence than previously reported. As Gram-negative bacilli are one of the notable bacterial groups that are post-cataract surgery pathogens causing endophthalmitis, these findings support the notion that nasolacrimal duct obstruction could be a risk factor of this infection.

Although *Corynebacterium* species is one of the most frequently detected bacterial species in normal bacterial flora in human conjunctiva, it was reported that it causes infection in corneas treated with topical corticosteroid therapy after penetrating keratoplasty [19]. Postoperative infectious endophthalmitis is quite rare, presumably because the aqueous humor contains low levels of lipid components that are required for *Corynebacterium* species to grow. *Corynebacterium* in the conjunctiva is sensitive to cephem antibiotics and aminoglycosides, while the bacterium is frequently resistant to new quinolones [6]. We successfully eliminated *Corynebacterium* that newly appeared after the elimination of Gram-negative bacilli by adding the aminoglycoside in case 7. The phenomenon observed in case 7 was considered to be a form of microbial substitution.

Conclusions

In summary, nasolacrimal duct obstruction was observed in 125 eyes of 90 patients (3.3%; 42 eyes of 30 male individuals, and 83 eyes of 60 female individuals) from a total of 3754 eyes of 2384 patients by using samples from syringing of the nasolacrimal duct with normal saline. Each case with positive microorganisms cultured from conjunctival swabs was treated with topical antibiotics based on the results of susceptibility tests. After results from culturing of cotton swab samples from the conjunctiva, and by direct micrography for bacteria every 2 or 3 days (consecutively for three times) were negative, the patients received cataract surgery. Normalization of bacterial flora in the conjunctiva with nasolacrimal duct obstruction reportedly requires 4–5 weeks after dacryocystorhinostomy [20]. Another report showed that dacryocystorhinostomy decreased the percentage of conjunctival sac Gram positive cases from 82% to 36% [21] We successfully eliminated bacterial contamination of the conjunctiva in 94.4% of the patients with nasolacrimal duct obstruction at 3 weeks before cataract surgery, and eventually also eliminated bacterial contamination in all the other cases. In our series, no patient required tubing or dacryocystorhinostomy to eliminate bacterial contamination in the conjunctiva following topical antibiotic therapy. No patient developed infectious endophthalmitis for at least 1-year post-cataract surgery who received topical antibiotic treatment, although previous reports already suggested that nasolacrimal duct obstruction is a potential risk factor of post-cataract surgery infectious endopthalmitis.

Abbreviations
ABK: Arbekacin; CEZ: Cefazolin; CMX: Cefmenoxime; CNS: Coagulase-negative *Staphylococcus*; DKB: Dibekacin; GFLX: Gatifloxacin; IOL: Intraocular lens; LVFX: Levofloxacin; MRSA: methicillin-resistant *Staphylococcus aureus*; MSSA: Methicillin-susceptible *Staphylococcus aureus*; TOB: Tobramycin; VCM: Vancomycin

Acknowledgments
The authors thank Dr. Peter S. Reinach for editing English.

Funding
This study was supported by the Department of Ophthalmology, Wakayama Medical University.

Authors' contributions
All authors participated in obtaining the results as well as in writing and revising the manuscript. Specific additional contributions include: YH, SF, KT, NI, MK, and TS participated in the examination of the syringed nasolacrimal duct samples and in taking the conjunctival swab samples from the patients. TM, YO, and SS participated in the interpretation of the results. All authors read and approved the final manuscript.

Competing interest
The authors declare that they have no competing interests and no financial competing interests.

Consent for publication
Not applicable (no identifying patient data).

Author details
[1]Department of Ophthalmology, Wakayama Medical University, 811-1 Kimiidera, Wakayama 641-0012, Japan. [2]Department of Ophthalmology, Wakayama Medical University Kihoku Hospital, 219 Myoji, Katsuragi-cho, Itogun, Wakayama 649-7113, Japan.

References
1. Wong TY, Chee SP. The epidemiology of acute endophthalmitis after cataract surgery in an Asian population. Ophthalmology. 2004;111:699–705.
2. Lalitha P, Rajagopalan J, Prakash K, Ramasamy K, Prjana NV, Srinivasan M. Post-cataract endophthalmitis in South India: incidence and outcome. Ophthalmology. 2005;112:1884–9.
3. Miller JJ, Scot IU, Flynn Jr HW, Smiddy WE, Newton J, Miller D. Acute onset endophthalmitis after cataract surgery (2000–04) incidence, clinical settings and visual acuity outcomes, after treatment. Am J Ophthalmol. 2005;139:983–7.
4. Peyman GA. Endophthalmitis diagnosis and management 102–107. London and New York: Taylor & Fransis; 2004.
5. Major Jr JC, Engelbert M, Flynn Jr HW, Miller D, Smiddy WE, Davis JL. Staphylococcus aureus endophthalmitis: antibiotic susceptibilities, methicillin resistance, and clinical outcomes. Am J Ophthalmol. 2010;149:278–83.
6. Scott IU, Loo RH, Flynn Jr HW, Miller D. Endophthalmitis caused by enterococcus feacalis: antibiotic selection and treatment outcomes. Ophthalmology. 2003;110:1573–7.
7. Schmidt ME, Smith MA, Levy CS. Endophthalmitis caused by unusual Gram-negative bacilli: three case reports and review. Clin Infect Dis. 1993;17:686–90.
8. Hartikainen J, Lehtonen OP, Saari KM. Bacteriology of lacrimal duct obstruction in adults. Br J Ophthalmol. 1997;81(1):37–40.
9. Kam JK, Cheng NM, Allen PJ, Brooks AM. Nasolacrimal duct screening to minimize post-cataract surgery endophthalmitis. Clin Experiment Ophthalmol. 2014;42:447–51.
10. Lopez PF, Beldavs RA, al-Ghamdi S, Wilson LA, Wojno TH, Sternberg Jr P, Aaberg TM, Lambert HM. Pneumococcal endophthalmitis associated with nasolacrimal obstruction. Am J Ophthalmol. 1993;116:56–62.
11. Speaker MG, Milch FA, Shah MK, Eisner W, Kreiswirth BN. Role of external bacterial flora in the pathogenesis of acute postoperative endophthalmitis. Ophthalmology. 1991;98:639–49.
12. Shigeta K, Takegoshi H, Kikuchi S. Sex and age differences in the bony nasolacrimal canal. Arch Ophthalmol. 2007;125:1667–81.
13. Hara J, Yasuda F, Higashitsutsumi M. Preoperative disinfection of the conjunctival sac in cataract surgery. Ophthalmologica. 1997;211 suppl 1:62–7.
14. Suto C, Morinaga M, Yagi M, Tsuji C, Toshida H. Conjunctival sac bacterial flora isolated prior to cataract surgery. Infect Drug Resist. 2012;5:37–41.
15. Keshav BR, Basu S. Normal conjunctival flora and their antibiotic sensitivity in Omanis undergoing cataract surgery. Oman Ophthalmol. 2012;5:16–8.
16. Arantes TE, Cavalcanti RF, Diniz Mde F, Severo MS, Lins N, Castro CM J. Conjunctival bacterial flora and antibiotic resistance pattern in patients undergoing cataract surgery. Arq Bras Ophthalmol. 2006;69:33–6.
17. Hoshi S, Urabe K. Risk factors for conjunctival bacterial colonization in preoperative cataract patients. Atarashii Ganka (J Eye). 2011;28:1313–9 (in Japanese).
18. Omatsu Y, Miyazaki D, Tominaga T, Matsuura K, Inoue Y. Bacterial flora in the conjunctival sac in eyes before cataract surgery cultured as routine procedure. Rinsho Ganka (Jpn J Clin Ophthalmol). 2014;68:637–43. in Japanese.
19. Eguchi H, Kuwahara T, Miyamoto T, Nakayama-Imaohji H, Ichimura M, Hayashi T, et al. High level fluoroquinolone resistance in ophthalmic clinic isolates belonging to the species corynebacterim macginleyi. J Clin Microbiol. 2008;46:527–32.
20. Owji N, Khalili MR. Normalization of conjunctival flora after dacryocystorhinostomy. Ophthal Plast Reconstr Surg. 2009;25:136–8.
21. Hamatsu Y, Gotoh Y, Tazawa Y. Changes in bacterial flora in the conjunctival sac following lacrimal drainage surgery. Rinsho Ganka (Jp J Clin Ophthalmol). 2003;57:249–52 (in Japanese).

12

Earliella scabrosa-associated postoperative Endophthalmitis after Phacoemulsification with intraocular lens implantation

Hong He[1], Xiaolian Chen[1], Hongshan Liu[1], Jiaochan Wu[1] and Xingwu Zhong[1,2]* 🄳

Abstract

Background: Postoperative endophthalmitis after cataract surgery is a severe eye infection that can lead to irreversible blindness in the affected eye. The characteristics, treatment and prognosis of this disease vary because of its association with different pathogens. Here, we report what is possibly the first case of endophthalmitis after cataract surgery to be associated with the rare pathogen *Earliella scabrosa*.

Case presentation: A 56-year-old man from Hainan Island (China) with a history of phacoemulsification and type II diabetes mellitus underwent intraocular lens (IOL) implantation. He later presented with progressive endophthalmitis in his right eye. IOL explantation with capsular bag removal and a 23G pars plana vitrectomy combined with a silicone oil tamponade was performed. The infection was cleared without recurrence, and the patient's visual acuity improved from light perception to 20/200 in the right eye. An in vitro culture determined that the causative pathogen was *Earliella scabrosa*, and this result was confirmed by an internal transcribed spacer (ITS) sequence analysis.

Conclusion: *Earliella scabrosa* has never been reported as an infectious agent in human eyes, and its clinical significance remains unknown. Here, we report a rare case of *Earliella scabrosa*-associated endophthalmitis after cataract surgery. The fungal infection presented as an acute attack and was successfully treated with vitrectomy.

Keywords: Postoperative Endophthalmitis, *Earliella scabrosa*, Ocular fungal infection

Background

Postoperative endophthalmitis is one of the most severe complications of cataract surgery and can result in extremely poor vision. However, its causative pathogens vary among different regions. Different fungi have been identified as a prime causative agents in developing countries with tropical and subtropical climates. For example, Anand et al. demonstrated that fungi accounted for 21.8% of 170 eyes with postoperative endophthalmitis in southern India [1]. Another large case series from India involved 124 eyes and revealed that over half of the cases involved a fungal infection [2]. The spectrum of fungi described in previous studies includes *Aspergillus* spp., *Candida* spp., *Acremonium falciforme*, *Paecilomyces* spp., *Fusarium* spp., and *Curvularia* spp. To the best of our knowledge, ours is the first reported case of endophthalmitis after cataract surgery to be associated with the rare pathogen *Earliella scabrosa*.

Case presentation

A 56-year-old male patient with a history of type II diabetes mellitus was referred to the Hainan Eye Hospital (Haikou, China) for a red and painful right eye with poor vision. One month before admission, the patient underwent phacoemulsification and IOL implantation in a local hospital. Within 72 h of this surgery, he presented at a private clinic with irritation, redness and reduced vision in the right eye. The patient was treated with antibacterial medications (levofloxacin eye drops, six

* Correspondence: xingzh88@hotmail.com
[1]Hainan Eye Hospital and Key Laboratory of Ophthalmology, Zhongshan Ophthalmic Center, Sun Yat-sen University, 19 Xiuhua Road, Haikou, China
[2]Zhongshan Ophthalmic Center and State Key Laboratory of Ophthalmology, Sun Yat-sen University, Guangzhou, China

times per day) for 3 days, and it was suggested that he present for a subsequent visit 3 days later. However, the patient missed this follow-up visit, and he applied the levofloxacin eye drops for 1 month. At 1 month after his presentation at the private clinic, his signs and symptoms had not improved. It was at this time that the patient was referred to the Hainan Eye Hospital (Haikou, China). Upon arrival, his visual acuity was light perception in the right eye and 20/20 in the left eye. A slit-lamp examination revealed conjunctival injection, a positive Tyndall effect (+) in the anterior chamber, and severe vitritis with no fundus view (Fig. 1a). Acute post-cataract endophthalmitis was suspected.

IOL explantation with capsular bag removal and a 23G pars plana vitrectomy combined with a silicone oil tamponade was performed. The intraocular irrigation solution used during surgery contained 1 mg/0.1 ml vancomycin to treat a possible bacterial infection. In addition, a vitreous biopsy was obtained for culture. Fortified tobramycin and levofloxacin eye drops were started after the vitrectomy and continued for 6 days. One week after surgery, the patient achieved a best-corrected visual acuity of 20/200. The intraocular silicon oil was removed after 6 months, and no recurrence was observed (Fig. 1b).

The vitreous fluid was cultured in Sabouraud dextrose agar (SDA). Seven days later, white colonies formed and were identified as *Earliella scabrosa* via internal transcribed spacer (ITS) sequence analysis. In addition, the vitreous fluid was further cultured on an SGA incubator plate at 28 °C for 2 weeks. Figure 2a presents the white filamentous mold colonies growing on this plate. The hyphae stained positive for acridine orange, exhibiting an extremely thick cell wall, sparse septae, and internal nuclei (Fig. 2b). The timeline for the patient's hospital course and treatment is presented in Fig. 3.

The isolates were identified by sequencing the ITS region as previously described [3]. Briefly, the genomic DNA was extracted from a mycelial mass using a Fungal Microbial DNA Isolation Kit (Solarbio Life Sciences

Laboratories, Beijing, PRC) in accordance with the manufacturer's instructions. For this test, 2 μl of fungal DNA and 12.5 μl of the Taq Master Mix (Vazyme Biotech Co., Ltd., Nanjing, PRC) with fungal specific primers were added to a 25-μl total reaction. The thermal cycling parameters were as follows: initial denaturation at 95 °C for 5 min; 35 cycles of denaturation at 95 °C for 30 s, annealing at 60 °C for 30 s, extension at 72 °C for 30 s; and a final extension at 72 °C for 10 min. The sequence of the amplified ITS PCR product that as obtained from the strain isolated in this study was analyzed using the National Center for Biological Information (NCBI) GenBank database and identified as *Earliella scabrosa* (KR706165, identity 99%). A sequence alignment revealed that this sequence shared 91% similarity with *Trametes* sp. and 89% similarity with *Ganoderma* sp.

Discussion and conclusion

Most acute post-cataract endophthalmitis cases reported worldwide are caused by bacterial infections [4, 5]. In this case, the patient complained of decreased vision and red eye within 72 h postoperatively. The patient was then suspected to suffer from acute endophthalmitis induced by bacterial infection. Therefore, empirical treatment consisting of a vitrectomy followed by intraocular irrigation with vancomycin was administered. However, *Earliella scabrosa*, a type of fungus, was isolated from the vitreous fluid and identified by sequencing the ITS region. In retrospect, this case is not the only acute endophthalmitis case associated with fungi. Although fungal-associated, acute, post-cataract endophthalmitis is rare, dozens of cases have been reported in tropical regions [6]. *Aspergillus* spp., *Acremonium falciforme* and *Candida* spp. are included in the spectrum of etiological agents.

Earliella scabrosa is a genus of fungi named by Gilbertson and Ryvarden in 1985 that belongs to the family Polyporaceae [7]. *Earliella scabrosa* is considered a plant pathogen, exhibiting a strong association with freshwater forested wetlands in tropical areas, such as Micronesia [8]. Notably, a recent case report published

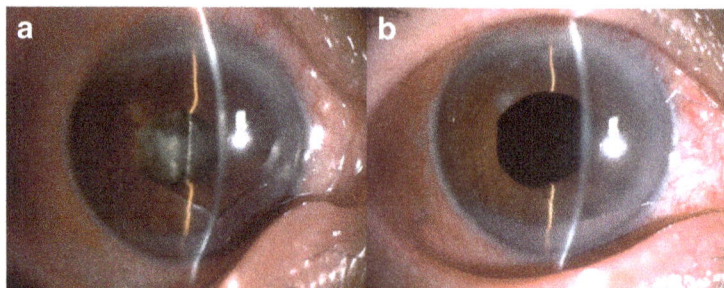

Fig. 1 Photographs of the infected ocular area. **a** The right eye (with the IOL) showed severe vitritis with no fundus view. **b** No recurrence was observed at 6 months after the IOL explantation was performed with capsular bag removal and 23G pars plana vitrectomy combined with a silicone oil tamponade

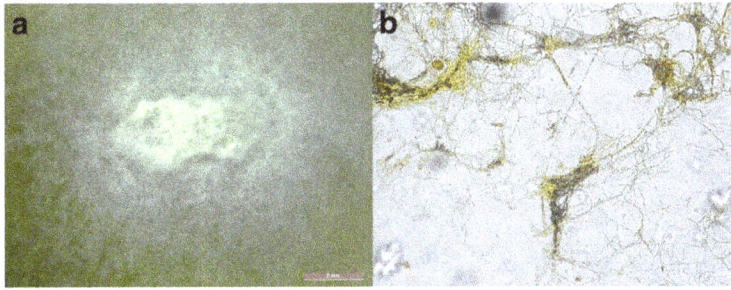

Fig. 2 The morphological characteristics of *Earliella scabrosa*. **a** The pathogen isolated from the patient was cultured in SDA and formed a white colony. **b** The hyphae stained positive for acridine orange, and the results indicated an extremely thick cell wall, sparse septae, and internal nuclei (200×)

by Desmond Shi-Wei Lim et al. was the first to document that this organism can infect humans [9]. In Lim's report, this pathogen caused cutaneous fungal septic emboli in an immunocompromised child, resulting in mortality. However, data regarding human disease remains limited.

Here, we report a case in which a human eye infection was associated with *Earliella scabrosa*. Several points should be noted in this report. First, *Earliella scabrosa* appears to be a novel opportunistic pathogen that can cause endophthalmitis after a cataract extraction. In this case, the patient had suffered from type II diabetes mellitus for 10 years. This disease can impair the immune response of a patient and increase the risk of infection after an operation [10]. Second, ITS sequence analysis is a reliable molecular method for fungal identification, especially for a rare pathogen [11]. As mentioned previously, data on

Earliella scabrosa are limited; therefore, the pathogen isolated from the patient in this case was considered to be an unidentified contaminant, given the lack of morphological characteristics and an absence of sporulation. This fungus was finally identified by genomic level evidence. Third, endophthalmitis induced by *Earliella scabrosa* may have a favorable prognosis. IOL explantation with capsular bag removal and a 23G pars plana vitrectomy combined with silicone oil tamponade seemed to be an effective treatment. In this case, the patient's vision post-operatively recovered from light perception to 20/200 without antifungal drug application. We noticed that there is considerable discrepancy between the prognoses described in Lim's and this report. In Lim's report, this pathogen resulted in death despite the use of massive antifungal treatment. However, in this case, the course was mild. One

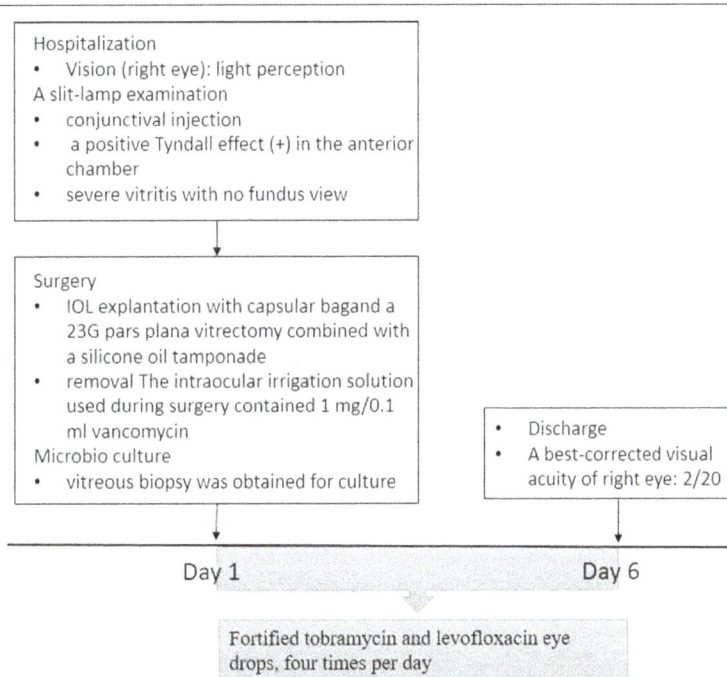

Fig. 3 Timeline of interventions and outcomes

potential reason for this discrepancy is that the characteristics of the site of initial presentation were different. In the child described in Lim's report, the skin was the initial site of infection. The vascular network within the skin may have facilitated the formation of vascular emboli by fungal hyphae, resulting in the dissemination of the infection and multi-organ involvement. On the contrary, the vitreous of the eye can, to some extent, restrict the dissemination of a pathogen because it contains no blood vessels and is a poor nutritional source for invading agents [12]. Another potential reason was that there were differences in the general physical condition of the two patients. The adult patient had type II diabetes but was in generally stable physical condition. However, the child described in Lim's case was in poor physical condition during the course of admission. In addition to the fungal infection, the child had severe idiopathic aplastic anemia and was suffering from graft failure, intracranial hemorrhage and multiple bacterial infections. The child's death may therefore have been the result of multiple diseases. Environmental risk factors were not assessed in our study because the surgery was performed in a local hospital before the patient was referred to Hainan Eye Hospital.

In conclusion, in this case, we reveal that *Earliella scabrosa*, a rare known fungal agent, was the underlying etiology in a human eye infection. These data reinforce the need to enhance awareness of fungal infections in acute endophthalmitis. Early diagnosis and prompt surgical treatment can improve the prognosis in affected patients.

Abbreviations

IOL: Intraocular lens; ITS: Internal transcribed spacer; NCBI: National Center for Biological Information; SDA: Sabouraud dextrose agar

Acknowledgements

Thanks American Journal Experts (AJE) supporting Premium Editing Service for this manuscript.

Funding

This research was supported by grants from Science and Technology Planning Project of Hainan Province (20168335, 817365) and Key Research and Development Program of Hainan Province (ZDYF2016111).

Authors' contributions

All authors made substantial contributions to conception and design. HH, XC and JW collected the data. XZ and HL were involved in the analysis. HH wrote the first draft of the manuscript. All authors were involved in revising the manuscript critically for important intellectual content. And XZ has given final approval of the version to be published. All authors read and approved final manuscript.

Consent for publication

Informed consent for publication were obtained from the patient before examination and surgery. All authors have seen the manuscript and approved to publish it to the journal.

Competing interests

The authors declare that they have no competing interests.

References

1. Anand AR, Therese KL, Madhavan HN. Spectrum of etiological agents of postoperative endophthalmitis and antibiotic susceptibility of bacterial isolates. Indian J Ophthalmol. 2000;48:123–8.
2. Gupta A, Gupta V, Gupta A, Dogra MR, Pandav SS. Spectrum and clinical profile of post cataract surgery endophthalmitis in north India. Indian J Ophthalmol. 2003;51:139–45.
3. Badenoch P, Wetherall B, Woolley M. Coster D. Newer emerging pathogens of ocular non-sporulating molds (NSM) identified by polymerase chain reaction (PCR)-based DNA sequencing technique targeting internal transcribed spacer (ITS) region. Curr Eye Res 2008; 33:139–147.
4. Kocak I, Kocak F, Teker B, Aydin A, Kaya F. Evaluation of bacterial contamination rate of the anterior chamber during phacoemulsification surgery using an automated microbial detection system. Int J Ophthalmol. 2014;7:686–8.
5. Panda A, Pangtey MS, Deb M, Garg V, Badhu BP. Bacterial contamination of the anterior chamber during phacoemulsification. J Cataract Refract Surg. 2003;29:1465–6. author reply 1446
6. Sharma S, Sahu SK, Dhillon V, Das S, Rath S. Reevaluating intracameral cefuroxime as a prophylaxis against endophthalmitis after cataract surgery in India. J Cataract Refract Surg. 2015;41:393–9.
7. Gilbertson RL, Ryvarden L. Some new combinations in Polyporaceae. Mycotaxon. 1985;22:2.
8. Gilbert GS, Gorospe J, Ryvarden L. Host and habitat preferences of polypore fungi in Micronesian tropical flooded forests. Mycol Res. 2008;112:674–80.
9. Lim DS, Tan PL, Jureen R, Tan KB. Cutaneous emboli of invasive Basidiomycosis in a child with Aplastic anemia. Am J Dermatopathol. 2017;39:204–7.
10. Jabbarvand M, Hashemian H, Khodaparast M, Jouhari M, Tabatabaei A. Endophthalmitis occurring after cataract surgery: outcomes of more than 480,000 cataract surgeries, epidemiologic features, and risk factors. Ophthalmology. 2016;123:295–301.
11. Bejdak P, Lengerova M, Palousova D, Volfova P, Kocmanova I. Detection and identification of filamentous fungi causing mycoses using molecular genetic methods. Klin Mikrobiol Infekc Lek. 2012;18:109–14.
12. Irving Fatt, Barry A. Weissman. The Vitreous Body. In: Fatt I, Barry A. Weissman. Physiology of the Eye An Introduction to the Vegetative Functions. Second Edition. Stoneham: Butterworth-Heinemann; 1992. p. 77–84.

13

Descemet membrane detachment in femtosecond laser-assisted cataract surgery

Peiqing Chen*, Yanan Zhu and Ke Yao

Abstracts

Background: Femtosecond laser-assisted cataract surgery (FLACS) has grown in popularity among ophthalmologists as a novel technique. However, descemet membrane detachment (DMD) began to be found as the complication after FLACS. We report a case of serious DMD following FLACS due to the inappropriate incision design.

Case presentation: An 85-year-old man with apparent cornea arcus senilis underwent femtosecond laser-assisted cataract surgery in his right eye. A biplanar model was chosen for the main incision. A serious descemet membrane detachment (DMD) occurred at the end of phacoemulsification, which was connected with the main incision. However, the surgeon confused it with the transient swelling of corneal endothelium, and did not treated DMD timely. DMD was confirmed by anterior segment optical coherence tomography (AS-OCT) at the postoperative 1-month follow-up. Eventually DMD was resolved by intracameral perfluropropane (C3F8) gas injection.

Conclusions: This case suggests that a careful incision separation and a triplanar incision design in FLACS may reduce the incidence of DMD in cataract surgery.

Keywords: Descemet Membrane Detachment, Femtosecond Laser, Cataract Surgery

Backgrounds

Femtosecond laser-assisted cataract surgery (FLACS) has become increasingly common since its introduction in 2008. Many benefits have been reported, including consistent and reproducible capsulotomy creation, watertight triplanar incisions, ability to correct astigmatism, less ultrasound energy, less endothelial cell loss, less macular edema, and better intraocular lens centration. However, some adverse effects have begun to be recognized, such as capsule tags and bridges, suction break, conjunctival hemorrhage, intraoperative miosis, and, less frequently, endothelial damage [1].

Descemet membrane detachment (DMD) is an infrequent complication following phacoemulsification. It can occur as a discontinuity or tear of the Descemet membrane, usually at or near the corneal incision. Reports established an incidence of 0.044% to 0.52% with the

manual technique [2]. Recently, DMD was found to occur after FLACS [3]. Ricardo reported four cases of peri-incisional DMD due to air bubbles around the secondary incision. Here, we report on one case of serious DMD in FLACS that resulted from the incomplete incision and the inappropriate design of the main incision [4].

Case presentation

An 85-year-old man with apparent cornea arcus senilis underwent FLACS in the right eye. He had no systematic disease. The degree of nuclear hardness was IV, and his pre-operative best-corrected visual acuity (BCVA) was 20/1000. In the process of femtosecond laser-assisted cataract surgery (LenSx Laser; Alcon Laboratories, Inc., Fort Worth, TX, USA), the surgeon chose a biplanar model for the main incision; the outer turning point was located at the 40% layer of cornea, while the inner turning point was located at the endothelium layer (Fig. 1). After the laser, the surgeon used a separator to separate the incision; however, it was somewhat difficult. Phacoemulsification was performed after separating the incision. A Stellaris phacoemulsificator

---

* Correspondence: qingqinghz@163.com
Eye Center of the 2nd Affiliated Hospital, School of Medicine, Zhejiang University, #88 Jiefang Road, Hangzhou, Zhejiang 310009, China

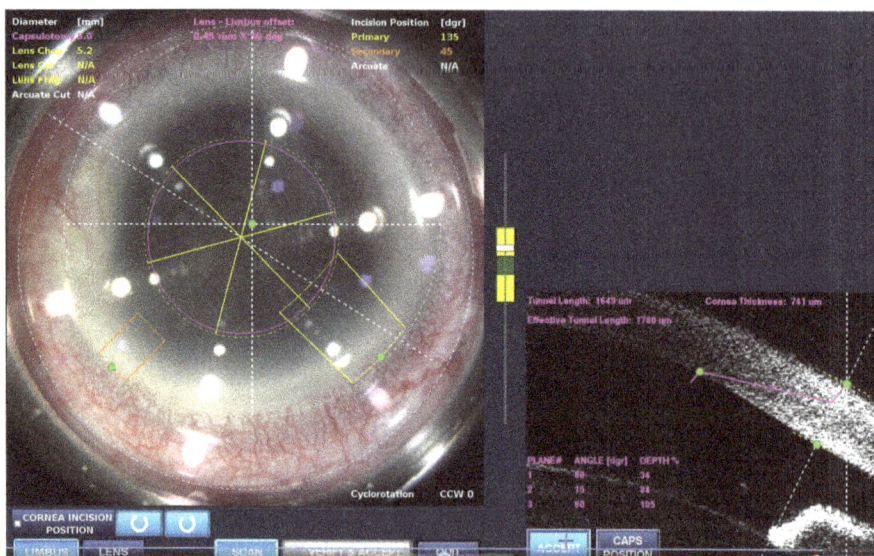

Fig. 1 The main incision design of the patient in FLACS DMD occurred during surgery. Model: biplanar; laser energy:6 μJ; angulation:135°; focal spot separation: 5 μm; length: 1620 μm; width: 2 mm

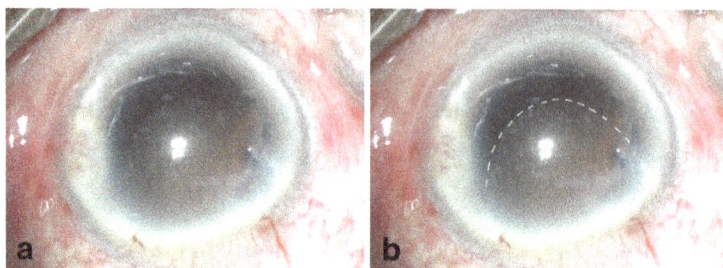

Fig. 2 DMD happened during the surgery. **a** Status of DMD at the end of inspiration. **b** The dotted line shows the range of DMD

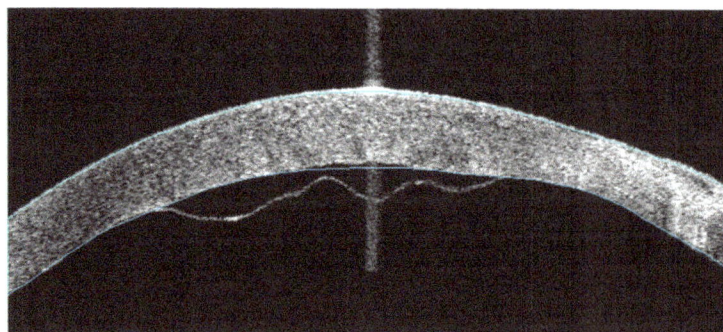

Fig. 3 AS-OCT of planar DMD 1 month after phacoemulsification surgery

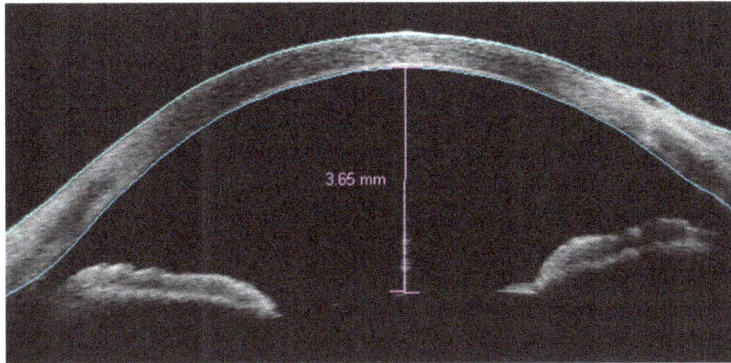

Fig. 4 AS-OCT of resolved DMD after intracameral C3F8 gas injection

(Bausch + Lomb Laboratories, Rochester, NY, USA) was used. The cumulative dissipated energy (CDE) was 35 s. DMD occurred at the end of phacoemulsification, which was located in the upper cornea and connected with the main incision. During aspiration, the range of DMD became larger (Fig. 2). Unfortunately, the surgeon confused it with the transient swelling of corneal endothelium, which could have resulted from the phacoemulsification energy. Therefore, the DMD was not treated during the surgery. The patient experienced severe corneal edema postoperatively. His BCVA was hand motion at the first day postoperatively, and 20/200 at the one-week follow-up. Considering that the corneal edema resulting from the phacoemulsification energy would last for a long time postoperatively, the surgeon did not perform anterior segment optical coherence tomography (AS-OCT) on the patient at the early postoperative stage (1 day and 1 week). A topical steroid (dexamethasone) and a nonsteroidal anti-inflammatory drug (NSAID) were prescribed for the patient, and each drug was given four times a day. However, after 1 month, limited corneal edema persisted in the central cornea, and her BCVA was 20/100. The AS-OCT (Carl Zeiss Meditec, Dublin, CA, USA) confirmed a typical DMD (Fig. 3). Therefore, we did an intracameral perfluoropropane (C3F8) gas (14%) injection for her. In the surgery, 0.3 mL C3F8 gas was injected into the anterior chamer through the inferior temporal incision (5 o' clock), and the aqueous humor was drained out through the inferior nasal incision (8 o' clock) at the same time. Both of incisions were located at the transparent cornea area. Finally, the normal intraocular pressure was ensured at the close of surgery. The patient was informed and signed his consent according to the institutional guidelines and in compliance with the Helsinki Declaration. After gas injection for 1 month, the cornea was transparent, and the BCVA increased to 20/40 (Figs. 4, 5). The patient achieved a BCVA of 20/30 by the time the 6 month follow-up visit occurred.

Discussion

DMD is an unusual complication of phacoemulsification surgery. In manual phacoemulsification surgery, the described surgical risk factors are three: first, incision-related, such as the use of dull blades [5], inappropriate incisions (oblique, excessively anterior, shelved incisions) [6], tight main incisions that do not fit the phaco probe [7]; second, instrument-related, such as the use of blunt instruments [8], inadvertent insertion of instruments between the corneal stroma and the Descemet membrane [9]; and, third, surgeon-related, such as engagement of the Descemet membrane during the irrigation/aspiration stage, unexpected injection of antibiotics, saline, or viscoelastic into the space between the deep stroma and the Descemet membrane [10], and surgeon inexperience [11]. After femtosecond laser was applied in cataract surgery, Ricardo first reported four localized DMD cases in FLACS that occurred because of an encapsulated bubble that did not spread into the anterior chamber (AC) and had formed when the incision was created [4]. Our eye center began to perform femtosecond laser-assisted cataract surgery in 2014. To date, we have performed more than 2000 of these surgeries. This was the first DMD case seen in our center.

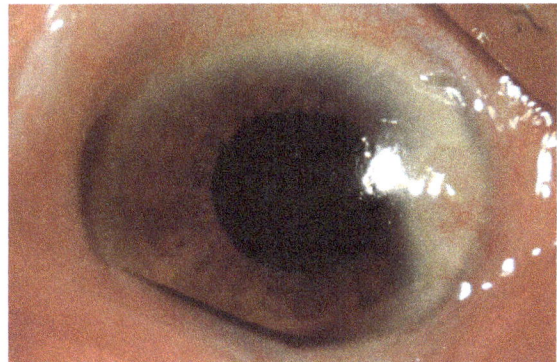

Fig. 5 Anterior segment photograph of the patient 1 month after intracameral C3F8 gas injection

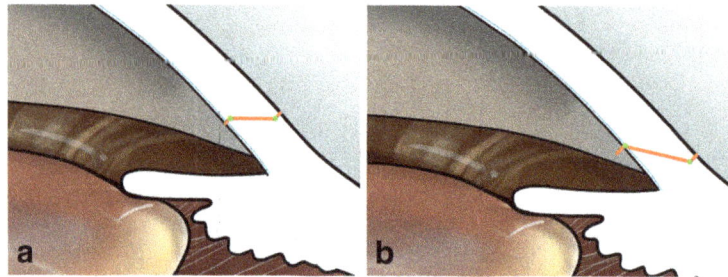

Fig. 6 a Ideal triplanar incision design in FLACS. **b** Incision design in our case. Blue curve indicates Descemet membrane

Our case was a serious DMD after FLACS, and we analyzed the cause of the DMD. First, the patient had apparent cornea arcus senilis that may have influenced the laser penetration. In addition, the mild difficulty in separating the incision indicated the possibility of incomplete endothelium penetration. Also, the blunt force of the separation possibly made tiny dotted tears at the inner side of corneal incision. Furthermore, during phacoemulsification process, the weak endothelium became a support point for the phaco probe due to the biplanar incision design. Because of the frequent movement of the phaco probe and the irrigation, a serious DMD occurred at the end of the phacoemulsification. Moreover, a patient age of more than 65 years and the dense cataract of this case were also significant DMD risk factors, which have previously been seen [12].

Previous studies showed that inadequate docking, cornea arcus senilis, and corneal pannus may lead to incomplete laser corneal incisions in the femtosecond laser process [13, 14]. Here, our patient had apparent cornea arcus senilis, which rendered the incision imperfect. In the Chinese population, cornea arcus senilis is common. Thus, we suggest that the surgeons should be more aware when separating the incision in this type of patient.

Additionally, we compared our biplanar incision with the ideal triplanar incision (Fig. 6). When a triplanar incision is performed, the endothelium and part of the stroma would be affected by a well-distributed force of instruments during the irrigation/aspiration stage (Fig. 7). However, in the current case, because of the biplanar incision design, only the endothelium was affected by the force, so the DMD readily occurred when the tiny tear existed. We therefore suggest that an ideal triplanar incision would reduce the incidence of DMD and make the incision watertight. The triplanar incision might be more suitable in FLACS; however, more clinical studies are required to confirm this.

DMDs usually arise from tears at the incision site that progress to the central cornea as aqueous humor enters the predescemetic space, and shallowness of the anterior chamber has been considered a predisposing factor [15]. It is particularly important that surgeons are aware of this. Sometimes, however, DMD is insidious. In our surgery, although the senior surgeon was highly experienced and had performed more than 10,000 surgeries, during the surgery, she mistook the DMD for transient corneal endothelial edema.

AS-OCT is a very useful tool in the diagnosis and classification of DMD and is becoming the standard method

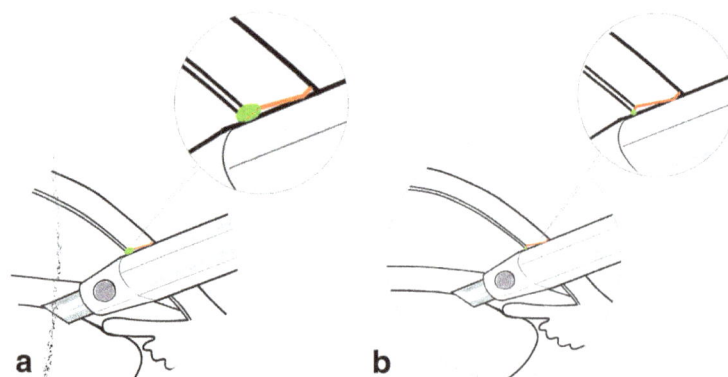

Fig. 7 a The sketch shows that the endothelium and part of the stroma were affected by a well-distributed force of the instrument when a triplanar incision was made. **b** The sketch shows that the endothelium was affected by the force of the instrument only in our case. Green dots indicate the instrument's support points

for diagnosis [16]. Unfortunately, considering that the corneal edema was due to the serious postoperative inflammation, we did not perform AS-OCT for the patient on the first postoperative day or at the one-week follow-up. However, at the 1-month follow-up, the patient was diagnosed with DMD by AS-OCT. Therefore, using AS-OCT at the early postsurgical stage could very possibly help the surgeon understand the status of the cornea, realize DMD as early as possible, and enable the patient to be treated in a timely manner. We suggest that in the presence of corneal edema in the postoperative setting, AS-OCT should be performed if it is available as slit-lamp examination of the posterior cornea and if DM may be unsatisfactory or incomplete due to opacification.

There is no gold standard for the treatment of DMDs. Many options have been described, such as medical treatment, manual reattachment with or without suturing, descemetopexy with air or expansible gases such as sulfur hexafluoride (SF6) or C3F8, and corneal transplantation, which could be penetrating keratoplasty, Descemet stripping endothelial keratoplasty, and, more recently, DMEK.2 In our case, considering that DMD existed for a long time (1 month), we used the intracameral C3F8 gas injection and were able to achieve a positive prognosis.

Conclusion

Our case showed that the incomplete incision and inappropriate incision design became new risk factors for DMD in FLACS. It is important to carefully separate the incision and design a triplanar incision in FLACS to reduce the incidence of DMD in cataract surgery.

Abbreviations
AC: Anterior chamber; AS-OCT: Anterior segment optical coherence tomography; BCVA: Best-corrected visual acuity; CDE: Cumulative dissipated energy; DMD: Descemet membrane detachment; FLACS: Femtosecond laser-assisted cataract surgery; NSAID: Nonsteroidal anti-inflammatory drug

Acknowledgements
Not applicable.

Authors' contributions
PC did the surgery, drafted the article and analyze the data, ZY acquired data, drafted the article and obtained funding, YK provided conception. All authors reviewed the manuscript. All authors read and approved the final manuscript.

Consent for publication
Written informed consent was obtained from the patient for publication of this case report and any accompanying images. A copy of the written consent is available for review by the Editor of this journal.

Competing interests
The authors declare that they have no competing interests.

References
1. Nagy Z, Takes A, Filkorn T, et al. Complications of femtosecond laser assisted cataract surgery. J Cataract Refract Surg. 2014;40:20–8.
2. Banitt M, Malta J, Shtein M, et al. Delay onset isolated central Descemet membrane Blister detachment following phacoemulsification. J Cataract Refract Surg. 2008;34:1601–3.
3. Nosé RM, Rivera-Monge MD, Forseto AS, Nosé W. Descemet Membrane Detachment in Femtosecond Laser-Assisted Cataract Surgery. Cornea. 2016; 35(4):562–4.
4. Mohammadpour M, Jabbarvand M, Nikdel M, et al. Effect of preemptive topical diclofenac on postoperative pain relief after photorefractive keratectomy. J Cataract Refract Surg. 2011;37:633–7.
5. John ME, Noblitt RL, Boleyn KL, et al. Effect of a superficial and a deep scleral pocket incision on the incidence of hyphema. J Cataract Refract Surg. 1992;18:495–9.
6. Wang Y, Guan H. A case of Descemet's membrane detachments and tears during phacoemulsification. Ther Clin Risk Manag. 2015;11:1727–9.
7. Bhatia HK, Gupta R. Delayed-onset descemet membrane detachment after uneventful cataract surgery treated by corneal venting incision with air tamponade: a case report. BMC Ophthalmol. 2016;16:35.
8. Scheie HG. Stripping of Descemet's membrane in cataract extraction. Trans Am Ophthalmol Soc. 1964;62:140–52.
9. Bhattacharjee H, Bhattacharjee K, Medhi J, Altaf A. Descemet's membrane detachment caused by inadvertent vancomycin injection. Indian J Ophthalmol. 2008;56:241–3.
10. Samarawickrama C, Beltz J, Chan E. Spontaneously resolving Descemet's membrane detachment caused by an ophthalmic viscosurgical device during cataract surgery. Saudi J Ophthalmol. 2015;29:301–2.
11. Ti SE, Chee SP, Tan DTH, et al. Descemet membrane detachment after phacoemulsification surgery: risk factors and success of air bubble tamponade. Cornea. 2012;32:454–9.
12. Talamo JH, Gooding P, Angeley D, et al. Optical patient interface in femtosecond laser-assisted cataract surgery: contact corneal applanation versus liquid immersion. J Cataract Refract Surg. 2013;39(4):501–10.
13. Tian F, Zhang H, Li X. Early experience of femtosecond laser assisted cataract surgery. Zhonghua Yan Ke Za Zhi. 2014;50(2):133–6.
14. Gatzioufas Z, Schirra F, Löw U, et al. Spontaneous bilateral late-onset Descemet membrane detachment after successful cataract surgery. J Cataract Refract Surg. 2009;35:778–81.
15. Sharma N, Gupta S, Maharana P, et al. Anterior segment optical coherence tomography-guided management algorithm for descemet membrane detachment after intraocular surgery. Cornea. 2015;34:1170–4.
16. Benatti CA, Tsao JZ, Afshari NA. Descemet membrane detachment during cataract surgery: etiology and management. Curr Opin Ophthalmol. 2017; 28(1):35–41.

14

Iris reconstruction using autologous iris preserved in cold balanced salt solution for 8 hours in iatrogenic total iridodialysis during cataract surgery

Seung Pil Bang and Jong Hwa Jun[*]

Abstract

Background: A large iris defect or extensive iridodialysis can be an intractable cause of visual disturbance, photophobia, glare, monocular diplopia, or cosmetic deformity. The implantation of an artificial iris substitute could be an effective option, but this can cause a reduction in endothelial cell density. We succeeded in the anatomical restoration of iris tissue that was totally dialyzed out of the eye, and was preserved in cold balanced salt solution for 8 h. Engrafted iris tissue was maintained within the aqueous humor.

Case presentation: A 71-year-old man was referred to our clinic for management of an iatrogenic total iridodialysis. The totally dialyzed iris tissue was immediately preserved in sterile cold balanced salt solution and packed in a sterile biopsy bottle that was surrounded with ice cubes. Under general anesthesia, a pars plana vitrectomy was performed to remove the remaining lens cortex and vitreous fiber anterior to the equator. A sulcus-positioned intraocular lens (IOL) was repositioned and fixed by *ab externo* scleral sutures. Preserved iris tissue was inserted and ironed using both iris spatula and ocular viscoelastic devices. Five-point *ab interno* scleral sutures were made 1.0 mm posterior to the limbus.

Conclusions: The engrafted iris was successfully maintained for 6 months and did not undergo any atrophic change or depigmentation, which may be caused by primary implantation failure due to a blocked blood supply.

Keywords: Balanced salt solution, Iatrogenic, Iris reconstruction, Total iridodialysis

Background

The iris functions as a light-limiting diaphragm. Iris defects, whether traumatic or iatrogenic, can cause deterioration in visual acuity, photophobia, glare, as well as diplopia if the edge of the phakic or pseudophakic lens is involved [1]. In addition, an extensive defect can be a significant cosmetic concern [2]. Various techniques to overcome partial or total iris defects have been described, including iridoplasty, coloured contact lenses, and corneal tattooing [3]. Implantation of an artificial iris substitute is a new and effective therapeutic option, but can cause significant reduction of endothelial cell density or even corneal decompensation after surgery [4]. Thus, a widespread defect could be a vision-threatening situation. We encountered a case of iatrogenic total iridodialysis during cataract surgery. We restored the structure of the autogenous iris, which had been preserved in cold balanced salt solution for 8 h.

Case presentation

A 71-year-old man was referred to our clinic for treatment of an iatrogenic total iridodialysis. Just before the referral, his iris had been totally torn out and jammed into the hinge of a prechopper during the removal of an instrument during cataract surgery. Examination revealed a visual acuity (VA) of hand-motion in the left eye. A complete iris defect with remaining lens cortex, a ruptured posterior lens capsule with radial tear of the capsule, and an intraocular lens (IOL) implanted in the

* Correspondence: junjonghwa@gmail.com
Department of Ophthalmology, Keimyung University School of Medicine, #56, Dalseong-ro, Jung-gu, Daegu 700-712, Korea

sulcus were noted (Fig. 1a). The totally dialyzed iris was sent to our clinic preserved in sterile cold balanced salt solution, packed in a sterile biopsy bottle surrounded by a towel to prevent direct contact with ice cubes, and was transported in an icebox.

We decided to perform surgery under general anesthesia considering the patient's poor cooperation due to dementia. To minimize IOL decentration during scleral fixation, we used a toric axis marker and marked the fixation axis (Fig. 1b). After the scleral flaps were in two positions 180° apart, a 10–0 polypropylene suture was passed through the bed of half-thickness scleral flaps 2.0 mm posterior to the limbus (Fig. 1c). A sulcus positioned IOL (PC-60 AD, HOYA Corporation, Tokyo, Japan) was repositioned and fixed by *ab externo* scleral sutures (Fig. 1d). We conducted a pars plana vitrectomy to remove the remaining lens cortex material and vitreous fibre anterior to the equator to avoid trapping the vitreous during the iris-fixating suturing (Fig. 1e). The preserved iris was examined. It did not show any signs of necrosis but kept its own color and morphology soundly (Fig. 1f). We spread out the iris on the patient's cornea to estimate the range of damage and locate a wider part of the iris inferiorly to minimize the glare after iridopexy (Fig. 1g). A 10–0 Prolene on a CIF4 needle (Ethicon, Somerville, New Jersey, USA) was consecutively passed through the iris (Fig. 1h) and sclera 1.0 mm posterior to the limbus at the 6' O/C position (Fig. 1i). Properly using both an iris spatula and ocular viscoelastic devices (OVDs), we inserted the iris into the anterior chamber completely and unfolded it to its proper position (Fig. 1j, k). The estimated cool-to-anterior chamber insertion time of the preserved iris was 8 h. Four more points of *ab interno* scleral sutures (4', 1:30, 10:30 and 8' O/C positions in sequence) were made

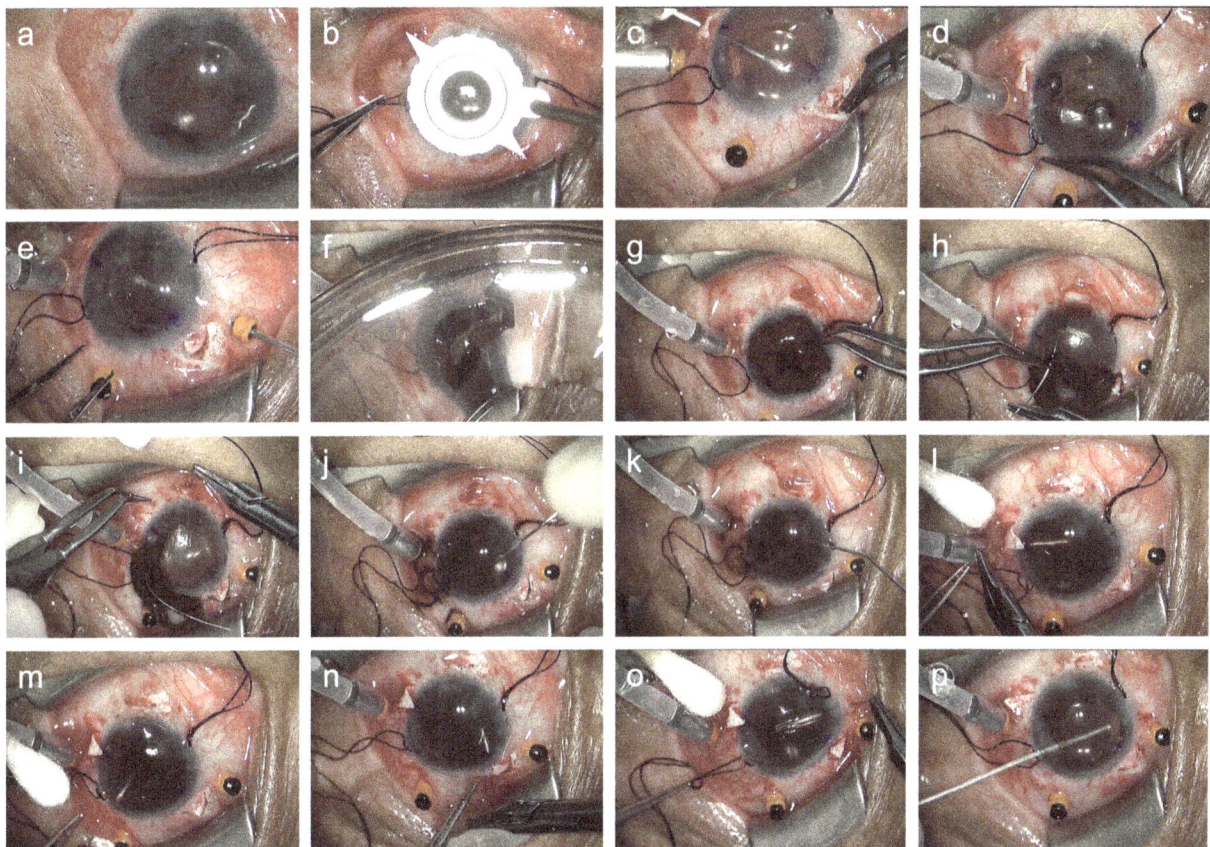

Fig. 1 Intraoperative photographs of the iridopexy of an autologous iris in iatrogenic total iridodialysis. **a** A complete iris defect with remaining lens cortex, a ruptured posterior capsule of the lens with a radial tear and an intraocular lens (IOL) implanted in the sulcus position were observed. **b** A toric axis marker was used to indicate the fixation axis. **c** After scleral flaps were prepared in 2 positions 180° apart, a 10–0 Prolene suture was passed through the bed of half-thickness scleral flaps 2.0 mm posterior to the limbus. **d** Implanted IOL was repositioned using transscleral fixation using an *ab externo* method. **e** Pars plana vitrectomy was performed to remove the remaining lens cortex material and vitreous fiber anterior to the equator. **f** The transferred iris was examined and showed no signs of necrosis. **g** The iris was spread out; the wider part of the iris was located inferiorly. **h, i** A 10–0 Prolene suture was consecutively passed through the iris and sclera. **j, k** Using an iris spatula and ocular viscoelastic devices (OVDs), the iris was inserted into the anterior chamber completely. **l-o** Four more iridopexies were performed. **p** The remaining vitreous, OVDs, and dispersed iris pigments were removed using a vitreous cutter

(Fig. 1l-o). Then, the remaining vitreous, OVDs, and dispersed iris pigments were removed using a vitreous cutter (Fig 1p).

One week postoperatively, intraocular pressure (IOP) increased up to 30 mmHg because of hyphema from the torn root of the iris (Fig. 2a); however, 3 weeks postoperatively, hyphema decreased with improved VA (20/200) and lowered IOP (15 mmHg) (Fig. 2b). At 4 weeks postoperatively, a much improved VA (20/100) and lowered IOP (14 mmHg) were detected (Fig. 2c). At 7 weeks postoperatively, VA was 20/63, IOP was 14 mmHg and there were no signs of inflammation in the anterior chamber (Fig. 2d). Until 6 months postoperatively, the engrafted iris did not have any signs of atrophic change, depigmentation, or inflammation; the patient complained of minimal glare, and the uncorrected VA was 20/25 with the IOP of 13 mmHg (Fig. 2e).

Discussion

An intact iris diaphragm is essential for accurate visual function as it decreases the aberrations arising from the crystalline lens and increases the depth of focus [3]. Coloured contact lenses may not be acceptable or tolerated. Corneal tattooing leaves a permanent opacity in the cornea, and the results are unpredictable. In the absence of readily available iris prosthetic devices in many areas of the world, including the USA, an approach must be tailored appropriately for the surgical challenge. For that reason, we decided to perform a

remodeling of the autologous iris. Reconstruction of a totally dialyzed iris was a technical challenge because the forces applied by the sutures often leave the iris and pupil with an irregular and distorted appearance. To the best of our knowledge, this is the first report of restoration of an autologous iris in iatrogenic total iridodialysis. Iris tissue defects can also be cosmetically upsetting for the patient, and an aesthetically pleasing surgical outcome is often a key concern. Fortunately, our patient expressed satisfaction with the cosmetic appearance of his left eye.

We were concerned that even if we could do the reconstruction successfully, a primary implantation failure with atrophic change or depigmentation of the engrafted iris and severe inflammation of the anterior chamber would be inevitable. However, the iris maintained its own morphological stability without a direct blood supply from ciliary vessels for 6 months postoperatively; conceivably, it might have been sustained through the nutrition supply from the aqueous by principle of diffusion. Additionally, the engrafted iris might have restored its vasculature near its remnant root after implantation. One animal study showed that isolated acapsular glomeruli transplanted into the anterior chamber of the mouse eye were capable of spontaneously regaining access to the recipient vasculature and retaining their structure and function [5], indicating the possibility of regrowth of the engrafted iris vessels in our case.

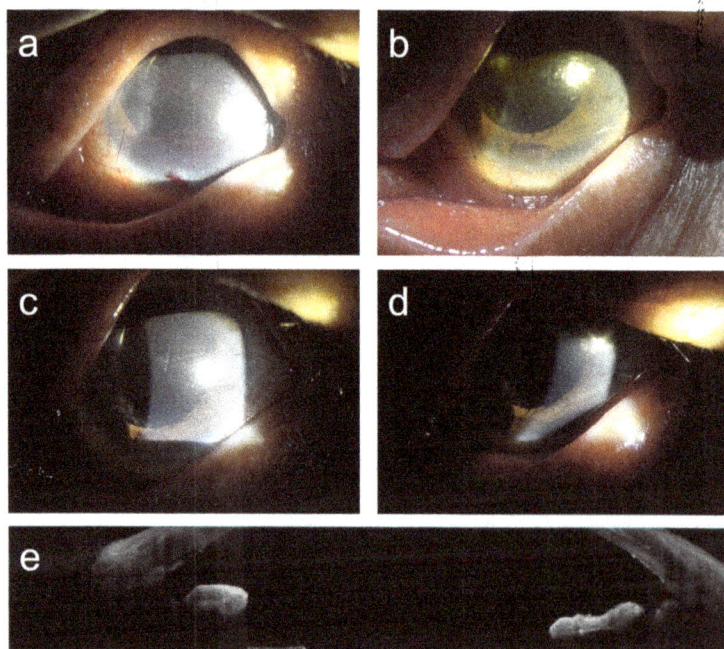

Fig. 2 Postoperative slit-lamp examination and tomographic image. **a** Bleeding from the torn root of the iris at 1 week postoperatively. **b** Hyphema decreased at 3 weeks postoperatively. **c, d** No atrophy or pigment loss and no signs of inflammation at 4 and 7 weeks postoperatively. **e**. Anterior optical coherence tomographic image showed morphologic stability of the iris

Though cases have been reported in the literature of traumatic iridodialysis following blunt injury to pseudophakic eyes [6–12], our case is unique in that it is the first case of iatrogenic iridodialysis during cataract surgery instead of trauma [13]; the iris reconstruction was also unique in using an autologous iris instead of prosthetic iris implantation [1, 3, 14]. Considering the short follow-up period of this case, long-term observation is planned to exclude the possibility of chronic atrophic change or depigmentation of the engrafted iris. It might also be necessary to conduct studies on the engrafted iris vasculature such as fluorescein angiography [15, 16], indocyanine green angiography [17] or optical coherence tomography angiography [18].

Conclusions

We successfully performed the reconstruction of a totally avulsed iris during cataract surgery and obtained cosmetically favourable morphology of the engrafted iris. Despite 8 h of extracorporeal preservation of the iris and depletion of a direct blood supply after reconstruction, the implanted iris maintained its own stability without any complication or graft failure.

Abbreviations

IOLs: Intraocular lens; IOP: Intraocular pressure; OVDs: Ocular viscoelastic devices; VA: Visual acuity

Acknowledgements

None.

Funding

This work was supported by a National Research Foundation of Korea (NRF) grant funded by the Korean government (Ministry of Science, ICT and Future Planning) (NRF-2015R1C1A1A02037062) and the NRF Grant funded by the Korea Government (MSIP) (No. 2014R1A5A2010008).

Authors' contributions

JHJ operated on the patient, initiated, supervised, and critically revised the manuscript and contributed to the manuscript with his expertise. SPB collected and analyzed data and wrote this manuscript. All authors have read and approved the final manuscript.

Competing interests

The authors declare that they have no competing interests.

Consent for publication

Written informed consent for publication of the clinical details and clinical images was obtained from a legal guardian of the patient.

References

1. Burk SE, Da Mata AP, Snyder ME, Cionni RJ, Cohen JS, Osher RH. Prosthetic iris implantation for congenital, traumatic, or functional iris deficiencies. J Cataract Refract Surg. 2001;27(11):1732–40.
2. Blackmon DM, Lambert SR. Congenital iris coloboma repair using a modified McCannel suture technique. Am J Ophthalmol. 2003;135(5):730–2.
3. Hanumanthu S, Webb LA. Management of traumatic aniridia and aphakia with an iris reconstruction implant. J Cataract Refract Surg. 2003;29(6):1236–8.
4. Mayer CS, Reznicek L, Hoffmann AE. Pupillary reconstruction and outcome after artificial iris implantation. Ophthalmology. 2016;123(5):1011–8.
5. Kistler AD, Caicedo A, Abdulreda MH, Faul C, Kerjaschki D, Berggren PO, Reiser J, Fornoni A. In vivo imaging of kidney glomeruli transplanted into the anterior chamber of the mouse eye. Sci Rep. 2014;4:3872.
6. Navon SE. Expulsive iridodialysis: an isolated injury after phacoemulsification. J Cataract Refract Surg. 1997;23(5):805–7.
7. Ball J, Caesar R, Choudhuri D. Mystery of the vanishing iris. J Cataract Refract Surg. 2002;28(1):180–1.
8. Walker NJ, Foster A, Apel AJ. Traumatic expulsive iridodialysis after small-incision sutureless cataract surgery. J Cataract Refract Surg. 2004;30(10):2223–4.
9. Sullivan CA, Murray A, McDonnel P. The long-term results of nonexpulsive total iridodialysis: an isolated injury after phacoemulsification. Eye (Lond). 2004;18(5):534–6.
10. Kahook MY, May MJ. Traumatic total iridectomy after clear corneal cataract extraction. J Cataract Refract Surg. 2005;31(8):1659–60.
11. Muzaffar W, O'Duffy D. Traumatic aniridia in a pseudophakic eye. J Cataract Refract Surg. 2006;32(2):361–2.
12. Eom Y, Kang SY, Song JS, Kim HM. Traumatic aniridia through opposite clear corneal incision in a pseudophakic eye. J Cataract Refract Surg. 2013;39(4):645–8.
13. Jovanovic M, Radosavljevic P. Reconstruction of the iris in iridodialysis after a contusion injury of the eye. Srp Arh Celok Lek. 1991;119(7–8):224–6.
14. Ozturk F, Osher RH, Osher JM. Secondary prosthetic iris implantation following traumatic total aniridia and pseudophakia. J Cataract Refract Surg. 2006;32(11):1968–70.
15. Brancato R, Bandello F, Lattanzio R. Iris fluorescein angiography in clinical practice. Surv Ophthalmol. 1997;42(1):41–70.
16. Craandijk A, Aan de Kerk AL. Fluorescence angiography of the iris. Br J Ophthalmol. 1970;54(4):229–32.
17. Goto T, Shimura M, Nakazawa M. Indocyanine green iris angiography of lung carcinoma metastatic to the iris. Graefes Arch Clin Exp Ophthalmol. 1999;237(9):787–9.
18. Skalet AH, Li Y, Lu CD, Jia Y, Lee B, Husvogt L, Maier A, Fujimoto JG, Thomas Jr CR, Huang D. Optical coherence tomography angiography characteristics of iris melanocytic tumors. Ophthalmology. 2017;124(2):197–204. doi: 10.1016/j.ophtha.2016.10.003. Epub 2016 Nov 14.

15

Outcomes of and barriers to cataract surgery in Sao Paulo State, Brazil

Gabriel de Almeida Ferreira, Luisa Fioravanti Schaal, Marcela Dadamos Ferro, Antonio Carlos Lottelli Rodrigues, Rajiv Khandekar and Silvana Artioli Schellini*

Abstract

Background: Cataract is the leading cause of blindness in developing countries and identification of the barriers to accessing treatment is essential for developing appropriate public healthcare interventions. To evaluate the barriers to cataract surgery after diagnosis and assess the postoperative outcomes in Sao Paolo State, Brazil.

Methods: This prospective study evaluated cataract patients from 13 counties in São Paulo State in 2014. Cataract was diagnosed in the community by a mobile ophthalmic unit and patients were referred to a hospital for management. Gender, age, distance to the hospital and local municipal health structure were evaluated as possible barriers. Data were analyzed for postoperative outcomes and the impact on blindness and visual impairment.

Results: Six hundred patients were diagnosed with cataract with a mean age of 68.8±10.3 years and 374 (62.3%) were females. Two hundred and fifty-four (42.3%) patients presented to the referral hospital. One hundred forty-four (56.7%) underwent surgery, 56 (22.0%) decided not to undergo surgery, 40 (15.7%) required only YAG-Laser and 14 (5.5%) required a spectacle prescription only. Visual acuity increased statistically significantly from 1.07±0.73 logMAR at presentation to 0.25±0.41 logMAR at the final visit after intraocular lens implantation (p=0.000). There was a statistically significantly decrease from 17 (11.8%) blind patients and 55 (38.2%) visually impaired patients at presentation to 2 (1.4%) and 5 (3.5%) patients respectively after treatment (p=0.000).

Conclusion: Less than half of the individuals with cataract presented to the hospital for surgery. Among the patients who underwent treatment, there was an overall decrease in the number of blind individuals and visually impaired individuals. The barriers to cataract surgery were older age, greater distance to the hospital, municipalities with fewer inhabitants and less ophthalmic services.

Keywords: Cataract, Blindness, Treatment Outcome, Health services accessibility

Background

Cataract surgery is a leading cause of blindness in developing countries [1]. In 2010, there were an estimated 39 million blind individuals and 285 million visually impaired individuals globally. Cataract was considered the primary cause of blindness, responsible for 51% of these cases [2]. In 1990, the World Health Organization (WHO) created "Vision 2020 – the right for sight" initiative, which aims to eliminate avoidable blindness by 2020 worldwide. Despite improvement in access to surgery, many regions worldwide do have adequate coverage for cataract surgery [3].

Barriers to access cataract surgery differ by regions and include, gender, fear of surgery, status of visual disability, educational level, visual needs, distance from the care provider, cost and lack of an escort/caretaker [4].

Brazil has a universal public health system (*Sistema Único de Saúde – SUS*) that provides surgery without cost to those in need [5]. Despite universal healthcare, cataract remains the major cause of blindness in Brazil [6, 7]. Appropriate public healthcare strategies can be developed to eliminate cataract as a source of blindness using data from studies of barriers to cataract surgery in

* Correspondence: sschellini@gmail.com
Universidade Estadual Paulista Julio de Mesquita Filho Faculdade de Medicina Campus de Botucatu Botucatu, Sao Paulo, Brazil

regions of Brazil. Currently there are no published studies of barriers to cataract surgery in a Brazilian population. The present study evaluates the barriers to cataract surgery and presents some suggestions to increase the uptake of cataract surgery.

Methods

A cross-sectional prospective survey was performed in the southwest region of São Paulo State, Brazil, involving patients who were screened at a Ophthalmic Mobile Unit (OMU) in 2014. SUS covered all the costs for treatment. Patients were screened in 13 municipalities (Table 1). The tertiary health reference center for the 13 municipalities was the Clinical Hospital of Botucatu Medical School (*Hospital das Clínicas da Faculdade de Medicina de Botucatu* – HCFMB*)*. This study was approved by the Ethics Committee of the Faculdade de Medicina de Botucatu – UNESP, Sao Paulo, Brazil and adhered to the tenets of the Declaration of Helsinki. All study subjects signed a consent form.

The UMO team was composed of ophthalmologists and local health workers from each municipality. Subjects underwent a comprehensive ocular exam. Visual acuity (VA) was evaluated using an illuminated Snellen E chart and the values were converted to the logarithm of the minimum angle of resolution (logMAR) for statistical analysis. The Snellen to logMAR conversion was as follows: counting fingers, hand movement, light perception and without light perception corresponded to 2.10, 2.40, 2.70 and 3.00, respectively [8]. The WHO definitions were used to classify vision as follows: blindness was defined as

VA<20/400 and visual impairment was 20/400<VA<20/60 in the better eye with the best optical correction [9].

All participants underwent an objective and subjective refraction with an autorefractor (Accuref-K; Shinn Nippon, Tokyo, Japan) and a manual refractor (RT 6000; Nidek Co. Ltd., Gamagori, Japan). Slit lamp biomicroscopy (Shinn Nippon, Tokyo, Japan) was performed to evaluate the anterior segment and the posterior segment using a 90 D Volk lens. For patients who did not achieve good vision with refraction, a dilated examination was performed (Mydriacyl; Alcon Inc., Fort Worth, TX, USA) for comprehensive evaluation of the lens and fundus. Intraocular pressure (IOP) was measured with air-puff tonometer (CT-60; Topcon Corp., Tokyo, Japan). For patients with IOP over 20 mmHg, Goldmann tonometry was performed to confirm the air-puff tonometry readings (Haag-Streit AG, Köniz, Switzerland).

To ensure consistency, survey staff were trained, periodically monitored and the equipment was calibrated regularly. All data collection sheets were pretested.

After the ophthalmic exam, patients diagnosed with cataract or pseudophakia with posterior capsule opacification (PCO) were referred to the HCFMB for further examination, YAG (yttrium aluminum garnet) laser or surgery and an appointment was scheduled. The municipalities provided transportation to the hospital on the day of the appointment.

At the hospital, the patient underwent another ophthalmic examination. Biometry was performed using the IOLMaster 500 (Carl Zeiss Meditec, Jena, Germany) and IOL calculations targeted emmetropia in all eyes. In eyes with dense cataracts that precluded optical biometry, the

Table 1 Characteristics of the municipalities served by the Ophthalmic Mobile Unit in 2014

	Total patient referred n (%)	Inhabitants n	Per capita income (R$)	M-HDI	Distance to the Hospital (km)	Number of ophthalmologists n
Agudos	42 (7.0)	34524	627.75	0.745	75.3	a
Barra Bonita	99 (16.5)	35246	1056.38	0.788	60.0	4
Boracéia	41 (6.8)	4268	708.05	0.754	106.0	a
Brotas	57 (9.5)	21580	807.88	0.817	92.3	1
Conchas	27 (4.5)	16288	830.35	0.736	56.8	1
Dois Córregos	13 (2.2)	24761	896.77	0.725	81.3	1
Iacanga	30 (5.0)	10013	758.67	0.779	150.2	2
Igaraçu do Tietê	81 (13.5)	23362	650.03	0.727	53.3	1
Macatuba	50 (8.3)	16259	1065.29	0.777	68.8	1
Óleo	19 (3.2)	2673	788.27	0.761	133.3	2
Piramboia	19 (3.2)	5653	549.16	0.681	44.2	a
Promissão	102 (17.0)	35674	714.65	0.724	217.0	a
Taquarituba	20 (3.3)	23163	721.89	0.741	137.4	1

[a]Information not provided by municipalities
n=number

axial length was measured with an ultrasonic biometer (SP-1000AP; Sonoptek, Beijing, China) and the IOL power was calculated with the IOLMaster.

Patients underwent phacoemulsification or extracapsular cataract extraction (ECCE) based on surgeon preference. All patients underwent IOL implantation.

Statistical analysis

To analyze demographics and outcomes after treatment, the data obtained at the OMU visit were transferred to an Excel spreadsheet (Microsoft Corp., Redmond, WA, USA). The electronic medical records from the hospital were used to collect data on the diagnosis, surgical procedure and postoperative outcome and transferred to an Excel spreadsheet.

National data were consulted to determine possible barriers for evaluation in this study relating to patient adherence to the proposed treatment. The socioeconomic and demographic data of the assisted municipalities, such as Human Development Index (HDI), *per capita* income and number of inhabitants, were obtained from the *Instituto Brasileiro de Geografia e Estatística* – 2010 (IBGE) [10]. Data on the infrastructure of the ophthalmic service of the participating municipalities were collected using a standardized questionnaire, answered by the official representative of Public Health Care for the municipality.

Data analysis was performed with SPSS 22.0 software (IBM Corp., Armonk, NY, USA). The frequency, mean and standard deviation were calculated. Normally distributed data were analyzed by the Kolmogorov-Smirnov and Shapiro-Wilk tests. Statistical significance was indicated by $p<0.05$.

Results

During the study period, 600 patients from 13 participating municipalities were diagnosed with cataract or PCO and referred to the HCFMB. The mean age of the patients was 68.8 ± 10.3 years, of which 374 (62.3%) were female, 46 (7.7%) were blind and 202 (33.7%) were visually impaired (Table 2).

Table 2 General characteristics of the six hundred individuals referred to the reference hospital in 2014

Age (years)	68.8±10.3[a]
Best Corrected Visual Acuity (logMAR)	0.60±0.53[a]
Gender	
Female	374 (62.3)
Male	226 (37.7)
Blindness	46 (7.7)
Visual Impairment	202 (33.7)
Attended to the reference center	254 (42.3)

[a]mean± standard deviation n (%)

Two hundred and fifty-four (42.3%) patients presented for scheduled care. Presentation to the referral hospital varied between 16% to 63% among the municipalities. Younger patients had a statistically greater tendency to present to the referral hospital (67.4 ± 11.3 years vs. 70.0 ± 9.1 years, $p=0.004$) (Fig. 1), with no statistical influence of gender ($p>0.05$). Attendance was statistically associated with visual impairment ($p=0.000$) but not blindness ($p>0.05$) (Table 3).

Of the 254 patients who attended the hospital, 144 (56.7%) underwent surgery in at least one eye, 56 (22.0%) did not undergo surgery due other ophthalmic comorbidities or because the patient refused surgery, 40 (15.7%) were pseudophakic with PCO that required YAG capsulotomy, and 14 (5.5%) had milder lens opacities and reasonable VA with spectacle correction and remained under observation.

YAG capsulotomy was performed in 65 eyes of 40 patients, resulting in a statistically significant improvement in VA from 0.93 ± 0.73 logMAR before capsulotomy vs 0.25 ± 0.46 logMAR after capsulotomy, $p<0.000$). Prior to YAG laser treatment there were four (10.0%) blind patients and 11 (27.5%) visually impaired patients. After YAG capsulotomy there was a statistically significant reduction in the number of blind patients to zero and visually impaired patients to 2 (2.0%) ($p<0.000$, both comparisons).

Of the 56 patients who did not undergo surgery, 27 (48.2% of those who did not undergo surgery and 10.7% of all patients) had surgery postponed due to mild lens opacity, 17 (30.4) were lost to follow-up before surgery and 9 (16.1%) refused surgery.

A total of 253 surgeries were performed, of which 245 were phacoemulsification and 8 were extracapsular cataract extraction (ECCE), all with IOL implantation. There was a statistically significant increase in VA from 1.07 ± 0.73 logMAR (20/225 Snellen acuity) preoperatively to 0.25 ± 0.41 logMAR (20/32 Snellen acuity) at last postoperative visit ($p=0.000$). The mean improvement is VA was -0.86 logMAR, which is equivalent to 8 lines on an early treatment of diabetic retinopathy study (ETDRS) chart.

Of the patients who underwent surgery, 37 (14.6%) had an associated ocular comorbidity and, in 32 (12.6%) of these patients the comorbidity caused the low VA. The most common comorbidity was, age-related macular degeneration (AMD) in 11 (33.4%) cases. Comparison of groups with and without comorbidities justifying the low VA indicated, statistically significant differences in the preoperative VA (1.40 ± 0.80 logMAR vs 0.83 ± 0.70 logMAR; $p=0.000$) and the postoperative VA (1.05 ± 0.82 logMAR vs 0.21 ± 0.40 logMAR; $p=0.000$).

Preoperatively 17 (11.8%) patients who underwent phacoemulsification in at least one eye were classified as blind and 55 (38.2%) were considered visually impaired. There was a statistically significant decrease after phacoemulsification to 2 (1.4%) blind patients and 5 (3.5%)

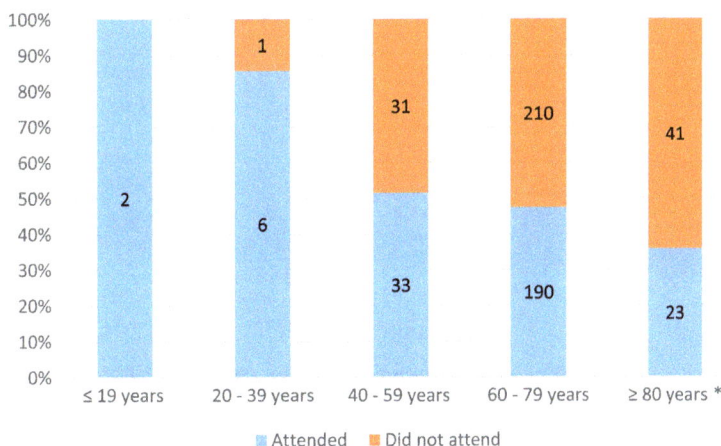

Fig. 1 Comparison between age groups who attended or did not attend the scheduled visit to the referral hospital

patients who were visually impairment (p=0.000). Of those who remained blind or visually impaired after phacoemulsification, 4 (57.1%) the low VA could be explained by an ocular comorbidity.

The final postoperative refraction was available for 154 (60.9%) eyes. At the final postoperative visit the mean spherical was -0.32 ± 1.13 D (range, -3.75 D to +2.75 D), the mean cylindrical was -1.02 ± 1.02 D (range -9.00 D to 0.00 D) and the mean spherical equivalent was -0.83±1.11 D (range -3.88±2.13).

There were 209 patients who underwent cataract surgery and YAG capsulotomy, of whom 21 (10.0%) were blind and 16 (7.6%) were visually impaired prior to treatment. After treatment, there was a statistically significant decrease in the number of blind patients to 2 (0.9%) and 7 (3.3%) remained visually impaired (p<0.000).

Data on local demographics and municipal health services was provided by 9 of the 13 municipalities covered in the study. Hence data on 396 patients could be analyzed for attendance and determination of possible barriers (Table 4).

For patients who did not present for their scheduled visits, the municipal HDI was statistically significantly higher (0.772±0.029 versus 0.763±0.034, p=0.034), there was a statistically greater distance to the hospital (83.2±32.9 km vs 73.6±28.9 km, p=0.00), a statistically higher per capita income (R$890.6±156.1 vs R$836.6±164.1, p=0.000) and statistically lower population (21,923.7±9,642.4 inhabitants vs 24,287.9± 8,349.1 inhabitants, p=0.000).

Regarding the municipality health structure, 84.2% of patients who did not present for the scheduled visit had ophthalmologists in their municipality of origin, compared to 92.3% of those who attended (p=0.016). Additionally, patients who did not attend had statistically significantly more blindness prevention programs (18.4% vs 4.8%, p=0.000), statistically better local coverage by ophthalmic surgeons (18.4% vs 4.8%, p=0.000), statistically greater availability of ophthalmic equipment at municipal primary healthcare facilities (50.9% vs 39.3%, p=0.022) and statistically better municipal hospital services and infrastructure to perform phacoemulsification (23.7% vs 9.5%, p=0.000).

Discussion

The outcomes of this cross-sectional study of cataract patients indicated that those who presented to the referral hospital were younger and mainly females. This observation is similar to other Brazilian studies [11–13] and is likely due to the characteristics of the Brazilian population which has a greater number of elderly women (IBGE – 2010) [10]. Although the current study reported greater female presentation to the referral hospital, there was no statistical difference between genders (p>0.05).

In the current study, a relatively low number of patients (42.3%) diagnosed with cataract (based on the OMU screening) presented to the specialized hospital for phacoemulsification or YAG capsulotomy.

Table 3 Comparison of individuals who attended or did not present to the reference hospital in 2014

	Attended (n=254) - n(%)	Did not present (n=346) - n (%)	p
Age (years)	67.4±11.3[a]	70.0±9.1	**0.004**
Best Visual Acuity (logMAR)	0.62±0.55[a]	0.59±0.52	0.631
Gender			
Female	155 (61.0)	219 (63.3)	0.571
Male	99 (39.0)	127 (36.7)	
Blindness	24 (9.4)	22 (6.4)	0.160
Visual Impairment	106 (41.7)	96 (27.7)	**<0.001**

[a]mean ± standard deviation
n=number; p<0.05 is statistically significant (bold values)

Table 4 Demographic data of 396 individuals and the municipalities of origin based on attendance in 2014

	Attended (n=168); (%)	Did not attend (n–228), n (%)	p
Age (years)	69.3±9.2[a]	67.3±12.0[a]	0.081
Best Visual Acuity (logMAR)	101 (60.1)	151 (66.2)	0.245
Gender			
Female	67 (39.9)	77 (33.8)	
Male	9 (5.4)	21 (9.2)	0.181
Blindness	46 (27.4)	59 (25.9)	0.818
HDI	0.763±0.034	0.770±0.029	**0.034**
Distance to the specialized hospital (km)	73.6±28.9	83.2±32.9	**0.000**
Per capita income (R$)	836.6±164.1	890.6±156.1	**0.000**
Inhabitants	24287.9±8349.1	21923.7±9642.4	**0.000**
Patients with blindness prevention program	8 (4.8)	42 (18.4)	**0.000**
Patients with ophthalmologist in county of origin	155 (92.3)	192 (84.2)	**0.020**
Hospital with structure for facectomy	16 (9.5)	54 (23.7)	**0.000**
Ophthalmic Apparatus in the basic health	66 (39.3)	116 (50.9)	**0.025**
Cataract campaign in the last five years	154 (91.7)	209 (91.7)	1.000
Total	168 (%)	228 (%)	

[a]mean±standard deviation
n=number; p<0.05 is statistically significant (bold values)

In the entire study sample, 10.0% of patients were blind and 7.6% were visually impaired at presentation. After treatment, there was a statistically significant decrease in blindness to 0.9% of patients and 3.3% of the patients were visually impaired (p<0.000). Hence, despite the low patient presentation rate for referral, the treatment was effective and achieved the WHO criteria. The WHO recommends a maximum of 5.0% of patients with best corrected visual acuity less than 20/400 (blindness) after cataract surgery.

A British study of 127,658 patients reported an improvement in VA from 0.63 logMAR at baseline to 0.16 ±0.30 logMAR after cataract surgery [8]. The VA outcomes of the current study are lower than the British study [8]. The differences in outcomes between studies are like because the British study was performed in a developed country, on a larger sample size and with earlier diagnosis. In the current study, many patients had associated ocular comorbidity that resulted in the low VA at final visit. However, the postoperative VA in patients without comorbidities in the current study was similar to the British study [8]. A recent study from São Paulo, Brazil reported a decrease from 17.6% blind patients and 23.5% visually impaired at baseline, to 5.9% and 11.8% respectively, after cataract surgery [14]. The VA outcomes from the current study are well within or exceed the range reported from other developing countries. For example, a study of cataract surgery in a rural province in Laos reported 9.5% blind and 44.3% visually impaired postoperatively [15]. In Nigeria, 58.5% remained blind

and 16.1% remained visually impaired after surgery [16]. In Nepal, 8.0% of patients remained blind and 22.0% remained visually impaired after surgery [17]. In Pakistan, 36.8% remained blind and 22.0% remained visually impaired [18]. The poorer VA outcomes at final postoperative visit from some of the other developing countries are likely due to the uncertain surgical conditions, often treating cases where biometry was difficult to perform, or patients were aphakic. Additionally, in some of the other developing countries standard cataract surgery techniques may not be possible the surgeons may need to improvise based on the surgical environment [19, 20]. However, in the current study cataract surgery was performed in a specialized tertiary hospital with good infrastructure with the option of IOL implantation in all patients which explains the good postoperative outcomes.

The number of surgeries, the quality of surgery and the final VA are all factors for achieving the goal of Vision 2020. Access to healthcare services is another barrier despite the strategy of approaching patients in their hometown using an OMU and detecting individuals who require surgery. For example, despite these initiatives, only 42.3% of the screened patients presented to the specialized hospital in the current study.

Our analysis of the social, economic and demographic characteristics and the health structure of the municipalities indicated that greater distance from the hospital, with higher HDI, higher per capita income and a lower municipal population were most unlikely to present to the referral hospital. These characteristics can be considered the barriers to treatment of cataracts in Sao Paolo State, Brazil. Interestingly the same barriers were reported in a rural region of China [21] and in central Ethiopia [22]. The factors "higher per capita income" and "higher HDI" differ from other studies, which described insufficient family income and an underdeveloped population as important barriers [21–23]. Perhaps patients with higher per capita income are able to undergo treatment in their hometown or elsewhere, bearing the expenses of the procedure. This observation may explain the lack of presentation to the referral hospital. Other factors that contribute to the low presentation rate for ophthalmic surgeries are, comorbidities, fear of the operation or of becoming blind postoperatively [4, 14].

There are an average 62 ophthalmologists per 1 million inhabitants in Latin America and this number is increasing. Therefore, there are an adequate number of ophthalmologists for coverage of cataract surgery [24]. However, the number of ophthalmologists that perform cataract surgery and how many surgeries each ophthalmologist performs remains unknown. Unlike a previous study [24], we found that the majority of patients who did not present to the referral hospital had a higher number of ophthalmologists in their hometown. Despite the unfavorable presentation, patients who did not attend can have their cataracts addressed in their own municipalities. These municipalities may have an adequate number of ophthalmologists, surgeons and hospital infrastructure for cataract surgery.

There are some limitations to the present study, including the lack of data on the best-corrected VA for all patients and that the barriers were not analyzed individually. Separate analyses of the barriers were not performed because we collected generalized data regarding the study population. However, there is a relative paucity of data from studies evaluating a Brazilian sample with an OMU. Hence, the outcomes of the current study provide data that can be used to allocate adequate resources and develop public healthcare initiatives.

The outcomes of the current study indicate that the elimination of cataract as a cause of blindness and/or visual impairment in Brazil requires greater coordination between the municipality and the regional tertiary hospital to ensure greater uptake of surgery.

Conclusion

Less than half of the patients diagnosed with cataract in municipalities using an OMU actually presented to a specialized hospital for treatment despite referral. However, the outcome of phacoemulsification was encouraging, resulting in a significant reduction of blind and visually impaired patients.

The main barrier to attendance were advanced age, greater distance to the specialized hospital and

municipalities with lower populations. However, the presence of blindness prevention programs, ophthalmic surgeons, available ophthalmic equipment at healthcare centers and hospital with the resources to perform phacoemulsification may be factors that reduce adherence to appointments at a specialized hospital.

Abbreviations
AMD: Age-related macular degeneration; ECCE: Extracapsular cataract extraction; ETDRS: Early treatment of diabetic retinopathy study; HCFMB: Hospital das Clínicas da Faculdade de Medicina de Botucatu; HDI: Human Development Index; IBGE: Instituto Brasileiro de Geografia e Estatística; IOL: Intraocular lens; IOP: Intraocular pressure; logMAR: logarithm of the minimum angle of resolution; OMU: Ophthalmic Mobile Unit; PCO: Posterior capsule opacification; SUS: Sistema Único de Saúde; VA: Visual acuity; WHO: World Health Organization; YAG: Yttrium aluminum garnet

Acknowledgements
None.

Funding
None.

Authors' contributions
GAF was the main writer and data analyzer. LFC and MFR realized the data collection. ACLR and SAS concepted and corrected the paper and suggested changes. RK collaborated with the data analysis and english spelling. All authors read and approved the final manuscript.

Consent for publication
Not applicable

Competing interests
The authors declare that they have no competing interests.

References
1. Allen D, Vasavada A. Cataract and surgery for cataract. Br J Ophthalmol. 2006;333(7559):128–32.
2. Pascolini D, Mariotti SP. Global estimates of visual impairment: 2010. Br J Ophthalmol. 2012;96(5):614–8.
3. Foster A. Cataract and "Vision 2020-the right to sight" initiative. Br J Ophthalmol. 2001;85(6):635–7.
4. Lewallen S, Courtright P. Recognising and reducing barriers to cataract surgery. Community Eye Health. 2000;13(34):20–1.
5. Kara-Júnior N, Dellapi R Jr. Espíndola RFd. Dificuldades de acesso ao tratamento de pacientes com indicação de cirurgia de catarata nos Sistemas de Saúde Público e Privado. Arq Bras Oftalmol. 2011;74:323–5.
6. Araújo Filho A, Salomão SR, Berezovsky A, Cinoto RW, Morales PHÁ, Santos FRG, et al. Prevalence of visual impairment, blindness, ocular disorders and cataract surgery outcomes in low-income elderly from a metropolitan region of São Paulo - Brazil. Arq Bras Oftalmol. 2008;71:246–53.

7. Salomão SR, Mitsuhiro MRKH, Belfort R Jr. Visual impairment and blindness: an overview of prevalence and causes in Brazil. An Acad Bras Ciênc. 2009;81:539–49.

8. Day AC, Donachie PH, Sparrow JM, Johnston RL, Royal College of Ophthalmologists' National Ophthalmology D. The Royal College of Ophthalmologists' National Ophthalmology Database study of cataract surgery: report 1, visual outcomes and complications. Eye (Lond). 2015;29(4):552–60.

9. Tabin G, Chen M, Espandar L. Cataract surgery for the developing world. Curr Opin Ophthalmol. 2008;19(1):55–9.

10. Instituto Brasileiro de Geografia e Estatística. Censo Demográfico 2010. Avalible from: http://www.ibge.gov.br/home/estatistica/populacao/censo2010/. [Last accessed on: 29 dez 2016]

11. Gomes BAF, Biancardi AL, Fonseca Netto C, FFP G, HVD MJ. Perfil socioeconômico e epidemiológico dos pacientes submetidos à cirurgia de catarata em um hospital universitário. Rev Bras Oftalm. 2008;67:220–5.

12. LMPD S, Muccioli C, Belfort R Jr. Perfil socioeconômico e satisfação dos pacientes atendidos no mutirão de catarata do Instituto da Visão - UNIFESP. Arq Bras Oftalmol. 2004;67:737–44.

13. Ventura LO, Brandt CT. Projeto Mutirão de Catarata em centro de referência oftalmológico, em Pernambuco: perfil, grau de satisfação e benefício visual do usuário. Arq Bras Oftalmol. 2004;67:231–5.

14. Mitsuhiro MH, Berezovsky A, Belfort R Jr, Ellwein LB, Salomao SR. Uptake, Barriers and Outcomes in the Follow-up of Patients Referred for Free-of-Cost Cataract Surgery in the Sao Paulo Eye Study. Ophthalmic Epidemiol. 2015;22(4):253–9.

15. Shields MK, Casson RJ, Muecke J, Laosern S, Louangsouksa P, Vannavong S, et al. Intermediate-Term Cataract Surgery Outcomes from Rural Provinces in Lao People's Democratic Republic. Ophthalmic Epidemiol. 2015;22(4):260–5.

16. Odugbo OP, Mpyet CD, Chiroma MR, Aboje AO. Cataract blindness, surgical coverage, outcome, and barriers to uptake of cataract services in Plateau State. Nigeria. Middle East Afr J Ophthalmol. 2012;19(3):282–8.

17. Thapa SS, Khanal S, Paudyal I, Twyana SN, Ruit S, van Rens GH. Outcomes of cataract surgery: a population-based developing world study in the Bhaktapur district. Nepal. Clin Experiment Ophthalmol. 2011;39(9):851–7.

18. Bourne R, Dineen B, Jadoon Z, Lee PS, Khan A, Johnson GJ, et al. Outcomes of cataract surgery in Pakistan: results from The Pakistan National Blindness and Visual Impairment Survey. Br J Ophthalmol. 2007;91(4):420–6.

19. Venkatesh R, Muralikrishnan R, Balent LC, Prakash SK, Prajna NV. Outcomes of high volume cataract surgeries in a developing country. Br J Ophthalmol. 2005;89(9):1079–83.

20. Lindfield R, Vishwanath K, Ngounou F, Khanna RC. The challenges in improving outcome of cataract surgery in low and middle income countries. Indian J Ophthalmol. 2012;60(5):464–9.

21. Zhang XJ, Jhanji V, Leung CK, Li EY, Liu Y, Zheng C, et al. Barriers for poor cataract surgery uptake among patients with operable cataract in a program of outreach screening and low-cost surgery in rural China. Ophthalmic Epidemiol. 2014;21(3):153–60.

22. Mehari ZA, Zewedu RT, Gulilat FB. Barriers to cataract surgical uptake in central ethiopia. Middle East Afr J Ophthalmol. 2013;20(3):229–33.

23. Dhaliwal U, Gupta SK. Barriers to the uptake of cataract surgery in patients presenting to a hospital. Indian J Ophthalmol. 2007;55(2):133–6.

24. Batlle JF, Lansingh VC, Silva JC, Eckert KA, Resnikoff S. The cataract situation in Latin America: barriers to cataract surgery. Am J Ophthalmol. 2014;158(2):242-250 e1.

16

Evaluation of biometry and corneal astigmatism in cataract surgery patients

Ji-guo Yu[†], Jie Zhong[†], Zhong-ming Mei, Fang Zhao, Na Tao and Yi Xiang[*]

Abstract

Background: To evaluate the distribution of biometric parameters and corneal astigmatism using the IOLMaster device before phacoemulsification in cataract patients in Central China.

Methods: Consecutive cataract patients were recruited at the Central Hospital of Wuhan between January 2015 and June 2016. Ocular axial length (AL), keratometry values, anterior chamber depth (ACD) and horizontal corneal diameter (white to white [WTW]) of each cataract-affected eye were measured with the IOLMaster device.

Results: The study evaluated 3209 eyes of 2821 cataract patients. The mean AL, ACD, and WTW were 24.38 ± 2.47 mm, 3.15 ± 0.48 mm, and 11.63 ± 0.43 mm, respectively. Corneal astigmatism of 0.51–1.00 diopters (D) was the most common range of values (34.96%). A total of 10.56% patients exhibited a corneal astigmatism greater than 2.0 D. The flat and steep keratometry values gradually increased with age. The mean ACD and WTW showed increasing trends as the AL increased ($P < 0.001$). When the AL was shorter than 26.0 mm, the keratometry decreased as AL increased. The against-the-rule (ATR) astigmatism proportion increased with age and the with-the-rule (WTR) astigmatism proportion decreased with age.

Conclusions: The profile of ocular biometric data and corneal astigmatism may help ophthalmologists improve their surgical procedures and make an appropriate IOL choice to gain a high quality of postoperative vision.

Keywords: Biometry, Corneal astigmatism, Cataract, IOLMaster device, Central China

Background

Cataract is the leading cause of blindness and the only form of treatment is surgery. Phacoemulsification is the most commonly used and effective surgical method for the treatment of cataract worldwide. Accurate measurement of ocular axial length, keratometry, anterior chamber depth and corneal diameter before cataract surgery is crucial for obtaining the precise degree of implanted intraocular lens (IOL) to control the postoperative diopter (D) value plus or minus 0.50 D as well as to achieve satisfactory postoperative refractive results and improve the visual quality for cataract patients [1, 2].

Partial coherence interferometry (IOLMaster, Carl Zeiss Meditec, Germany) is a type of optical coherent biological measuring instrument that utilizes non-contact

technology to measure axial length, keratometry, anterior chamber depth and corneal diameter. With its ultra-high precision (5 mm or less) and good resolution (12 mm), it is widely used in evaluating the ocular parameters and IOL calculations in cataract patients before surgery. Through its innovative and accurate measurement of ocular parameters, the degree of intraocular lens can be accurately calculated before implantation [3]. Corneal astigmatism is also a major factor affecting postoperative visual quality. The IOLMaster can measure preoperative corneal astigmatism and predict the residual corneal astigmatism after cataract surgery [4].

However, most previous studies of preoperative ocular biometry and corneal astigmatism on cataract patients focused on the European and American populations [5–8]. Although there have been some domestic related studies, they aimed to evaluate the Southern, Northern, and Eastern Chinese populations [1, 9, 10]. However, the epidemiological investigation of ocular biometry and

* Correspondence: xyyanke@163.com

[†]Equal contributors

Department of Ophthalmology, the Central Hospital of Wuhan, Tongji Medical College, Huazhong University of Science and Technology, No, 26 Shengli Street, Wuhan, Hubei Province 430014, China

corneal astigmatism of cataract patients in the Central China region has yet to be investigated. Therefore, the aim of our study was to evaluate the distribution of biometric parameters, and determine the prevalence of corneal astigmatism using the IOLMaster measurement device before phacoemulsification in cataract patients in Central China, to provide some reference for improving cataract surgical procedures and designing an intraocular lens to meet eye characteristics of the Central Chinese population.

Methods

Subjects

This study was approved by the institutional ethics committee of the Central Hospital of Wuhan (Hubei, Central China), and followed the tenets of the Declaration of Helsinki. Consecutive cataract patients scheduled for phacoemulsification and foldable IOL implantation were recruited at the Central Hospital of Wuhan between January 2015 and June 2016. All patients who were local residents of Central China, had cataract, and were older than 30 years were included. Exclusion criteria included a history of ocular surgery, such as refractive surgery, corneal diseases, ocular inflammation, and trauma; patients from other areas of China were also excluded. Routine eye examinations were performed before surgery, including visual acuity, refraction, tonometry, slit lamp evaluation, and dilated fundus evaluation. The procedures were fully explained to each patient, and they provided written informed consent.

Biometry examination

Ocular axial length (AL), keratometry values, anterior chamber depth (ACD) and horizontal corneal diameter (white to white [WTW]) of each cataract-affected eye were measured with the IOLMaster (Carl Zeiss Meditec, Germany, software version 5.4). Keratometry was measured in 2 meridians: that is, flat keratometry (K1) and steep keratometry (K2). The K value was calculated as the mean of K1 and K2. The patients were divided into 7 groups on the basis of age as follows: 30–40 years, 41–50 years, 51–60 years, 61–70 years, 71–80 years, 81–90 years, and 90 years and older. All eyes were stratified into 4 groups based on AL as follows: shorter than 22.0 mm, 22.0–24.5 mm, longer than 24.5 mm–26.0 mm, and longer than 26.0 mm.

Statistical analysis

All data were recorded in Microsoft Excel spreadsheets, and analyzed using the Kolmogorov-Smirnov test for normal distribution. Continuous variables were expressed as the mean ± standard deviation for those displaying normal distribution. One-way analysis of variance and the Kruskal-Wallis test were applied for the comparison of variance for normally and non-normally distributed data among the different age groups, respectively. Statistical analysis was performed using SPSS PASW Statistics Version 18.0 software (IBM Corporation, Armonk, NY, USA). *P*-values less than 0.05 were considered statistically significant.

Results

Distribution of ocular biometry

This study evaluated 3209 eyes of 2821 cataract patients. The patient demographics are shown in Table 1, which also shows a comparison of these demographics with 4 other published papers that studied populations from the different regions in China. The histograms of the frequency distribution of corneal astigmatism for all patients are shown in Fig. 1. Corneal astigmatism of 0.51–1.00 D was the most common range of values (34.96%), followed by 1.01–1.50 D (21.72%), 0.0–0.50 D (21.19%), and 1.51–2.0 D (11.56%). A total of 10.56% patients exhibited a corneal astigmatism greater than 2.0 D.

Different age groups

Table 2 shows the mean and standard deviation values of all measured biometric parameter values in the 7 different age groups. The flat and steep keratometry values gradually increased with age. Most eyes in this cohort were between 71 and 80 years old (34.66%), followed by 61 and 70 years old (33.04%). In addition, the AL, ACD, and WTW values showed a gradually decreasing trend with age; corneal astigmatism showed first a decline and then a rising trend (Fig. 2).

Distribution of axial length

Table 3 shows the distribution of ocular biometry for different ALs. The AL in the majority of eyes was between 22.0 and 24.5 mm (63.63%). The mean ACD and WTW showed increased as the AL increased (*P* < 0.001). When the AL was shorter than 26.0 mm, the keratometry values (K1, K2, and K) decreased with an increase in AL. However, this trend seemed to revert in patients with an AL of more than 26.0 mm. The smallest mean corneal astigmatism (1.03 D) was in eyes with an AL between 22.0 and 24.5 mm, and the largest (1.26 D) was in eyes with a longer AL than 26.0 mm.

Distribution of corneal astigmatism

Corneal astigmatism was with-the-rule (WTR, the steepest meridian of the cornea being within 90 ± 30 degrees) in 1186 eyes (36.96%), against-the-rule (ATR, the steepest meridian of the cornea being within 180 ± 30 degrees) in 1535 eyes (47.83%), and oblique (steepest meridian between 30 and 60 degrees or 120 and 150 degrees) in 488 eyes (15.21%). The ATR astigmatism proportion increased with age and the WTR astigmatism

Table 1 Comparison of demographic features between the present study and 4 other published studies

Parameters	Present	Cui [1]	Chen [11]	Yuan [9]	Guan [10]
Location	Central China	Southern China	Southern China	Northern China	Eastern China
Eyes/patients	3209/2821	6750/4561	4831/2849	12,449/6908	1430/827
Age (y)					
Mean ± SD	70.51 ± 9.81	70.4 ± 10.5	70.56 ± 9.55	69.80 ± 11.15	72.27 ± 11.59
Range	32, 95	40, 101	40, 95	30, 97	16, 98
Male/female	1071/1750	2026/2535	1090/1759	3199/3709	359/468
Keratometry (D)					
Mean ± SD	1.09 ± 0.77	0.90(Median)	1.01 ± 0.69	1.15 ± 0.84	1.07 ± 0.73
Range	0.0, 6.21	NR	0.05, 6.59	0.0, 6.63	0.06, 5.52
K1 mean ± SD	43.75 ± 1.59	43.57 ± 1.69	43.76 ± 1.53	43.93 ± 1.67	43.57 ± 1.56
K2 mean ± SD	44.84 ± 1.65	44.69 ± 1.69	44.76 ± 1.56	45.08 ± 1.73	44.64 ± 1.65
K mean ± SD	44.29 ± 1.58	44.13 ± 1.63	NR	NR	NR
Corneal astigmatism (%)					
≤ 0.5D	21.19%	NR	23.14%	20.76%	21.2%
≥ 1.0D	43.85%	43.9%	41.3%	47.27%	45.46%
≥ 2.0D	10.56%	11.6%	8.22%	13.16%	10.42%
≥ 3.0D	2.80%	3.4%	1.68%	3.75%	2.31%
axis	88.82 ± 49.63	NR	NR	NR	NR
AL (mm)	24.38 ± 2.47	24.07 ± 2.14	23.58 ± 1.13	NR	NR
ACD (mm)	3.15 ± 0.48	3.01 ± 0.57	NR	NR	NR
WTW (mm)	11.63 ± 0.43	11.68 ± 0.45	NR	NR	NR

D diopter, *K1* flat keratometry, *K2* steep keratometry, *K* mean keratometry, *SD* standard deviation, *AL* axial length, *ACD* anterior chamber depth, *WTW* white to white, *NR* not reported

proportion decreased with age. The proportion of oblique astigmatism changed little with increasing age. The percentages of WTR, ATR, and oblique corneal astigmatisms in the 7 groups are shown in Fig. 3.

Discussion

This study evaluated the distribution of ocular biometric parameters and characteristics of corneal astigmatism measured using the IOLMaster device in cataract patients residing in Central China. Studies of corneal

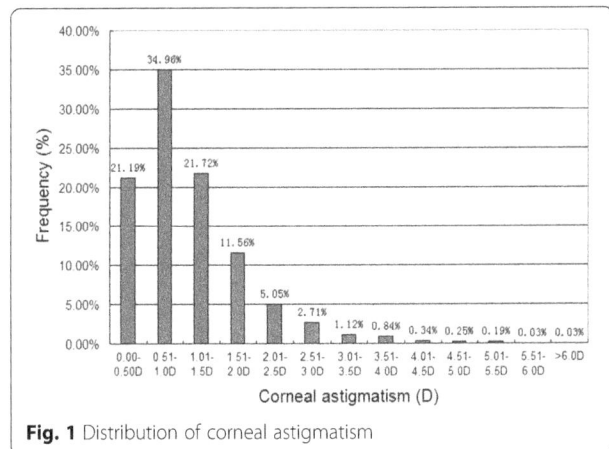

Fig. 1 Distribution of corneal astigmatism

astigmatism in cataract patients from Southern [1, 11], Northern [9] and Eastern [10] China have previously been published. We compared these previous results with those in the present study and found that the corneal power in patients from Northern China was greater than that in other different regions, while the difference among other areas was not obvious. The highest astigmatism in patients from the four areas did not exceed 7.00 D, but the percentage of cataract patients with astigmatism higher than 1.00 D was the greatest in Northern China. This is probably attributed to a regional difference in the populations, as well as different environmental and life style factors [12].

Corneal astigmatism across all age groups showed a similar distribution pattern compared to previous studies [6, 8, 9, 13]. The vast majority of eyes with cataract had a corneal astigmatism between 0.5 D and 1.0 D. In contrast, only a small percentage of eyes with corneal astigmatism greater than 3.0 D were observed. Understanding the distribution of astigmatism is important to help ophthalmologists choose first-line treatment that will be most effective and reduce the occurrence of postoperative astigmatism. This includes procedures such as limbal relaxing incisions [14], opposite clear corneal incisions [15], excimer laser refractive procedures [16, 17],

Table 2 Descriptive statistics for the 7 age groups

Age Group (Y)	AL (mm)	ACD (mm)	WTW (mm)	Astigmatism (D)	K1 (D) mean ± SD	K2 (D) mean ± SD	K (D) mean ± SD	Eyes (%)
30–40	26.50 ± 2.58	3.57 ± 0.22	11.79 ± 0.41	1.21 ± 0.45	42.86 ± 1.52	44.07 ± 1.74	43.47 ± 1.62	13(0.41%)
41–50	25.10 ± 2.70	3.42 ± 0.36	11.77 ± 0.36	1.08 ± 0.71	42.87 ± 1.33	43.95 ± 1.43	43.41 ± 1.33	61(1.90%)
51–60	25.41 ± 3.42	3.36 ± 0.44	11.70 ± 0.45	1.01 ± 0.69	43.74 ± 1.74	44.75 ± 1.76	44.24 ± 1.71	422(13.15%)
61–70	24.68 ± 2.66	3.22 ± 0.47	11.68 ± 0.39	1.01 ± 0.72	43.81 ± 1.56	44.82 ± 1.64	44.32 ± 1.55	1060(33.04%)
71–80	23.95 ± 1.89	3.06 ± 0.44	11.57 ± 0.44	1.13 ± 0.82	43.78 ± 1.56	44.91 ± 1.62	44.35 ± 1.53	1112(34.66%)
81–90	23.74 ± 1.69	2.95 ± 0.52	11.58 ± 0.43	1.22 ± 0.76	43.68 ± 1.60	44.89 ± 1.65	44.29 ± 1.58	514(15.99%)
>90	23.50 ± 1.33	2.70 ± 0.27	11.67 ± 0.49	1.75 ± 1.00	43.67 ± 2.07	45.42 ± 1.93	44.54 ± 1.93	27(0.85%)
P-value	< .001	< .001	< .001	< .001	< .001	< .001	< .001	

Y years, mm millimeter, D diopter, K1 flat keratometry, K2 steep keratometry, K mean keratometry, SD standard deviation, AL axial length, ACD anterior chamber depth, WTW white to white

femtosecond laser-assisted astigmatic keratotomy [18], and toric IOL implantation [19–22]. At present, toric IOL implantation is highly recognized and it can be used to correct up to 8.0 D of corneal astigmatism after cataract surgery [23, 24]. In the present study, 21.28% of cataract patients in Central China had corneal astigmatism values between 1.5 D and 4.0 D, most of which could be effectively corrected with toric IOLs. Therefore, the use of toric IOLs in Central China is still required, and that is not less than the demand in other parts of China.

The mean AL, ACD and WTW in the present study are consistent with that reported by Cui et al. [1], who reported on biometry characteristics of the Southern China population. Unfortunately, the data mentioned

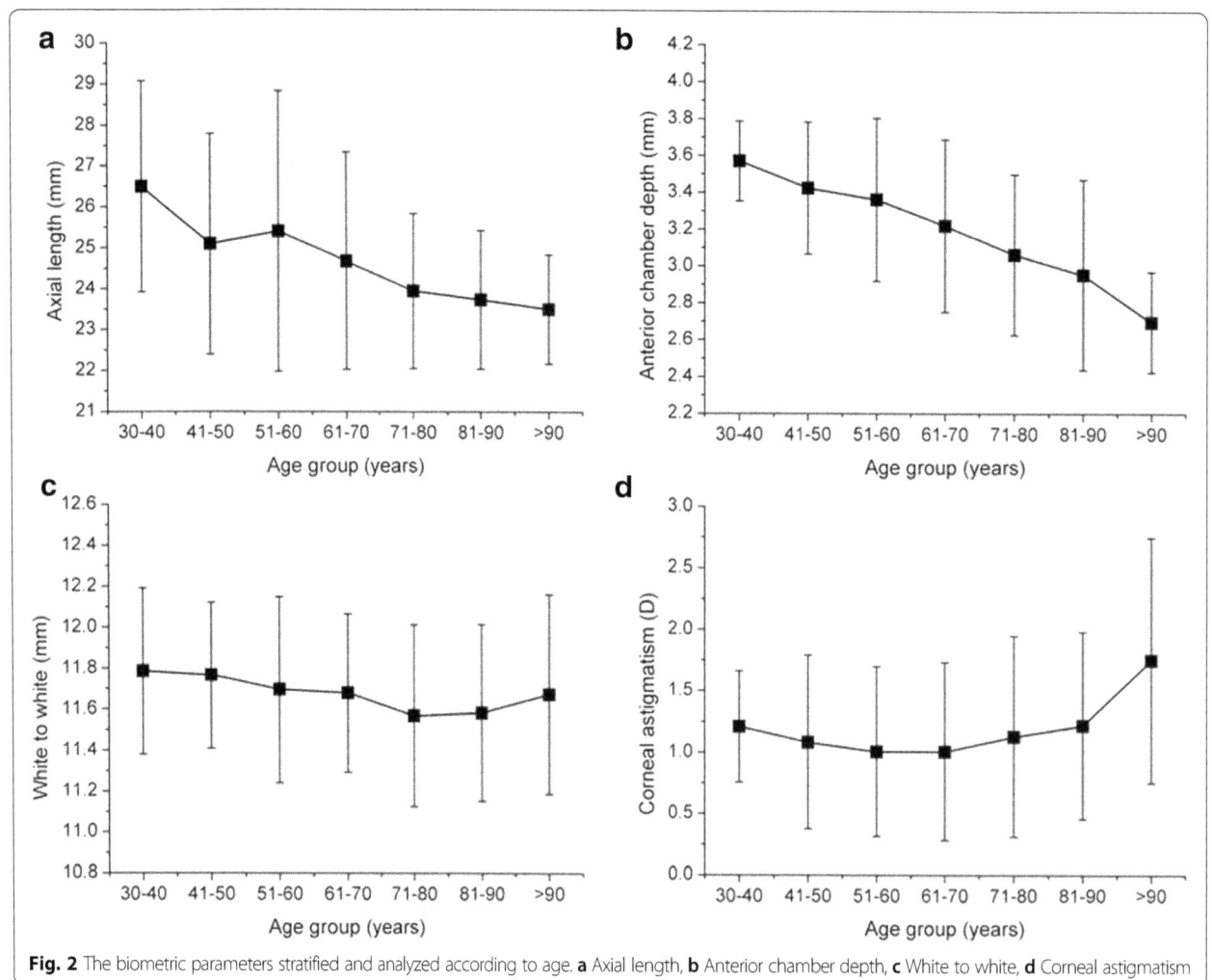

Fig. 2 The biometric parameters stratified and analyzed according to age. **a** Axial length, **b** Anterior chamber depth, **c** White to white, **d** Corneal astigmatism

Table 3 The distribution of ocular biometry for different ALs

AL (mm)	Eyes, n (%)	Mean ± SD						
		ACD (mm)	WTW (mm)	Keratometry (D)			Astigmatism (D)
				K1	K2	K	
Shorter than 22.0	218 (6.80%)	2.79 ± 0.48	11.38 ± 0.46	45.39 ± 1.40	46.51 ± 1.41	45.95 ± 1.36	1.12 ± 0.75
22.0–24.5	2042 (63.63%)	3.01 ± 0.44	11.62 ± 0.42	43.85 ± 1.41	44.88 ± 1.45	44.37 ± 1.39	1.03 ± 0.72
Longer than 24.5–26.0	390 (12.15%)	3.35 ± 0.37	11.66 ± 0.44	43.00 ± 1.70	44.14 ± 1.97	43.57 ± 1.79	1.15 ± 0.87
Longer than 26.0	559 (17.42%)	3.50 ± 0.40	11.72 ± 0.37	43.32 ± 1.71	44.58 ± 1.78	43.95 ± 1.69	1.26 ± 0.83
Total	3209 (100%)	3.15 ± 0.48	11.63 ± 0.43	43.75 ± 1.59	44.84 ± 1.65	44.29 ± 1.58	1.09 ± 0.77
P-value		< .001	< .001	< .001	< .001	< .001	< .001

mm millimeter, *D* diopter, *K1* flat keratometry, *K2* steep keratometry, *K* mean keratometry, *SD* standard deviation, *AL* axial length, *ACD* anterior chamber depth, *WTW* white to white

above were not reported for the Northern and Eastern China populations; therefore, we were unable to make a comparison with those studies. All biometric parameters that were measured using the IOLMaster device were presented as significant differences between age groups. The AL, ACD, and WTW values gradually decreased with age; corneal astigmatism showed an initial decline and then subsequently an increase. This suggests that the human eye biometric parameters change with age. This might be related to the occurrence of lens opacity and thickening, accommodative lags, cornea arcus senilis, extraocular muscle relaxation and orbital fat prolapse generating compression on the eye.

Ocular axial length affects other components of the biometric parameters in eyes. In the present study, we found that as the AL increased, ACD and WTW also increased. Additionally, the keratometry values (K1, K2, and K) decreased when the AL was between 20.0 and 26.0 mm. These results are consistent with the findings reported in previous studies [1, 6, 25, 26]. This suggests that the cornea becomes flatter when the AL increases, accompanied by a larger horizontal WTW. However,

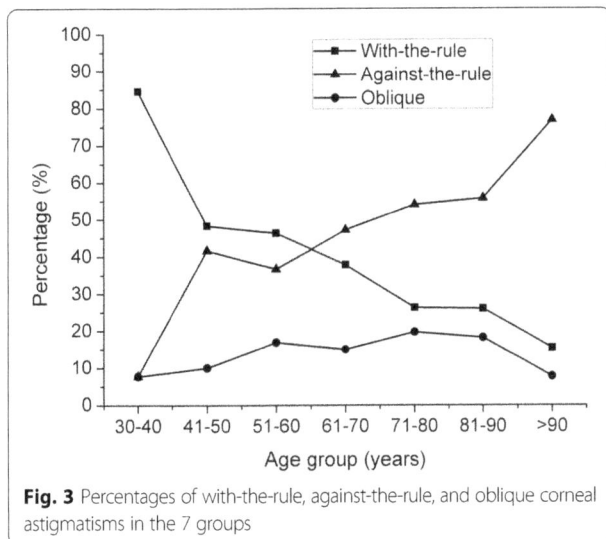

Fig. 3 Percentages of with-the-rule, against-the-rule, and oblique corneal astigmatisms in the 7 groups

this characteristic was not observed when the AL was greater than 26.0 mm. ATR astigmatism accounted for the majority of the cataract population, and the prevalence increased with age. By contrast, the percentage of WTR astigmatism decreased with age. These findings are consistent with the characteristics seen in populations from different countries and regions [6, 9, 27, 28]. These changes have been found to be due to a discrepancy in eyelid morphology and power [29].

It is well known that a toric IOL is indicated when there is a corneal astigmatism of 1.50 D or more. Although the IOLMaster measures six points of the central corneal surface within a 2.3 mm range, it is unable to reflect the entire corneal surface curvature. The pupil is only approximately 2.0–3.0 mm wide during the day, and considering the long duration of daytime eye use in most people, the IOLMaster mainly reflects the results of the central corneal astigmatism; therefore, the IOLMaster measurements also have reference values. Corneal topography can measure the total corneal astigmatism, and is more accurate for distinguishing between regular and irregular astigmatism. Therefore, we believe that for the selection of toric IOLs, one should consider both the corneal topography and IOLMaster measurements in order to make a comprehensive judgment. The current study found that a total of 710 (22.13%) eyes in our study were potential candidates, however when considering implantation of toric IOLs, other factors such as the surgical techniques, economic feasibility for the patient, and rotation of the optical axis should also be taken into account. Total astigmatism is determined by corneal astigmatism, which is the major factor affecting postoperative visual quality; therefore it is crucial to select a reasonable and economical operative procedure to correct corneal astigmatism [1]. The most cost-effective methods to reduce corneal astigmatism are to make smaller incision and choose the most appropriate location for the corneal incision. Our study reported that ATR astigmatism accounted for the majority of the cataract population, and that prevalence increased with age. The characteristics of corneal astigmatisms in our study suggest that when considering large-scale cataract surgery for patients with a low socioeconomic status in Central China, smaller and temporal corneal incisions should be used frequently to reduce preexisting corneal astigmatism, especially in the underdeveloped areas in China.

Our study has some limitations. First, the ocular biometric data drawn from the cataract patients in our hospital do not completely represent the data of the whole population in Central China. Second, we did not make a comparative analysis of eye biometric parameters with data reported abroad because previous studies reported much more detail, and we did not compare findings between men and women. Furthermore, we did not assess the relationship between biometric parameters and genetics, diet, education, occupation, and the severity of the cataract due to lack of relevant data.

Conclusions

In conclusion, our study determined the distribution of ocular biometric parameters and the characteristics of corneal astigmatism as well as their variation among different age groups in Central China. The profile of ocular biometric data and corneal astigmatism may help ophthalmologists improve their surgical procedures including appropriate IOL choice and more accurate corneal incision made to gain a high quality of postoperative vision.

Abbreviations
ACD: Anterior chamber depth; AL: Axial length; ATR: Against-the-rule; D: Diopter; IOL: Intraocular lens; K: Mean keratometry; K1: Flat keratometry; K2: Steep keratometry; Mm: Millimeter; NR: Not reported; SD: Standard deviation; WTR: With-the-rule; WTW: White to white; Y: Years

Acknowledgements
Not applicable.

Funding
This study was supported by the Health and Family Planning Commission Fund of Wuhan, China (Grant WX16E28).

Authors' contributions
JY and JZ contributed to research design, data collection, analysis, and interpretation as well as preparation of the manuscript. ZM and FZ contributed to data analysis and interpretation and provided major revisions to the manuscript. NT contributed to the data collection as well as the data interpretation. YX contributed to study design, study analysis and discussion, and revision of the manuscript. All authors read and approved the final manuscript.

Competing interests
The authors declare that they have no competing interests.

Consent for publication
Not applicable.

References
1. Cui Y, Meng Q, Guo H, Zeng J, Zhang H, Zhang G, et al. Biometry and corneal astigmatism in cataract surgery candidates from Southern China. J Cataract Refract Surg. 2014;40:1661–9.
2. Olsen T. Improved accuracy of intraocular lens power calculation with the Zeiss IOLMaster. Acta Ophthalmol Scand. 2007;85:84–7.
3. Karunaratne N. Comparison of the Pentacam equivalent keratometry reading and IOL master keratometry measurement in intraocular lens power calculations. Clin Experiment Ophthalmol. 2013;41:825–34.
4. Yong Park C, Do JR, Chuck RS. Predicting postoperative astigmatism using Scheimpflug keratometry (Pentacam) and automated keratometry (IOLMaster). Curr Eye Res. 2012;37:1091–8.
5. Fotedar R, Wang JJ, Burlutsky G, Morgan IG, Rose K, Wong TY, et al. Distribution of axial length and ocular biometry measured using partial coherence laser interferometry (IOL master) in an older white population. Ophthalmology. 2010;117:417–23.
6. Hoffmann PC, Hutz WW. Analysis of biometry and prevalence data for corneal astigmatism in 23,239 eyes. J Cataract Refract Surg. 2010;36:1479–85.
7. De Bernardo M, Zeppa L, Cennamo M, Iaccarino S, Rosa N. Prevalence of corneal astigmatism before cataract surgery in Caucasian patients. Eur J Ophthalmol. 2014;24:494–500.
8. Khan MI, Muhtaseb M. Prevalence of corneal astigmatism in patients having routine cataract surgery at a teaching hospital in the United Kingdom. J Cataract Refract Surg. 2011;37:1751–5.
9. Yuan X, Song H, Peng G, Hua X, Tang X. Prevalence of corneal astigmatism in patients before cataract surgery in Northern China. J Ophthalmol. 2014; 2014:536412.
10. Guan Z, Yuan F, Yuan YZ, Niu WR. Analysis of corneal astigmatism in cataract surgery candidates at a teaching hospital in shanghai. China J Cataract Refract Surg. 2012;38:1970–7.
11. Chen W, Zuo C, Chen C, Su J, Luo L, Congdon N, et al. Prevalence of corneal astigmatism before cataract surgery in Chinese patients. J Cataract Refract Surg. 2013;39:188–92.
12. Meng W, Butterworth J, Malecaze F, Calvas P. Axial length of myopia: a review of current research. Ophthalmologica. 2011;225:127–34.
13. Ferrer-Blasco T, Montes-Mico R, Peixoto-de-Matos SC, Gonzalez-Meijome JM, Cervino A. Prevalence of corneal astigmatism before cataract surgery. J Cataract Refract Surg. 2009;35:70–5.
14. Ouchi M, Kinoshita S. AcrySof IQ toric IOL implantation combined with limbal relaxing incision during cataract surgery for eyes with astigmatism >2.50 D. J Refract Surg. 2011;27:643–7.
15. Mendicute J, Irigoyen C, Ruiz M, Illarramendi I, Ferrer-Blasco T, Montes-Mico R. Toric intraocular lens versus opposite clear corneal incisions to correct astigmatism in eyes having cataract surgery. J Cataract Refract Surg. 2009;35: 451–8.
16. Gunvant P, Ablamowicz A, Gollamudi S. Predicting the necessity of LASIK enhancement after cataract surgery in patients with multifocal IOL implantation. Clin Ophthalmol. 2011;5:1281–5.
17. Norouzi H, Rahmati-Kamel M. Laser in situ keratomileusis for correction of induced astigmatism from cataract surgery. J Refract Surg. 2003;19:416–24.
18. Ruckl T, Dexl AK, Bachernegg A, Reischl V, Riha W, Ruckhofer J, et al. Femtosecond laser-assisted intrastromal arcuate keratotomy to reduce corneal astigmatism. J Cataract Refract Surg. 2013;39:528–38.
19. Horn JD. Status of toric intraocular lenses. Curr Opin Ophthalmol. 2007;18: 58–61.
20. Bachernegg A, Ruckl T, Riha W, Grabner G, Dexl AK. Rotational stability and visual outcome after implantation of a new toric intraocular lens for the

correction of corneal astigmatism during cataract surgery. J Cataract Refract Surg. 2013;39:1390–8.

21. Bachernegg A, Ruckl T, Strohmaier C, Jell G, Grabner G, Dexl AK. Vector analysis, rotational stability, and visual outcome after implantation of a new aspheric Toric IOL. J Refract Surg. 2015;31:513–20.

22. Ferreira TB, Berendschot TT, Ribeiro FJ. Clinical outcomes after cataract surgery with a new transitional Toric intraocular lens. J Refract Surg. 2016;32:452–9.

23. Rubenstein JB, Raciti M. Approaches to corneal astigmatism in cataract surgery. Curr Opin Ophthalmol. 2013;24:30–4.

24. Kessel L, Andresen J, Tendal B, Erngaard D, Flesner P, Hjortdal J. Toric intraocular lenses in the correction of astigmatism during cataract surgery: a systematic review and meta-analysis. Ophthalmology. 2016;123:275–86.

25. Jivrajka R, Shammas MC, Boenzi T, Swearingen M, Shammas HJ. Variability of axial length, anterior chamber depth, and lens thickness in the cataractous eye. J Cataract Refract Surg. 2008;34:289–94.

26. Olsen T, Arnarsson A, Sasaki H, Sasaki K, Jonasson F. On the ocular refractive components: the Reykjavik eye study. Acta Ophthalmol Scand. 2007;85:361–6.

27. Nemeth G, Szalai E, Berta A, Modis L Jr. Astigmatism prevalence and biometric analysis in normal population. Eur J Ophthalmol. 2013;23:779–83.

28. Mohammadi M, Naderan M, Pahlevani R, Jahanrad A. Prevalence of corneal astigmatism before cataract surgery. Int Ophthalmol. 2016;36:807–17.

29. Read SA, Collins MJ, Carney LG. A review of astigmatism and its possible genesis. Clin Exp Optom. 2007;90:5–19.

17

Prospective study of bilateral mix-and-match implantation of diffractive multifocal intraocular lenses

Chan Min Yang[1†], Dong Hui Lim[1,2†], Sungsoon Hwang[1], Joo Hyun[3] and Tae-Young Chung[1*]

Abstract

Background: To evaluate monocular and binocular visual outcomes for near, intermediate, and far distance in patients implanted with diffractive multifocal intraocular lenses (IOLs) with different add power contralaterally.

Methods: This is a prospective contralateral study. Two diffractive multifocal IOLs with different added power were implanted bilaterally in twenty patients. TECNIS® ZKB00 (+ 2.75 D) was implanted in a dominant eye, and TECNIS® ZLB00 (+ 3.25 D) was implanted in a non-dominant eye. Uncorrected distance visual acuity (UDVA), uncorrected intermediate visual acuity (UIVA), uncorrected near visual acuity (UNVA), and manifest refraction (MR) values were measured at 1 month and 3 months postoperatively. At the 3-month follow-up, defocus curve, contrast sensitivity, and reading performance were evaluated. Quality of vision, overall satisfaction, and spectacle independence were evaluated by questionnaire.

Results: Postoperative binocular UDVA, visual acuity at 80 cm, 60 cm, 50 cm, 43 cm, 33 cm were − 0.08 ± 0.10, 0.12 ± 0.14, 0.09 ± 0.09, 0.07 ± 0.11, 0.14 ± 0.09, 0.25 ± 0.11 logMAR. The binocular defocus curve showed an extended range of good visual acuity with sharp vision being observed from 0 D to − 2.50 D defocus (logMAR≤0.1). Reading performance was significantly improved compared to baseline. All patients were spectacle-free at distance, and 94.74% of the patients did not require glasses for near and intermediate vision.

Conclusions: Mix-and-match implantation of diffractive multifocal IOLs with different add power provides an excellent wide range of vision, as well as high levels of visual quality and patient satisfaction.

Background

A monofocal intraocular lens (IOL) implanted after cataract extraction to replace the focusing power of the crystalline lens has a fixed focal length. Although patients can achieve a good uncorrected-distance visual acuity after monofocal IOL implantation, most patients need glasses for reading or other activities at close distance.

However, in recent years, the increasing use of smartphones and tablets and new leisure activities require a fast alternation of far and near distance tasks, also in elderly people. So spectacle dependence after cataract surgery can be inconvenient in the daily life of patients. In order to solve both cataract and presbyopia simultaneously, a variety of intraocular lenses have been developed. Diffractive bifocal IOLs with various levels of additional power have been widely used for correcting presbyopia after cataract surgery. The additional power of diffractive bifocal IOLs was selected according to patients' lifestyle. Although diffractive bifocal IOL implantation is an effective way to satisfy patients who want to stop using their glasses after cataract surgery, it often results in visual symptoms, including diminished contrast sensitivity and dysphotopsia due to the IOLs' diffractive surface [1, 2]. Other disadvantages of the implantation of bifocal IOLs is

* Correspondence: tychung@skku.edu
†Equal contributors
[1]Department of Ophthalmology, Samsung Medical Center, Sungkyunkwan University School of Medicine, #81 Irwon-ro, Gangnam-gu, Seoul 06351, South Korea
Full list of author information is available at the end of the article

a suboptimal intermediate visual acuity compared to near and distance visual acuities [3, 4].

Diffractive trifocal IOLs aim to provide a wider range of spectacle independence especially at an intermediate distance compared to bifocal IOLs. Trifocal IOLs provide three foci to enhance intermediate visual acuity. However, the distribution of light energy for a third focus could negatively affect near and distance visual acuity [5]. Decreased contrast sensitivity and unwanted visual symptoms may also occur after trifocal IOLs implantation [6, 7].

Recently, several methods of combining different types IOLs have been introduced to meet the diverse needs of the patients [8, 9]. And bilateral mix-and-match implantation of diffractive multifocal IOLs with different add power may be another option for enhancing intermediate visual acuity. However, previous studies of contralateral implantation of diffractive multifocal IOLs with different add power have used AcrySof IQ ReSTOR [10, 11].

The purpose of this study was to evaluate the clinical outcomes following bilateral mix-and-match implantation of the recently developed Tecnis diffractive bifocal IOLs with + 2.75 and + 3.25 add power.

Methods

This prospective, contralateral study comprised 20 patients affected by bilateral senile cataract. The study was approved by the Institutional Review Board of the Samsung Medical Center, and adhered to the tenets of the Declaration of Helsinki. Written informed consent was obtained from all patients.

The inclusion criteria were patients with bilateral senile cataract and the desire to be spectacle-free for all distances. Exclusion criteria were ages younger than 21 years, corneal astigmatism greater than 1.00 D, previous ocular surgery or trauma and ocular disease other than cataract. Hole-in-the card test was conducted in all patients for detection of dominant eye preoperatively.

The implanted IOLs were TECNIS ZKB00 (add power + 2.75 diopter [D], theoretical working distance 50 cm; Abbott Medical Optics, Santa Ana, California, USA) and TECNIS ZLB00 (add power + 3.25D, theoretical working distance 42 cm). The + 2.75D IOL was implanted in the dominant eye and that + 3.25D IOL in the non-dominant eye. Emmetropic intraocular lens power was selected from SRK/T, SRKII, Haigis, or Hoffer Q formulas according to corneal curvature, axial length and anterior chamber depth measured by IOLMaster version 5.4 (Carl Zeiss Meditec, Jena, Germany).

Surgical technique

One experienced surgeon (T.Y.C) performed all surgical procedures under topical anesthesia using a standardized sutureless phacoemulsification with a 2.75 mm clear corneal incision. Steep axis corneal incision was created in eyes with corneal astigmatism of more than 0.5D, and temporal corneal incision was made in eyes with corneal astigmatism less than 0.5D. The non-dominant eye was operated first. After that contralateral surgery was performed at an interval of one week. Postoperative gatifloxacin and fluometholone 0.1% eye drops were used 4 times a day for 1 month.

Patient evaluation

Preoperatively, all patients underwent a complete ophthalmologic examination including corrected and uncorrected visual acuity, manifest refraction, slit-lamp bio-microscopy, and fundus examination.

Patients were evaluated postoperatively at 1 day, 1 week, and 1 and 3 months. At 1 and 3 months after surgery, corrected and uncorrected visual acuity, manifest refraction, defocus curve, contrast sensitivity, reading performance, and subjective satisfaction were examined.

All patients underwent measurement of corrected and uncorrected distance visual acuity at 5 m (CDVA and UDVA). Uncorrected intermediate visual acuities (UIVA) were measured at 60 cm and 80 cm and uncorrected near visual acuities (UNVA) at 33 cm, 43 cm, and 50 cm using the ETDRS chart. All visual acuity were measured monocularly and binocularly.

Defocus curves were plotted by measuring the visual acuity under photopic condition at 5 m, adding lenses in 0.5D increments from − 4.0 to + 2.0D.

Contrast sensitivity at 3, 6, 12, and 18 cycles per degree was measured using a CSV-1000 chart (Vector Vision, Greenville, OH) under photopic (85 cd[cd]/m^2) and mesopic ($\sim$ 3 cd/m^2) conditions at 3 months after surgery. Results were converted in log units for statistical analysis using a specific table for the CSV-1000 [12].

At baseline and 3 months postoperatively, reading performance was measured using an iPad application at 50 cm [13]. The print size of the reading chart ranges from 1.0 to 0 logarithm of the minimal angle of resolution (logMAR). Average reading speed in words per minute (wpm) was calculated with the iPad application. Critical print size was defined as the last acuity measured before the reading speed was reduced below the 95% confidence interval of that individual's average reading speed [14]. Threshold print size was determined as the smallest print size that could be read and expressed in logarithm of the reading acuity determination (logRAD).

One and three months after surgery, all patients were asked to complete the questionnaire regarding overall satisfaction, presence of visual artifacts, and dependency on spectacles for near, intermediate and far vision. Overall satisfaction was evaluated using 5 levels (very satisfied, satisfied, neither satisfied nor dissatisfied, unsatisfied, very unsatisfied). Severity of visual artifacts, divided into 4 levels (none, minimal, moderate and severe), were assessed using a Quality of Vision questionnaire [15]. Furthermore, patients were asked if they would choose the same IOL again.

Statistical analysis

All data are presented as mean ± standard deviation. The statistical analysis was performed using SPSS software version 18.0 (SPSS, Inc., Chicago, IL). Measured decimal visual acuities were converted to logMAR for data analysis. Because the variables did not follow a normal distribution, non-parametric statistical analysis was used. The Wilcoxon signed-rank test was applied to assess the difference between preoperative and postoperative data. The Mann-Whitney U test was used to compare the dominant and non-dominant eyes. A sample size of 17 patients would allow the detection of a minimum clinical relevant difference in depth of focus with a standard deviation of 5.8. The sample sizes took into account a significance level of 5% and a power of 80% for a 2-sided test. Assuming an proportion of withdrawal of 10%, 20 patients were included.

Results

A total of 20 patients were enrolled, of which 19 completed the study. Patient recruitment was from August 2015 to January 2016. The study was finished after 3 months postoperative follow-up visit was completed for all patients in April 2016. All patients received regular follow-up examinations for at least 3 months. The mean age was 60.1 ± 6.61 years (range: 45 to 70 years), 63.1% (12 of 19) of the patients were female. Preoperative mean axial length was 24.74 ± 1.43 mm (range: 22.19 mm to 27.87 mm), mean keratometric value was 43.18 ± 1.25 D (range: 40.91 D to 45.18 D). Preoperative mean anterior chamber depth was 3.15 ± 0.49 mm (range: 2.42 mm to 4.53 mm). The mean IOL power implanted was 18.5 ± 4.4 D (range: 7.5 D to 25.5 D). Table 1 shows preoperative and postoperative monocular refractive results and visual acuities. At 3 months, there were statistically significant improvements in CDVA, UDVA, UIVA, and UNVA ($p < 0.001$). However, UNVA at 33 cm of eye with ZKB00 was not significantly different compared to the preoperative value ($p = 0.178$). No significant differences between eyes implanted with ZKB00 and eyes implanted with ZLB00 were found in uncorrected and corrected visual acuity at all distances ($p > 0.05$).

Table 2 shows preoperative and postoperative binocular visual acuities. Postoperative binocular visual acuities were significantly better than preoperative values, except for binocular UNVA at 33 cm. Cumulative binocular UNVA, UIVA, and UDVA at 1 and 3 months after surgery are shown in Figs. 1, 2 and 3.

Monocular and binocular defocus curves are shown in Fig. 4. Eyes implanted with ZKB00 and ZLB00 had two peaks at 0 and – 2 D. When comparing both eyes,

ZKB00 eyes had a slightly better visual acuity from – 1.0 to – 2.0 D. However, these differences were not statistically significant ($p = 0.84$, $p = 0.103$ and $p = 0.908$, respectively). Eyes with ZLB00 showed significantly better visual acuity at – 2.5, – 3.0, and – 3.5D compared to eyes implanted with ZKB00 ($p = 0.003$, $p = 0.022$ and p = 0.022, respectively). The binocular defocus curve also showed two peaks and overlapping curves with monocular defocus curves, as well as a wider range of good visual acuity from 0 to – 3.0 D (log MAR < 0.2 [range; – 0 ~ – 3.0 D], logMAR< 0.1 [range: 0–2.5 D]) Eyes with ZKB00 had a slightly better visual acuity from – 1.0 to – 2.0 diopters (D) compared to eyes with ZLB00. Eyes with ZLB00 showed significantly better visual acuity at – 2.5, – 3.0, and – 3.5 D (Mann-Whitney U test, p values < 0.05). Binocular defocus curve showed good visual acuity better than 0.1 logMAR from 0 to – 2.5 D.

Postoperative contrast sensitivity at 3 months was statistically significantly better at some spatial frequencies than that measured preoperatively (Fig. 5).

The mean reading speed increased from 76.93 ± 17.47 wpm (range: 44.33 to 106.17 wpm) at baseline to 86.83 ± 17.45 wpm (range: 64.99 to 123.53 wpm) at 3 months after surgery. The mean critical print size decreased from 0.65 ± 0.22 logRAD (range: 0.1 to 0.8 logRAD) at baseline to 0.24 ± 0.13 logRAD (range: 0 to 0.5 logRAD) at 3 months after surgery. The threshold print size also decreased from 0.35 ± 0.22 logRAD (range: 0 to 0.8 logRAD) at baseline to 0.14 ± 0.13 logRAD (range: 0 to 0.4 logRAD) at 3 months after surgery. There were statistically significant differences in mean reading speed, critical print size, and threshold print size between baseline and 3 months after surgery ($p = 0.07$, $p = 0.01$ and $p = 0.03$, respectively).

Overall satisfaction, visual symptoms and spectacle dependence are summarized in Table 3. Postoperative overall satisfaction with distance vision was statistically significant regarding the improvement achieved compared to preoperative ($p < 0.05$). Although halo and starburst were increased at 1 and 3 months after surgery, there were no significant differences compared to baseline (halo: $p = 0.108$ and $p = 0.301$, respectively; starburst: $p = 0.890$ and $p = 0.209$, respectively). All patients reported complete spectacle independence for distance after surgery. One patient required spectacles for near vision and another one patient sometimes for intermediate vision after surgery. A total of 94.7% of the patients (18 of 19) answered that they would choose the same IOLs again and 89.4% (17 of 19) did not feel dizzy and recognized the difference between both eyes.

Discussion

In this prospective study, the clinical outcomes of mix-and-match implantations of ZKB00 and ZLB00

Table 1 Monocular refractive results and visual acuities in patients implanted with ZKB00 and ZLB00 multifocal IOLs at preoperative, 1 month and 3 months after surgery

Measurement	Preoperative		1 month				3 months			
	Dominant eye	non-dominant eye	Dominant eye	P value[a]	non-dominant eye	P value[b]	Dominant eye	P value[c]	non-dominant eye	P value[d]
Spherical equivalent (D)	−1.61 ± 3.71	−1.69 ± 3.92	−0.01 ± 0.32		0.00 ± 0.30		−0.03 ± 0.22		0.06 ± 0.27	
CDVA at 5 m	0.09 ± 0.13	0.21 ± 0.24	−0.04 ± 0.08	0.005	−0.04 ± 0.07	< 0.001	−0.06 ± 0.07	< 0.001	−0.06 ± 0.07	< 0.001
UDVA at 5 m	0.53 ± 0.45	0.62 ± 0.45	−0.03 ± 0.09	< 0.001	−0.02 ± 0.10	< 0.001	−0.02 ± 0.10	< 0.001	−0.01 ± 0.10	< 0.001
UIVA at 80 cm	0.61 ± 0.27	0.67 ± 0.32	0.26 ± 0.17	0.002	0.27 ± 0.16	0.001	0.19 ± 0.14	< 0.001	0.19 ± 0.12	< 0.001
UIVA at 60 cm	0.66 ± 0.15	0.66 ± 0.27	0.12 ± 0.12	0.003	0.18 ± 0.14	0.005	0.16 ± 0.12	0.003	0.25 ± 0.13	< 0.001
UNVA at 50 cm	0.62 ± 0.23	0.65 ± 0.26	0.13 ± 0.12	< 0.001	0.14 ± 0.12	< 0.001	0.14 ± 0.13	< 0.001	0.16 ± 0.12	< 0.001
UNVA at 43 cm	0.58 ± 0.21	0.69 ± 0.18	0.24 ± 0.15	< 0.001	0.22 ± 0.13	< 0.001	0.21 ± 0.11	< 0.001	0.16 ± 0.10	< 0.001
UNVA at 33 cm	0.46 ± 0.29	0.53 ± 0.31	0.41 ± 0.21	0.441	0.30 ± 0.20	0.005	0.36 ± 0.18	0.178	0.30 ± 0.13	0.008

CDVA Corrected distance visual acuity, UDVA Uncorrected distance visual acuity, UIVA Uncorrected intermediate visual acuity, UNVA Uncorrected near visual acuity
[a]Dominant eye: Preoperative to 1 month after surgery
[b]Nondominant eye: Preoperative to 1 month after surgery
[c]Dominant eye: Preoperative to 3 months after surgery
[d]Nondominant eye: Preoperative to 3 months after surgery

Table 2 Binocular visual acuities in patients implanted with ZKB00 and ZLB00 multifocal IOLs at preoperative, 1 month and 3 months after surgery

Measurements	Preoperative	1 month	p value[a]	3 months	p value[b]
CDVA at 5 m	0.03 ± 0.12	−0.11 ± 0.08	0.001	−0.12 ± 0.08	0.001
UDVA at 5 m	0.36 ± 0.27	−0.10 ± 0.10	< 0.001	−0.08 ± 0.10	< 0.001
UIVA at 80 cm	0.50 ± 0.27	0.21 ± 0.23	0.013	0.12 ± 0.14	< 0.001
UIVA at 60 cm	0.51 ± 0.18	0.10 ± 0.14	0.003	0.09 ± 0.09	0.003
UNVA at 50 cm	0.43 ± 0.19	0.10 ± 0.10	< 0.001	0.07 ± 0.11	< 0.001
UNVA at 43 cm	0.45 ± 0.17	0.16 ± 0.15	< 0.001	0.14 ± 0.09	< 0.001
UNVA at 33 cm	0.31 ± 0.30	0.27 ± 0.23	0.491	0.25 ± 0.11	0.348

CDVA Corrected distance visual acuity, UDVA Uncorrected distance visual acuity, UIVA Uncorrected intermediate visual acuity, UNVA Uncorrected near visual acuity
[a]Preoperative to 1 month
[b]Preoperative to 3 months

were showed good UCVA and UNVA as well as UIVA and high satisfaction without visual disturbance such as glare and halo. Although there was previous study comparing ZMB00, ZKB00 and ZLB00, we could confirm that depth of focus was increased through contralateral mix-and-match implantation of ZKB00 and ZLB00. Compared with previous studies using the trifocal diffractive IOLs, our results revealed that contrast sensitivity was not reduced and visual disturbance was less. The previous version, ZMB00 Tecnis multifocal IOLs with + 4.0 D add power has the same design as the studied IOLs; however, the study IOLs have a relatively lower add power of + 2.75 D and + 3.25 D. All IOLs of this platform have a refractive zone on the anterior surface to provide distance vision and a full diffractive posterior surface for near vision. The fewer diffractive rings of ZKB00 and ZLB00 compared to ZMB00 are considered to reduce unwanted visual symptoms [16].

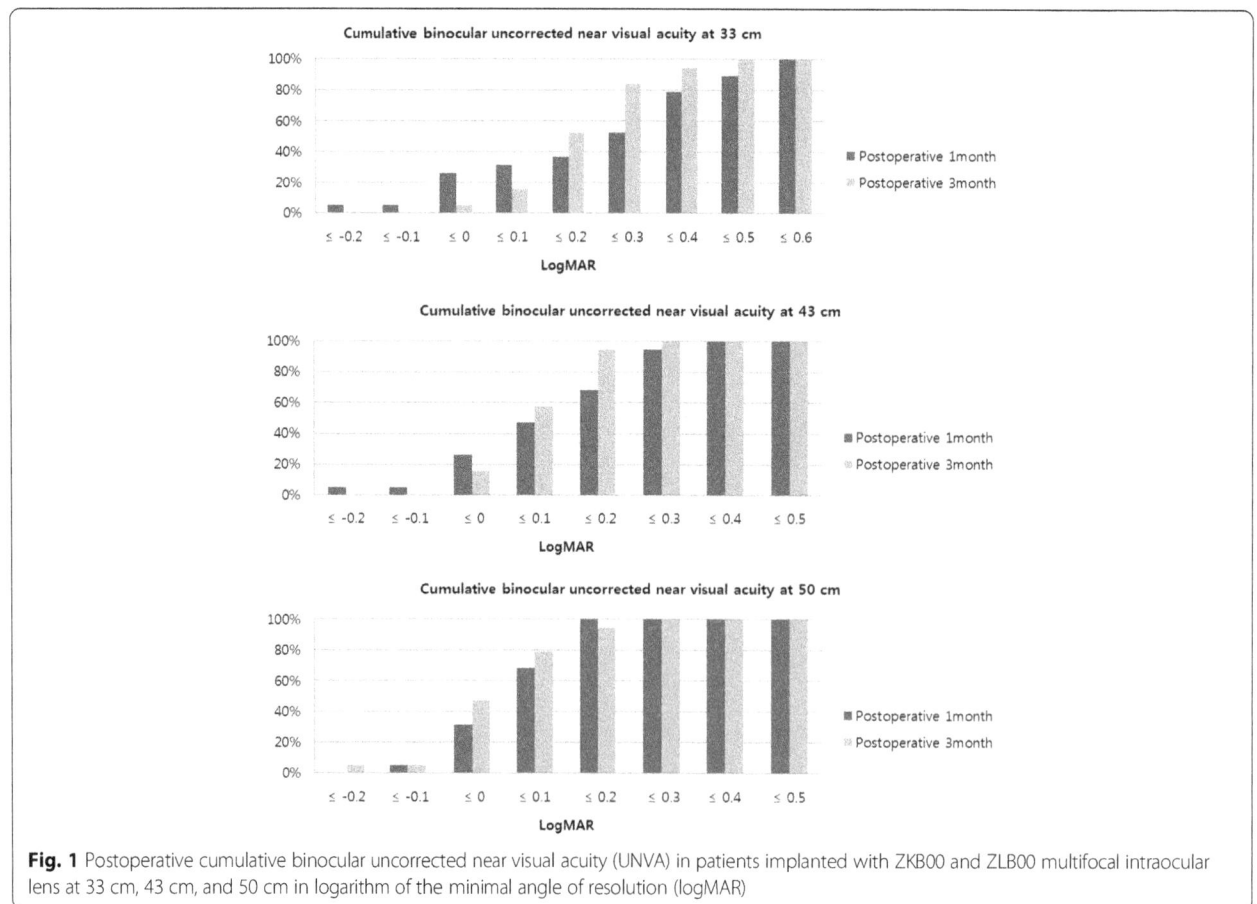

Fig. 1 Postoperative cumulative binocular uncorrected near visual acuity (UNVA) in patients implanted with ZKB00 and ZLB00 multifocal intraocular lens at 33 cm, 43 cm, and 50 cm in logarithm of the minimal angle of resolution (logMAR)

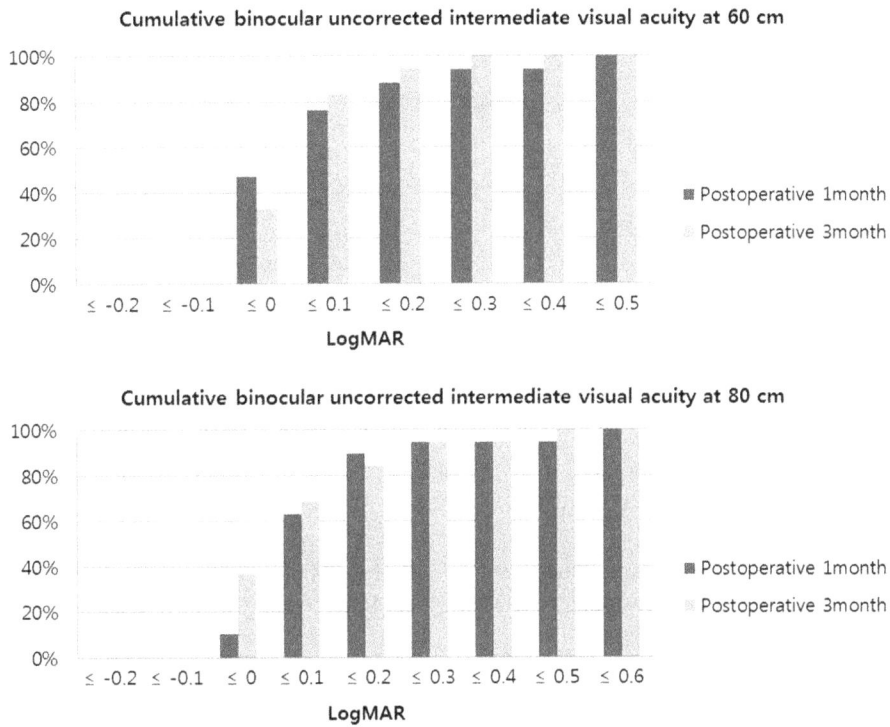

Fig. 2 Postoperative cumulative binocular uncorrected intermediate visual acuity (UIVA) in patients implanted with ZKB00 and ZLB00 multifocal intraocular lens at 60 cm and 80 cm in logarithm of the minimal angle of resolution (logMAR)

Regardless of pupil size, the light is evenly distributed between distance and near foci. Other optical principles of multifocal IOLs are dependent on pupil size [17].

Other studies with ZKB00 and ZLB00 IOL implantation report that subjects implanted with low add power bifocal IOLs had good intermediate and distance visual acuity with a high level of satisfaction [16, 18, 19]. Kretz et al. [19] reported 63.3% of the patients implanted with ZKB00 in both eyes achieved a binocular UIVA at 80 cm of 0.1 logMAR or better. In this study, the percentage of patients with binocular logMAR UIVA better than 0.1 logMAR at 80 cm was 68.5%. Kretz et al. [18] reported that bilaterally implantation of the ZLB00 IOL revealed a

binocular UIVA of 0.06 ± 0.09 logMAR at 60 cm. In our study, we found comparable results with 0.09 ± 0.09 logMAR. However, previous studies did not include the defocus curve which makes it difficult to compare the achieved visual acuity at various distances directly. Previous studies of bilateral mix-and-match implantation of diffractive bifocal IOLs reported a better visual acuity over a wider range compared to bilateral implantation of IOLs with the same add power [11]. Our study with mix-and-match implantations of Tecnis ZKB00 and ZLB00 found a 0.1 logMAR or better visual acuity in the 0 to – 2.5 D range of the defocus curve. We could speculate that outcomes of mix-and-match implantation

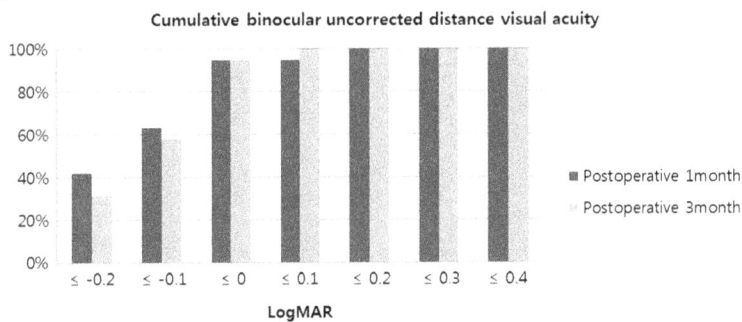

Fig. 3 Postoperative cumulative binocular uncorrected distance visual acuity (UDVA) in patients implanted with ZKB00 and ZLB00 multifocal intraocular lens in logarithm of the minimal angle of resolution (logMAR)

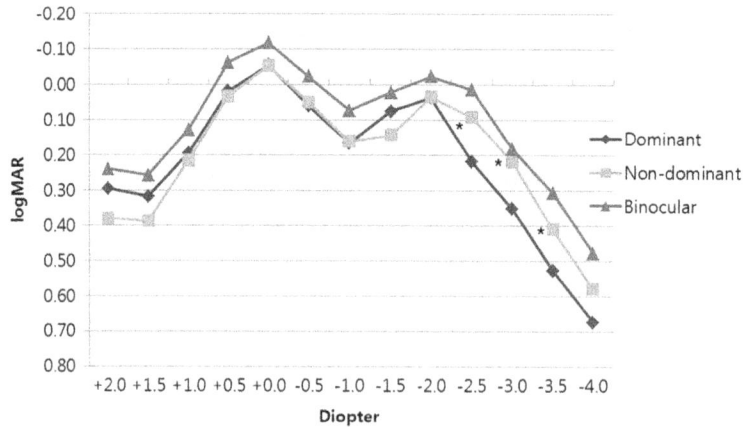

Fig. 4 Monocular and binocular defocus curve plotted in logarithm of the minimal angle of resolution (logMAR) in patients implanted with ZKB00 and ZLB00 multifocal intraocular lens at 3 months postoperatively. (*: $p < 0.05$, between dominant and non-dominant eye)

of Tecnis ZKB00 and ZLB00 might be better visual acuity at a broader range than bilateral implantation of IOLs with the same add power (ZKB00 or ZLB00).

This study is the first prospective study applying the bilateral mix-and-match implantation of Tecnis ZKB00 and ZLB00. All previous studies on mix-and-match implantations of diffractive bifocal IOLs used the AcrySof ReSTOR IOL [10, 11]. Nakamura et al. [10] reported that contralateral implantation of ReSTOR IOLs with +

3.0 and + 4.0 D addition was an effective way to get a broad range of good uncorrected visual acuity in the defocus curve. Mastropasqua R et al. [11] also reported that patients, implanted with ReSTOR IOLs with contralateral + 2.5 and + 3.0 D additions, had good uncorrected visual acuity over a wide range, and contrast sensitivity and visual quality did not decrease compared to bilateral implantation of diffractive multifocal IOLs with the same additional power. Compared with the

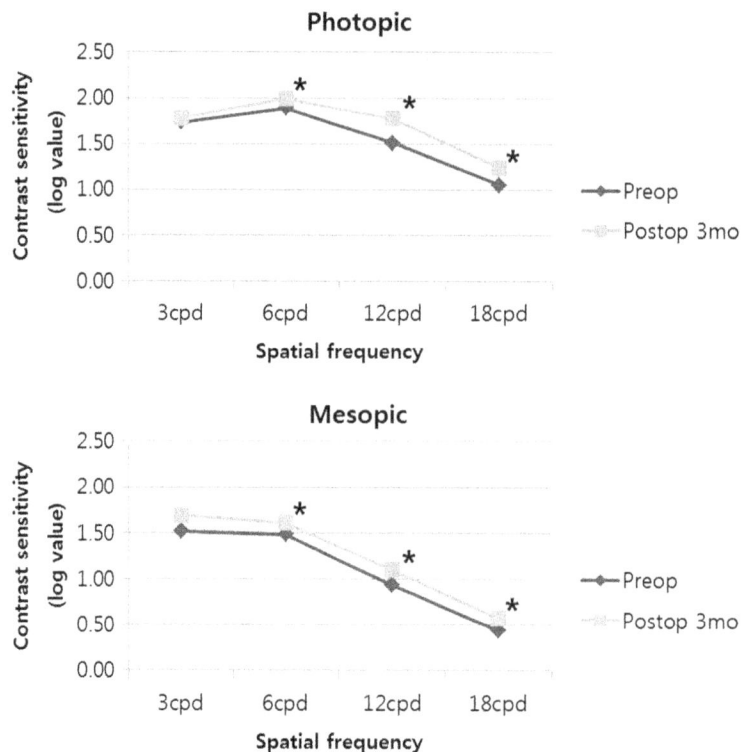

Fig. 5 Mean binocular photopic (Top) and mesopic (Bottom) contrast sensitivity in patients implanted with ZKB00 and ZLB00 multifocal intraocular lens

Table 3 Overall satisfaction, visual artifact questionnaire response and spectacle dependence in patients implanted with ZKB00 and ZLB00 multifocal IOLs at preoperative, 1 month and 3 months after surgery

	Preoperative	1 month	p value[a]	3 months	p value[b]
Overall satisfaction					
Far	2.68 ± 0.89	4.37 ± 0.50	< 0.001	4.42 ± 0.51	0.001
Intermediate	2.68 ± 0.89	3.95 ± 1.13	0.003	4.11 ± 0.81	0.001
Near	2.84 ± 1.01	3.84 ± 0.90	0.013	3.89 ± 0.88	0.008
Visual artifact					
Glare	0.47 ± 1.02	0.58 ± 1.07	0.777	0.21 ± 0.71	0.334
Halo	0.47 ± 1.02	1.11 ± 1.33	0.108	0.84 ± 1.12	0.164
Starburst	0.37 ± 0.96	0.32 ± 0.75	0.890	0.79 ± 1.13	0.179
Spectacle use					
Far	73.68%	0.00%	< 0.001	0.00%	< 0.001
Intermediate	78.94%	5.26%	< 0.001	5.26%	< 0.001
Near	63.16%	5.26%	< 0.001	5.26%	< 0.001

Overall satisfaction: 1 = very dissatisfied; 2 = dissatisfied; 3 = neither satisfied nor dissatisfied; 4 = satisfied; 5 = very satisfied
Visual artifacts: 0 = none; 1 = minimal; 2 = moderate; 3 = severe
Visual artifact was assessed using the Quality of Vision questionnaire
[a]Preoperative to 1 month
[b]Preoperative to 3 months

defocus curve of Mastropasqua et al., our study revealed 0.1 logMAR or better vision from 0 to − 2.5 D, whereas Mastropasqua et al. report 0.1 logMAR or better in the range from 0D and − 1.5 ∼ − 2.5D. In the range of intermediated distance from − 0.5D to − 1.5D, the results of ours study appear better than those of Mastropasqua et al. Although the add power differs slightly between studies, it seems that the IOL design is responsible for the better intermediate vision. And it may be due to differences in clinical characteristics of patients, such as axial length that can affect effective lens position.

Recently, trifocal diffractive IOLs were developed to provide better intermediate visual acuity. So far, no direct comparative study between bilateral implantation of diffractive trifocal IOLs and contralateral implantation of diffractive bifocal IOLs has been published. Ours study shows 0.1 logMAR or better visual acuity in the range from 0 to − 2.5D in the defocus curve and it was comparable to or slightly better than that reported in previous studies on trifocal diffractive IOLs [20].

Multifocal IOLs had a drawback in decreasing contrast sensitivity However, for Tecnis multifocal IOLs it was known as the prolate anterior surface could improve the mesopic contrast sensitivity [17, 21]. Gierek-Ciaciura et al. [22] reported that eyes with ZM900 Tecnis multifocal IOLs had better contrast sensitivity than eyes with other diffractive multifocal IOLs or refractive multifocal IOLs. Kim et al. [16] found that contrast sensitivity was higher in subjects with ZKB00 or ZLB00 than subjects with ZM900. This study, using ZKB00 and ZLB00, also showed improvement of contrast sensitivity compared

with preoperative contrast sensitivity, and statistically significant improvement in some spatial frequency.

Diffractive multifocal IOLs with fewer diffractive rings and lower add power could theoretically improve the quality of vision after cataract surgery. Trifocal IOLs need it split more light energy to form the third focal point compared to bifocal IOLs and more diffractive rings are used for the trifocal IOLs compared to the IOLs used in our study. This might have an effect on the quality of vision for near and distance [5–7]. Montes-Mico R et al. [5] used optical bench testing to confirm the quality of the apodized trifocal IOL (Finevision Micro F, Phys-IOL, Liege, Belgium), and report a worse quality of vision compared bifocal diffractive IOLs. Kohnen T et al. [7] reported that halo and glare appeared in 60% and 28% of patients, respectively, after the implantation of AT LISA tri839MP, another trifocal IOL (Carl Zeiss Meditec, Jena, Germany). Our study showed halo and glare in 31.5% and 5.3% of patients, respectively, less visual artifacts compared to the results of Kohnen et al. Jonker et al. [6] also reported that mesopic contrast sensitivity was slightly decreased in eyes with diffractive trifocal IOLs compared to diffractive bifocal IOLs. Future studies should compare the quality of vision between groups with bilaterally implanted with diffractive trifocal IOLs and contralaterally implanted diffractive bifocal IOLs.

Reading performance, such as reading speed, critical print size, and threshold print size, were significantly improved postoperatively compared to baseline. Alfonso et al. [14] reported critical print size and threshold size after bilateral implantation of AcrySof + 3.0 toric multifocal IOLs were

0.28 ± 0.12 logRAD and 0.08 ± 0.08 logRAD, respectively. Schmickler et al. [23] reported that critical print size was 0.27 ± 0.12 logRAD in patients after bilateral implantation of Tecnis ZMB00 + 4.0 diffractive multifocal IOLs. Our results of critical print size and threshold print size were 0.24 ± 0.13 logRAD and 0.14 ± 0.13 logRAD, respectively, and comparable to previous studies [14, 23]. In our study, postoperative reading speed was 86.83 ± 17.45 wpm. Alfonso et al. [14] reported a reading speed of 132.68 ± 23.69 wpm after the implantation of diffractive multifocal IOLs. Reading speed in our study is slightly lower compared to results from Western regions [14, 24]. One study using the same application as in our study to test reading speed in Koreans reported a reading speed of 129.7 ± 25.9 wpm for adults in their 20s and 30s [13]. Considering that the reading speed of young adults without presbyopia is faster than that of the older adults with presbyopia, it is possible that the difference in the testing method and characteristics of the languages are the reason for the variance between the results [6, 14, 24].

When the overall satisfaction was evaluated on a five-point scale, satisfaction with distance, intermediate and near vision was 4.42 ± 0.51, 4.11 ± 0.81, and 3.89 ± 0.88, respectively. The results showed that most patients were satisfied. When patients were asked if they would choose the same IOLs again and if they would recommend the IOLs to others, 68.4% of the patients (13 of 19) would choose the same IOLs and recommend it to others.

In this study, ocular dominance was tested prior to cataract surgery, and ZKB00 (add power + 2.75D) was implanted in the dominant eyes and ZLB00 (add power + 3.25D) was implanted in the non-dominant eyes. We assumed that the 'relatively far' near focus (ZKB00) in the dominant eye and 'relatively near' near focus (ZLB00) in the non-dominant eye would benefit according to the classic monovision trial. However, due to conflicting results with cross monovision results, it may be necessary to conduct additional research to compare the results with cross monovision [25]. Although both eyes of each patient were implanted with different add power, visual acuities of the dominant and non-dominant eyes at each distances were not statistically different. This may be due to the fact that difference in add power between the two IOLs was only 0.5 D. When patients were asked whether they could feel differences between eyes, 17 out of 19 patients did not perceive any difference between both eyes and they did not feel uncomfortable with it. It would be interesting to apply the mix-and-match technique using IOLs with an add power of + 2.75 D and + 4.00 D.

The strength of this prospective contralateral study is the first study applying bilateral mix-and-match implantation of Tecnis multifocal IOLs. Second strength is visual acuities were measured at 6 different distances and that an objective measure of the expected vision at different distances was performed with a defocus curve. Previous studies measured intermediate and near visual acuity only at a single distance. And we comprehensively evaluate clinical outcomes including reading performance, contrast sensitivity and questionnaire. The limitation of this study is the missing direct comparison with bilaterally implanted IOLs with the same add power. However, the results of defocus curve of this study were good and not inferior to those of previous studies.

Conclusions

In conclusion, the mix-and-match technique using Tecnis multifocal IOLs with low add power is an effective way to achieve good visual acuity over a wide range without affecting quality of vision. The mix-and-match technique is an interesting option for patients who want to be spectacle-free after cataract surgery.

Abbreviations
CDVA: Corrected distance visual acuity; IOL: Intraocular lens; logMAR: Logarithm of the minimal angle of resolution; logRAD: Logarithm of the reading acuity determination; MR: Manifest refraction; UDVA: Uncorrected distance visual acuity; UIVA: Uncorrected intermediate visual acuity; UNVA: Uncorrected near visual acuity; WPM: Words per minute

Acknowledgements
None.

Funding
This research received no specific grant from any funding agency.

Authors' contributions
Involved in conception and design (DHL, T-YC) and conduct of the study (CMY, DHL, T-YC); collection, management and interpretation of data (CMY, DHL, SH, JH); data analysis (CMY, DHL); writing the article (CMY, DHL); and preparation, review, and approval of the manuscript (CMY, DHL, T-YC). CMY and DHL contributed equally to the manuscript as the first authors. T-YC contributed to the manuscript as the corresponding authors.

Consent for publication
Not applicable.

Competing interests
No conflicts of interest and have no proprietary interest in any of the materials mentioned in this article.

Author details
[1]Department of Ophthalmology, Samsung Medical Center, Sungkyunkwan University School of Medicine, #81 Irwon-ro, Gangnam-gu, Seoul 06351, South Korea. [2]Department of Preventive Medicine, Catholic University School of Medicine, Seoul, South Korea. [3]Department of Ophthalmology, Saevit Eye Hospital, Goyang, South Korea.

References

1. Packer M, Chu YR, Waltz KL, et al. Evaluation of the aspheric tecnis multifocal intraocular lens: one-year results from the first cohort of the food and drug administration clinical trial. Am J Ophthalmol. 2010;149:577–84e1.
2. Ang R, Martinez G, Cruz E, et al. Prospective evaluation of visual outcomes with three presbyopia-correcting intraocular lenses following cataract surgery. Clin Ophthalmol. 2013;7:1811–23.
3. Maxwell WA, Cionni RJ, Lehmann RP, et al. Functional outcomes after bilateral implantation of apodized diffractive aspheric acrylic intraocular lenses with a +3.0 or +4.0 diopter addition power Randomized multicenter clinical study. J Cataract Refract Surg. 2009;35:2054–61.
4. de Vries NE, Webers CA, Montes-Mico R, et al. Visual outcomes after cataract surgery with implantation of a +3.00 D or +4.00 D aspheric diffractive multifocal intraocular lens: comparative study. J Cataract Refract Surg. 2010;36:1316–22.
5. Montes-Mico R, Madrid-Costa D, Ruiz-Alcocer J, et al. In vitro optical quality differences between multifocal apodized diffractive intraocular lenses. J Cataract Refract Surg. 2013;39:928–36.
6. Jonker SM, Bauer NJ, Makhotkina NY, et al. Comparison of a trifocal intraocular lens with a +3.0 D bifocal IOL: results of a prospective randomized clinical trial. J Cataract Refract Surg. 2015;41:1631–40.
7. Kohnen T, Titke C, Bohm M. Trifocal intraocular lens implantation to treat visual demands in various distances following lens removal. Am J Ophthalmol. 2016;161:71–7 e1.
8. Yoon SY, Song IS, Kim JY, et al. Bilateral mix-and-match versus unilateral multifocal intraocular lens implantation: long-term comparison. J Cataract Refract Surg. 2013;39:1682–90.
9. Pepose JS, Qazi MA, Davies J, et al. Visual performance of patients with bilateral vs combination Crystalens, ReZoom, and ReSTOR intraocular lens implants. Am J Ophthalmol. 2007;144:347–57.
10. Nakamura K, Bissen-Miyajima H, Yoshino M, et al. Visual performance after contralateral implantation of multifocal intraocular lenses with +3.0 and +4.0 diopter additions. Asia Pac J Ophthalmol (Phila). 2015;4:329–33.
11. Mastropasqua R, Pedrotti E, Passilongo M, et al. Long-term visual function and patient satisfaction after bilateral implantation and combination of two similar multifocal IOLs. J Refract Surg. 2015;31:308–14.
12. Schmitz S, Dick HB, Krummenauer F, et al. Contrast sensitivity and glare disability by halogen light after monofocal and multifocal lens implantation. Br J Ophthalmol. 2000;84:1109–12.
13. Song J, Kim JH, Hyung S. Validity of Korean version reading speed application and measurement of reading speed: pilot study. J Korean Ophthalmol Soc DE - 2016-04-28. 2016;57:642–9.
14. Alfonso JF, Knorz M, Fernandez-Vega L, et al. Clinical outcomes after bilateral implantation of an apodized +3.0 D toric diffractive multifocal intraocular lens. J Cataract Refract Surg. 2014;40:51–9.
15. McAlinden C, Pesudovs K, Moore JE. The development of an instrument to measure quality of vision: the quality of vision (QoV) questionnaire. Invest Ophthalmol Vis Sci. 2010;51:5537–45.
16. Kim JS, Jung JW, Lee JM, et al. Clinical outcomes following implantation of diffractive multifocal intraocular lenses with varying add powers. Am J Ophthalmol. 2015;160:702–9 e1.
17. Gil MA, Varon C, Rosello N, et al. Visual acuity, contrast sensitivity, subjective quality of vision, and quality of life with 4 different multifocal IOLs. Eur J Ophthalmol. 2012;22:175–87.
18. Kretz FT, Koss MJ, Auffarth GU. Intermediate and near visual acuity of an aspheric, bifocal, diffractive multifocal intraocular lens with +3.25 D near addition. J Refract Surg. 2015;31:295–9.
19. Kretz FT, Gerl M, Gerl R, et al. Clinical evaluation of a new pupil independent diffractive multifocal intraocular lens with a +2.75 D near addition: a European multicentre study. Br J Ophthalmol. 2015;99:1655–9.
20. Sheppard AL, Shah S, Bhatt U, et al. Visual outcomes and subjective experience after bilateral implantation of a new diffractive trifocal intraocular lens. J Cataract Refract Surg. 2013;39:343–9.
21. Cillino G, Casuccio A, Pasti M, et al. Working-age cataract patients: visual results, reading performance, and quality of life with three diffractive multifocal intraocular lenses. Ophthalmology. 2014;121:34–44.
22. Gierek-Ciaciura S, Cwalina L, Bednarski L, et al. A comparative clinical study of the visual results between three types of multifocal lenses. Graefes Arch Clin Exp Ophthalmol. 2010;248:133–40.
23. Schmickler S, Bautista CP, Goes F, et al. Clinical evaluation of a multifocal aspheric diffractive intraocular lens. Br J Ophthalmol. 2013;97:1560–4.
24. Alio JL, Plaza-Puche AB, Pinero DP, et al. Optical analysis, reading performance, and quality of life evaluation after implantation of a diffractive multifocal intraocular lens. J Cataract Refract Surg. 2011;37:27–37.
25. Jain S, Ou R, azar DT. Monovision outcomes in presbyopic individuals after refractive surgery. Ophthalmology. 2001;108:1430–3.

18

Toric IOL implantation in a patient with keratoconus and previous penetrating keratoplasty

Karin Allard[1] and Madeleine Zetterberg[1,2*]

Abstract

Background: Cataract surgery in patients with keratoconus with or without previous penetrating keratoplasty (PKP) can be demanding due to difficulties in selecting the intraocular lens (IOL) and predicting the refractive outcome. We report a case of cataract surgery in a patient with keratoconus and previous PKP in one eye.

Case presentation: A 71-year-old man with bilateral cataract and advanced bilateral keratoconus and previous PKP in the left eye. Preoperatively, best corrected visual acuity (BCVA) was 20/150, with − 5.75 sph − 9.75 cyl 72°, in the right eye and 20/40, with − 0.25 sph − 5.0 cyl 50°, in the left eye. The patient was subjected to phacoemulsification with implantation of a spherical IOL in the right eye and a toric IOL in the left eye. BCVA postoperatively was 20/80 with + 1.25 sph − 3 cyl 65° in the right eye and 20/25 with − 0.5 sph − 3.25 cyl 80° in the left eye.

Conclusions: Correction of post-PKP astigmatism and cataract with phacoemulsification and implantation of a toric IOL can be an effective and safe choice. Predicting the refractive outcome in cataract surgery is difficult in patients with advanced keratoconus even when using non-toric IOLs, and the surgeon should be aware of different sources of biometric errors and the possible consequences.

Keywords: Cataract, Keratoconus, Penetrating keratoplasty, Phacoemulsification, Toric intraocular lens

Background

Keratoconus is a common corneal ectatic disorder characterized by corneal thinning and protrusion of the cornea, resulting in irregular astigmatism and decreased vision [1]. The disease usually begins at puberty, progresses and stabilizes in the late 30's [1]. Treatment is aimed at visual improvement and to prevent progress of the disease [1]. In the early stages of the disease the patients are treated with glasses or rigid contact lenses. Cross-linking with ultraviolet A (UVA) and riboflavin has emerged as an effective means of stabilizing the cornea and preventing progress of the disease. In more advanced stages, penetrating keratoplasty (PKP) may be needed [2, 3]. After PKP, corneal astigmatism

- both regular and irregular - frequently occurs [4]. Despite a clear graft the post-operative astigmatism may limit the visual function. Full correction with glasses is not always possible because of high astigmatism and anisometropia. Contact lenses may be an option but can be difficult to fit because of irregularities of the cornea. Several surgical approaches have been tried to manage postoperative astigmatism but it still remains a challenge [5–7]. Cataract surgery in patients with keratoconus with or without previous PKP can be demanding due to difficulties in selecting the intraocular lens (IOL) and predicting the refractive outcome. When the patient has both post-PKP astigmatism and cataract, a few small studies have reported phacoemulsification with implantation of a toric IOL as a feasible treatment alternative [8–10]. With a single procedure both defects are corrected simultaneously. In this report, management of a patient with keratoconus and previous PKP in one eye and bilateral cataract is described. A toric IOL was implanted in

---

* Correspondence: madeleine.zetterberg@gu.se
[1]Department of Ophthalmology, Sahlgrenska University Hospital, Mölndal, Sweden
[2]Department of Clinical Neuroscience/Ophthalmology, Institute of Neuroscience and Physiology, The Sahlgrenska Academy at University of Gothenburg, SE-431 80 Gothenburg, Sweden

the eye with post-PKP astigmatism and a spherical IOL was chosen in the other eye with advanced keratoconus. This report also provides a review of the current literature regarding implantation of a toric IOL after PKP.

Case presentation

A 71-year-old man with previously known keratoconus presented with bilateral cataract (Fig. 1). In the left eye, PKP had been performed when the patient was 25 years old because of keratoconus (Fig. 2). No surgery had been done in the right eye. Because of discomfort with contact lenses, the patient wore glasses both for near and far distance. The patient had a medical history of a transient ischemic attack and medicated with acetylsalicylic acid. The right eye presented with advanced keratoconus including Vogt striae (Fig. 3) in the cornea and moderate senile nuclear cataract but no other pathology. The left eye presented with a clear corneal graft and moderate senile nuclear cataract but no other pathology. First surgery was only planned in the left eye. After more than 1.5 years surgery was also performed

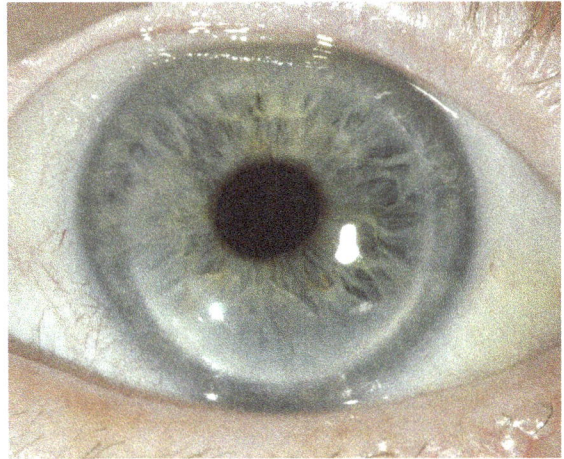

Fig. 2 In the left eye PKP was performed when the patient was 25 years old

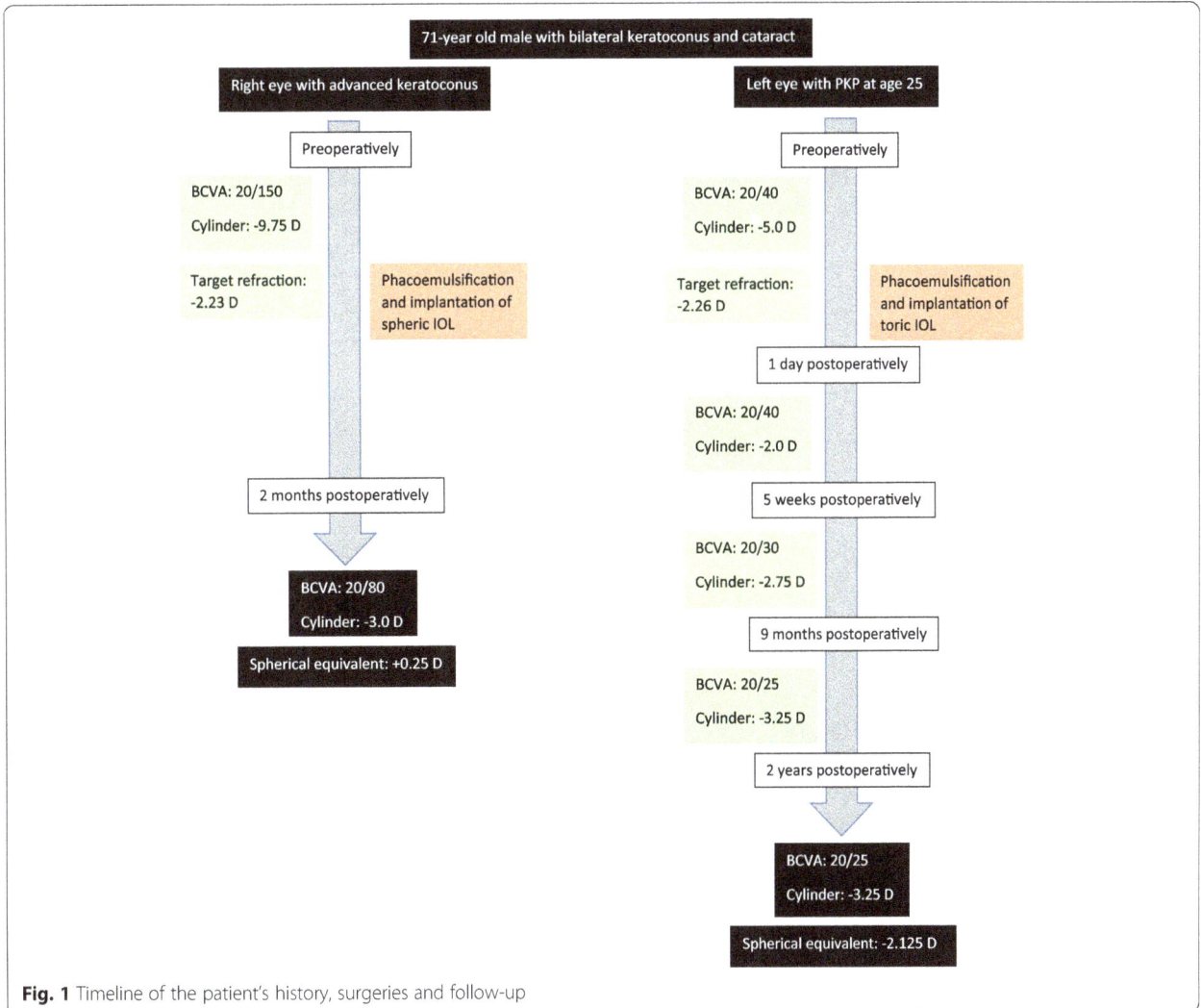

Fig. 1 Timeline of the patient's history, surgeries and follow-up

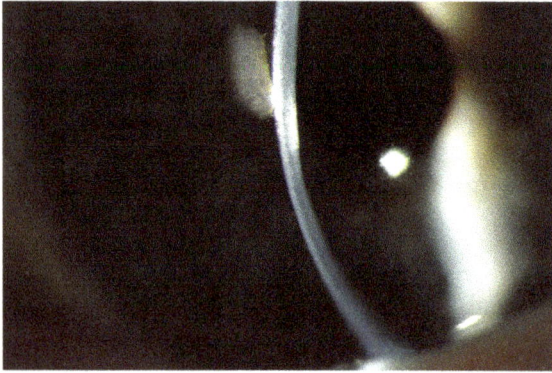

Fig. 3 Vogt striae in the right eye with advanced keratoconus

in the right eye. Written informed consent was acquired from the patient.

Left eye with previous PKP

Preoperatively, best corrected visual acuity (BCVA) was 20/40, with – 0.25 sph – 5.0 cyl 50°. The cornea exhibited regular astigmatism (K1 44.5 D, K2 48.5 D, astigmatism 3.9 D) (Fig. 4) based on corneal tomography performed with Scheimpflug imaging (Pentacam, Oculus, Germany). The toric IOL AcrySof IQ Toric SN6AT8 (Alcon, USA), 22 D was implanted with target refraction – 2.26 D. The target refraction was chosen to match the more myopic right eye. Biometry was performed with the IOLMaster (Carl Zeiss Meditec, Germany) and Haigis formula was used. Preoperative marking of the toric IOL axis was performed with the

patient in upright position to avoid misalignment due to cyclotorsion, using the RoboMarker (Surgilum, USA). Phacoemulsification and lens implantation were performed through a 2.2 mm limbal incision. One day postoperatively, BCVA was 20/40 with – 2.0 cyl 90°. Five weeks postoperatively BCVA was 20/30 with + 0.5 sph – 2.75 cyl 71°. Nine months postoperatively BCVA had improved to 20/25 with – 3.25 cyl 90° and the astigmatism was still regular (Fig. 5) based on corneal tomography performed with Scheimpflug imaging. Two years postoperatively BCVA was still 20/25 with – 0.5 sph – 3.25 cyl 80°. The spherical equivalent 2 years postoperatively only differed – 0.135 D from the intended target refraction. During all postoperatively controls the toric IOL only misaligned 1° (from 139° to 140°) from the implanted axis and the corneal graft remained clear. The patient was very satisfied with the visual result from day one postoperatively.

Right eye with advanced keratoconus

Preoperatively, BCVA was 20/150, with – 5.75 sph – 9.75 cyl 72° and the cornea had irregular astigmatism (K1 53 D, K2 57.7 D, astigmatism 4.7 D) (Fig. 6) based on corneal tomography performed with Scheimpflug imaging. In the right eye, the astigmatism was judged as being too irregular for toric IOL implantation and cataract surgery was performed with the spherical IOL Acrysof Multipiece MN60MA (Alcon, USA), 5 D. Conventional biometry (IOLMaster) and Haigis formula was used to calculate the power of the spherical IOL. Two months postoperatively, BCVA was 20/80 with + 1.25 sph – 3 cyl

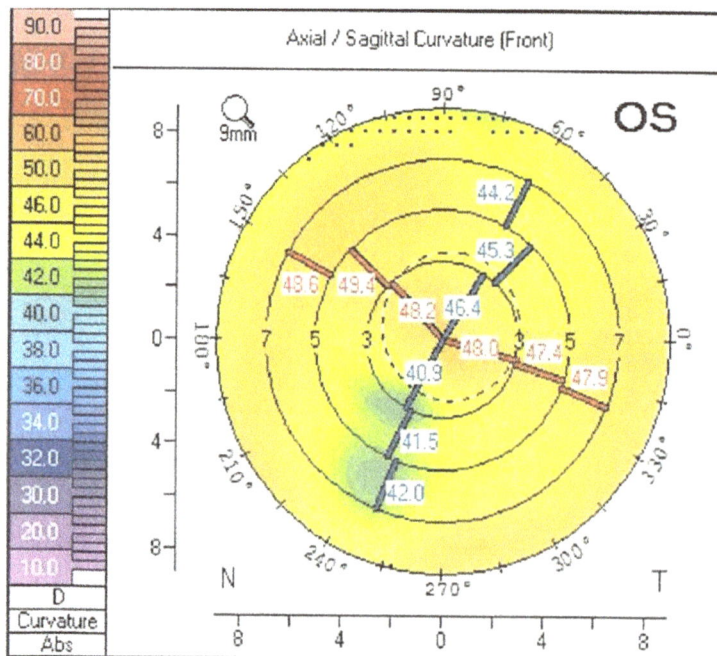

Fig. 4 Scheimpflug imaging (Pentacam, Oculus, Germany) of the corneal front surface of the left eye with previous penetrating keratoplasty

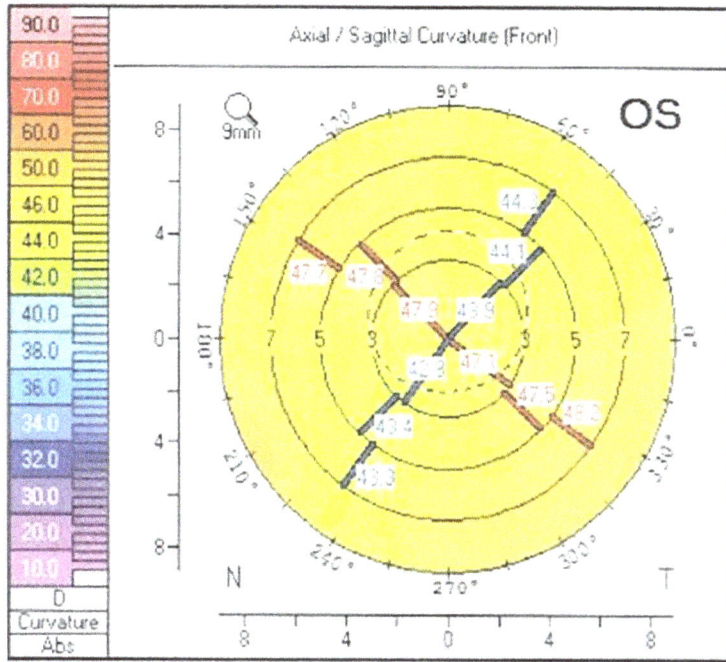

Fig. 5 Scheimpflug imaging (Pentacam, Oculus, Germany) postoperatively of the corneal front surface of the left eye with previous penetrating keratoplasty

65°, spherical equivalent – 0.25. Target refraction prior to surgery was – 2.33 D, however the patient was pleased with the obtained result. He continues to wear glasses for far distance but does not require glasses for near distance.

Discussion and conclusions

Our patient exhibited a decrease in astigmatism and increased BCVA after cataract extraction and implantation of a toric IOL in the left eye which had post-PKP astigmatism, with rotational stability of the IOL. The results remained stable during the follow-up time of 2 years. The patient was very pleased with the visual result even though we were not able to completely eliminate the corneal astigmatism (residual astigmatism of – 3.25 D). The residual astigmatism is somewhat surprising since preoperative Scheimpflug imaging showed regular astigmatism. However, it should be remembered that this eye

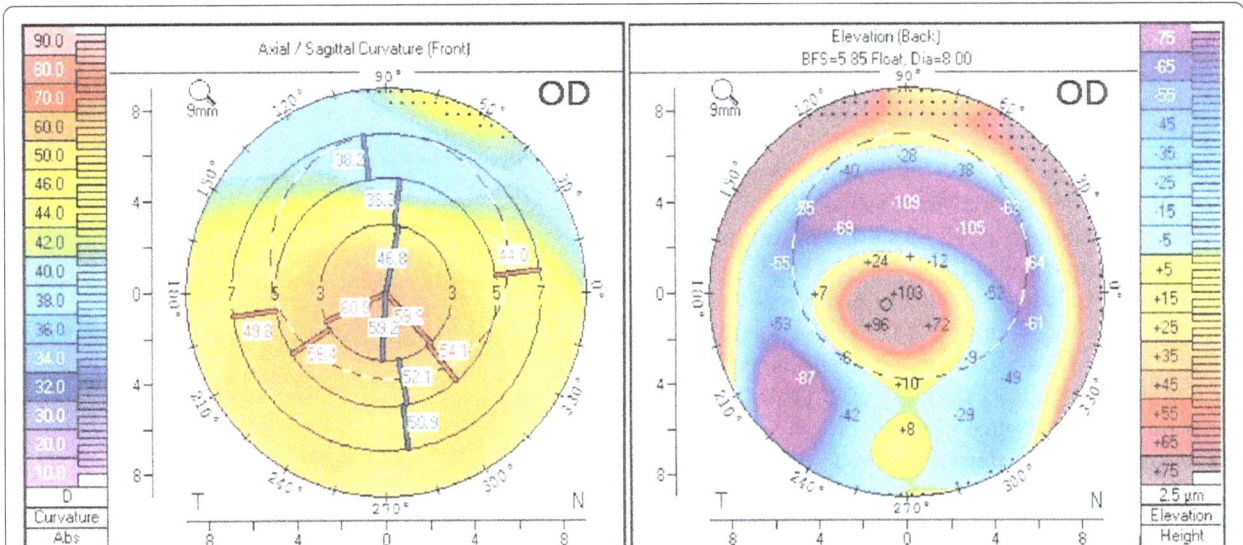

Fig. 6 Scheimpflug imaging (Pentacam, Oculus, Germany) of the corneal front and back surface of the right eye with advanced keratoconus

had been subjected to PKP, which may make the outcome more difficult to predict.

The good results in our case is in agreement with previously reported results [8–10]. Only small case-reports and case-series have been performed so far, the largest with 22 eyes is a retrospective case-series [8]. A concern with toric IOLs is rotational stability. Postoperative rotation of 10° reduces astigmatic correction by 30% and a rotation of 20° reduces astigmatic correction by 60% [11]. Our case and other studies [8–10] show stability of the toric IOL after implantation in a post-PKP eye. Another concern in cataract surgery is endothelial cell loss. In eyes with previous PKP the loss of endothelial cells during cataract surgery is even more pronounced [12]. For the present case we did not count endothelial cells preoperatively nor postoperatively since this is not standard procedure in our clinic but the patient's corneal graft showed no signs of decompensation even after 2 years follow-up. In our patient, post-PKP astigmatism was regular, but this is often not the case. One study found that 72% of patients had irregular astigmatism 12 months after PKP [13]. Irregular astigmatism is not suitable for correction with toric IOLs [10]. Therefore, toric IOLs should be reserved for those PKP-patients who have predominantly regular astigmatism.

In the present case, the second eye - which had advanced keratoconus but no previous PKP - astigmatism decreased and BCVA increased after cataract extraction and implantation of a spherical IOL. We believe that this was due to the surgical incisions. The follow-up time of this eye was only 2 months however. The spherical equivalent at follow-up differed – 2.08 D from the intended target refraction but the patient was very pleased with the outcome. Performing cataract surgery in patients with keratoconus needs planning and careful considerations. Accurate keratometry measurements are difficult which results in inaccurate corneal power estimates and difficulties in selecting the power of the IOL [14–16]. In eyes with keratoconus it cannot be assumed that the measured K-value is equal to the K-value at the visual axis nor that the effect of the measurement error is uniform for all keratometric values [16]. Typically, conventional biometry (IOLMaster) will overestimate the corneal power and underestimate the IOL power in eyes with keratoconus, resulting in postoperative hyperopia [16]. In eyes with mild (Kmax< 48 D) and moderate (Kmax = 48–55 D) keratoconus these effects are usually small and using K-values from the IOLMaster results in acceptable refractive outcomes [16].

In conclusion, correction of post-PKP astigmatism and cataract with phacoemulsification and implantation of a toric IOL can be an effective and safe choice. Prospective studies with larger cohorts are required to further investigate which patients may benefit from treatment with toric IOLs and to conclude on the efficacy. Predicting the refractive outcome in cataract surgery is difficult in patients with keratoconus even when using non-toric IOLs, and the surgeon should be aware of different sources of biometric errors and the possible consequences.

Abbreviations

BCVA: Best corrected visual acuity; IOL: Intraocular lens; PKP: Penetrating keratoplasty

Funding

The research was funded by the Swedish government ("Agreement concerning research and education of doctors"; ALF-GBG-145921) and Göteborg Medical Society.

Authors' contributions

MZ performed the cataract surgeries. KA was a major contributor in the pre- and postoperative examinations. Both authors contributed in writing the manuscript. Both authors read and approved the final manuscrip.

Consent for publication

Written consent for publication was obtained from the patient.

Competing interests

MZ is a member of the editorial board but did not participate in the handling of this manuscript. KA declares no competing interests.

References

1. Rabinowitz YS. Keratoconus. Surv Ophtalmol. 1998;42(4):297–319.
2. Tuft SJ, Moodaley LC, Gregory WM, Davison CR, Buckley RJ. Prognostic factors for the progression of keratoconus. Ophthalmology. 1994;101(3):439–47.
3. Fung SS, Aiello F, Maurino V. Outcomes of femtosecond laser-assisted mushroom-configuration keratoplasty in advanced keratoconus. Eye (Lond). 2016;30(4):553–61.
4. Fares U, Sarhan AR, Dua HS. Management of post-keratoplasty astigmatism. J Cataract Refract Surg. 2012;38(11):2029–39.
5. Bilgihan K, Özdek SC, Akata F, Hasanreisoglu B. Photorefractive keratectomy for post-penetrating keratoplasty myopia and astigmatism. J Cataract Refract Surg. 2000;26(11):1590–5.
6. Lindstrom RL. Surgical correction of postoperative astigmatism. Indian J Ophtalmol. 1990;38(3):114–23.
7. Kovoor TA, Mohamed E, Cavanagh HD, Bowman RW. Outcomes of LASIK and PRK in previous penetrating corneal transplant recipients. Eye Contact Lens. 2009;35(5):242–5.
8. Lockington D, Wang EF, Patel DV, Moore SP, McGhee CNJ. Effectiveness of cataract phacoemulsification with toric intraocular lenses in addressing astigmatism after keratoplasty. J Cataract Refract Surg. 2014;40(12):2044–9.
9. Wade M, Steinert RF, Garg S, Farid M, Gaster R. Results of toric intraocular lenses for post-penetrating keratoplasty astigmatism. Ophthalmology. 2014;121(3):771–7.
10. Kersey JP, O'Donnell A, Illingworth CD. Cataract surgery with toric intraocular lenses can optimize uncorrected postoperative visual acuity in patients with marked corneal astigmatism. Cornea. 2007;26(2):133–5.
11. Horn JD. Status of toric intraocular lenses. Curr Opin Ophtalmol. 2007;18(1):58–61.
12. Bourne WM, Hogde DO, Nelson LR. Corneal endothelium five years after transplantation. Am J Ophtalmol. 1994;118(2):185–96.

13. Karabatsas CH, COOK SD, Sparrow JM. Proposed classification for topographic patterns seen after penetrating keratoplasty. Br J Ophtalmol. 1999;83(4):403–9.
14. Thebpatiphat N, Hammersmith KM, Rapuano CJ, Ayres BD, Cohen EJ. Cataract surgery in keratoconus. Eye Contact Lens. 2007;33(5):244–6.
15. Leccisottie A. Refractive lens exchange in keratoconus. J Cataract Refract Surg. 2006;32(5):742–6.
16. Watson MP, Anand S, Bhogal M, Gore D, Moriyama A, Pullum K, et al. Cataract surgery outcome in eyes with keratoconus. Br J Ophtalmol. 2014;98(3):361–4.

19

Cataract surgery in patients with corneal opacities

Yi-Ju Ho[1]*, Chi-Chin Sun[2,3]* and Hung-Chi Chen[1]

Abstract

Background: Investigating the efficacy and safety of phacoemulsification with intraocular lens (IOL) implantation in corneal opacities.

Methods: This retrospective study was conducted in a tertiary medical center. Twenty-three eyes of 19 patients with cataracts and corneal opacities obscuring the pupillary center having received phacoemulsification with IOL insertion without any ancillary techniques were enrolled. The primary study outcome measures were uncorrected and best corrected visual acuity (BCVA), and complications. Backscatters of corneal scar lesions were evaluated by slit lamp-based haze grading, Scheimpflug Pentacam and anterior segment optical coherence tomography (ASOCT). Visual outcomes after cataract surgeries and improvement range were used to determine the safety and efficacy of cataract surgery for our patients.

Results: All patients underwent uneventful capsulorhexis and phacoemulsification. The mean age was 72.22 ± 10.1 years, and the mean follow-up period was 18.57 ± 15.42 months. The mean BCVA significantly improved from 1.45 ± 0.65 preoperatively to 0.94 ± 0.55 logMAR postoperatively ($p < 0.001$), and the number of eyes with a BCVA of 20/100 or better increased from 4 to 14. Complications included corneal edema in two eyes and reactivation of the previous corneal pathology in five eyes. Four eyes did not achieve an improvement in visual acuity after surgery, which may have been due to co-existing ocular co-morbidities. Both Pentacam corneal densitometry and ASOCT demonstrated no significant correlations with final visual outcome. However, a statistically significant relationship between the severity of corneal opacity and improvement range in BCVA ($r = -0.782$, $P = 0.001$) was found by our OCT grading method.

Conclusions: Phacoemulsification and IOL implantation in selected cases of coexisting cataracts and corneal opacities is safe that can provide suboptimal but long-term vision when penetrating keratoplasty is not possible or at high-risk of graft failure. ASOCT is a simple tool to predict visual outcomes after cataract surgery in opacified corneas.

Keywords: Corneal opacities, Cataract, Phacoemulsification, Anterior segment optical coherence tomography, Corneal densitometry

Background

Phacoemulsification is a standard cataract surgery with excellent outcomes. However, it is not unusual to encounter patients with coexisting corneal opacification and visually debilitating cataracts [1]. Corneal opacity can impede visualization during cataract surgery. There are two surgical options under such circumstances. The first is to perform simultaneous penetrating keratoplasty (PKP), cataract extraction and intraocular lens (IOL) implantation, which provides a shorter visual rehabilitation period [2]. However, the disadvantages include risk of expulsive hemorrhage, inadequate cortical cleaning and inaccuracy in IOL power calculation [3, 4]. The second option is to postpone cataract surgery after PKP to achieve refractive accuracy [5]. The drawbacks include a delay in visual rehabilitation and the risk of endothelial loss [4, 6]. In addition, factors such as graft rejection in high-risk recipients, poor patient compliance, meticulous follow-up and a paucity of good-quality

* Correspondence: arvin.sun@msa.hinet.net
[1]Department of Ophthalmology, Chang Gung Memorial Hospital, Linkou, Taiwan
[2]Department of Ophthalmology, Chang Gung Memorial Hospital, 6F, Mai-Jing Road, An-Leh District, Keelung, Taiwan, Republic of China
Full list of author information is available at the end of the article

donor corneas mean that immediate keratoplasty is often not possible. Therefore, cataract surgery alone can provide timely visual rehabilitation.

To enhance visibility during cataract surgery in opacified corneas, techniques such as capsule staining or alternative methods have been applied [7, 8]. However, toxicity of the staining dye should be taken into consideration, especially in a currently compromised cornea. Furthermore, uncontrolled dye dispersion through zonules can obscure the capsular anatomy [9]. With regards to modified illumination methods, transcorneal oblique illumination and endoscope-assisted phacoemulsification have been utilized, however, they are time consuming and require skilled clinicians [5, 10].

Variable outcomes have been reported after cataract surgery in eyes with corneal opacities [11, 12], and corneal opacity severity has been one of the major prognostic factors. Optical coherence tomography (OCT) has been used to investigate the histopathology of corneal opacities [13], and the degree of opacity has been reported a useful parameter in preoperative planning [14]. Corneal haze could hinder the light transmission resulting backward and forward scattering. Light-backscattering analysis with OCT seems to be a reliable method of detecting backscatter [15].

However, routine analysis has not been applied to evaluate the efficacy of cataract surgery in opacified corneas [16].

Recently, studies assessing the corneal pathology has included double-pass instrument for intraocular forward scattering [17], Scheimpflug rotating camera for backward scattering and corneal higher-order aberrations. Kamiya et al. suggested no significant correlations between visual performance and backward scattering in band keratopathy, while intraocular forward scattering maybe the only effective objective assessment for corneal pathology regarding visual acuity [18]. Although the correlation between reduced visual acuity and Scheimpflug corneal densitometry is not significant but still provide a quantitative value for backscatter in previous normative cohort study [19]; but in another study, significant level of correlations between visual performance was found in assessing granular corneal dystrophy [17]. Regarding backward scatter, previous study had demonstrated optical coherence tomography can precisely detect depth and visualize different corneal dystrophy in augment of treatment planning [20, 21]. But no quantitative analysis of the corneal opacities with visual performance was performed yet.

Therefore, the primary goal of this study was to report the visual outcomes and complications in patients undergoing cataract surgery in eyes with coexisting corneal opacities. The second aim was to evaluate whether anterior segment OCT can be used as an alternative objective modality to predict visual prognosis. To our knowledge, this is the first report to evaluate and compare non-transparent cornea with densitometry and new OCT grading methods.

Methods

Medical records of patients with cataracts and corneal opacities who underwent phacoemulsification and IOL implantation were reviewed. Inclusion criteria were a best-corrected visual acuity (BCVA) less than 20/40 and corneal opacification involving the visual axis and advanced cataracts. Only eyes with partially visible anterior capsules and pupillary margins were enrolled. The exclusion criteria were use of ancillary techniques or those who received simultaneous keratoplasty. No patients had previously ocular surgeries except for one who had PKP before cataract surgery.

Preoperative evaluation

The demographic and perioperative data were recorded. Visual acuity was expressed as logMAR. The severity of cataracts was categorized based on the Lens Opacity Classification System III [6]. Fundus examinations and B-scan ultrasonography were performed. Specular microscopy and anterior segment OCT were used to analyze the function and structure of the corneas.

Slit lamp-based haze grading

We scored corneal haze in accordance with modified VISX protocol as follow: 0 indicates clear cornea and no haze; 0.5 is barely detectable haze; 1 is mildly affecting visual performance; 2 is moderated haze; 3 is opaque area prevent refraction, anterior chamber visible; 4 indicates opacity hinder view of anterior chamber. The cornea haze was scored by two observers (YJH and CCS).

Corneal opacification grading

The boundary of corneal opacification was demarcated manually (Fig. 1a), and its size was measured using Image J software (National Institutes of Health, Maryland). The percentage of opacity occupying central corneal region was calculated. The central cornea was defined as a central ellipse with 50% corneal horizontal diameter as major axis and 50% vertical diameter as minor axis (Fig. 1a). To quantify the density of the opaque area, vertical and horizontal midline cross-sections were measured by anterior segment OCT (RT-100, Optovue, CA) and analyzed by Image J software (Fig. 1b). Detected signals were given a value ranging from 0 (plain black) to 255 (plain white) according to their reflectivity (Fig. 1b). The above value represented mean gray value of OCT (shown in below formula). Assumption was made that opacity density can be represented by average of mean gray value of vertical and horizontal cross sections. The objective severity of

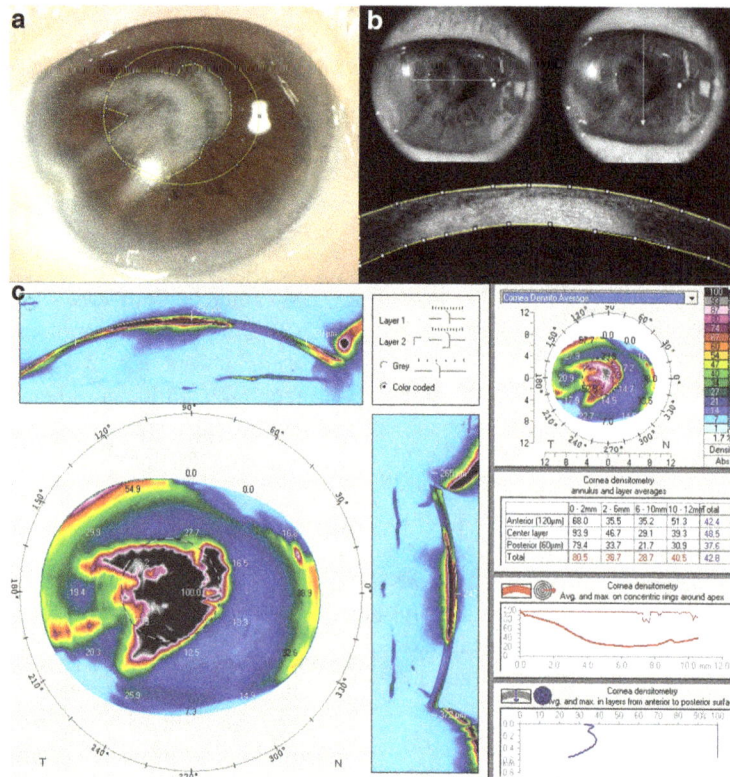

Fig. 1 Determination of the severity of corneal opacity by anterior segment OCT. **a** A pupillary-centered ellipse (50% corneal horizontal diameter as the major axis and 50% vertical diameter as the minor axis) was drawn, and the percentage of opacity occupying the central cornea was calculated. **b** To estimate the density of opacity involving the central cornea, OCT images with respect to central horizontal and vertical meridians (arrows in the upper figure) were taken to calculate the reflective signals of the cross-sectional images (lower figure). Corneal opacity density was defined as the mean value of the vertical and horizontal cross sectional signals. Corneal opacity severity = percentage of opacity in the central ellipse cornea x the density of opacity. **c** Standard output of Scheimpflug corneal densitometry of the same eye; the color coded topography map demonstrated the high density of opaque area, which is not irregular and non-homogenous; the right middle table provided the gray scale units including the central 2 mm and 2-6 mm annulus, which is area most relevant to visual performance

corneal opacification was calculated as the size multiplied by the density as followed:

$$\left(\frac{\text{Mean gray value of OCT vertical cross section} + \text{Mean gray value of OCT horizontal cross section}}{2} \right) = \text{Density of opacity}$$

$$\text{Corneal opacity severity} = \text{Percentage of opacity in central ellipse cornea} \times \text{Density of opacity}$$

Corneal densitometry

To measure the backscatter of the cornea, cornea densitometry was analyzed by rotating Scheimpflug camera (Pentacam AXL; Oculus, Wetzlar, Germany). This modality can demonstrate opaque area of entire cornea and express in color-scale units. And the scale is further calibrated by built-in software, which defines minimum light scatter of 0 (most transparent) and maximum light scatter of 100 (total opaque). Due to low repeatability and age-

related change effect measurement accuracy outside 6 mm-zone. We only analyzed area within 6 mm central zone diameter measured from corneal apex, and thickness of total corneal layer. Figure 1c demonstrated the result that Scheimpflug Pentacam analyzed corneal densitometry of corneal opacity shown in Fig. 1a.

Surgical technique

All surgeries were performed under topical anesthesia with same techniques. In brief, a side port was made, and a clear corneal tunnel was fashioned at the 11 o'clock. The viscoelastic device was injected into the anterior chamber, and continuous curvilinear capsulorhexis was performed without dye staining. Phacoemulsification was accomplished using a "divide and conquer" maneuver. Automated irrigation and aspiration were used to remove residual cortex. To calculate IOL power, a preoperative keratometry reading was taken in the ipsilateral eye or from the other eye. Emmetropic IOL power was calculated using the Sanders, Retzlaff and Kraff-T formula. A foldable acrylic lens was implanted. Stromal hydration was performed to seal the wounds. Topical gentamicin was applied to the ocular surface after surgery.

Postoperative follow-up

The patients were examined on postoperative days 1, 3 and 7, and then 1 month and every 3 to 4 months thereafter. During each follow-up visit, a complete ophthalmic examination including UCVA, BCVA, keratometry, tonometry, slit-lamp examination, endothelial cell density, central corneal thickness and fundus examination was performed.

Statistical analysis

All data was analyzed by commercially available SPSS statistical software (IBM Corp. Version 20.0, Armonk, NY). A P value of less than 0.05 was considered to be statistically significant.

The normality of all data samples was first checked by the Kolmogorov-Smirnov test. Because the data did not fulfill the criteria for normal distribution, the Spearman correlation coefficient was calculated to assess the relationships of clinical corneal haze score, corneal densitometry, and objective OCT corneal opacity grading with best corrected visual acuity. Linear regression was used to produce the line passing through the data.

Results

Preoperative and postoperative data

Table 1 summarizes the preoperative demographic features of the patients and characteristics of corneal pathologies. The study consisted of 23 eyes in 19 patients. The mean age at the time of surgery was 72.22 ± 10.1 years old. The most common cause of corneal opacity was infectious keratitis, followed by idiopathic keratopathy and bullous keratopathy. Among them, eleven eyes had posterior segment comorbidities. No perioperative complications were noted. Furthermore, none of the eyes shifted from phacoemulsification to extracapsular cataract extraction intraoperatively, and no intraoperative increase in the intensity of corneal haze was found.

Refractive and surgical outcomes

Table 2 summarizes the postoperative visual outcomes. The mean follow-up period was 18.57 ± 15.42 months. The preoperative mean UCVA and BCVA was 20/800 and 20/630, which significantly improved to 20/200 and 20/160, respectively ($P < 0.001$). All eyes had an improved UCVA except for three, including two with no change in UCVA and one with a decrease in UCVA from 20/285 to 20/2000. Figure 2a represent the true aim of our study, 92.3% cases achieved visual acuity were as good as or better than that preoperatively with correction. The BCVA improved for all

eyes except for four in which the BCVA was unchanged, and one, which lost BCVA postoperatively (Fig. 2b).

The causes of limited visual improvements could be either pre-existing posterior segment disorders such as macular degeneration and amblyopia, or exacerbation of OCP and reactivation of herpetic keratitis after surgery. PKP was performed 6 months after cataract surgery in 2 cases. Both corneal grafts remained clear at the last visit, with improvements in BCVA from 20/100 to 20/22 and from 20/66 to 20/22, respectively (Fig. 3).

Corneal condition after phacoemulsification

To investigate whether cataract surgery induced corneal decompensation, changes in corneal endothelial count were analyzed. The mean preoperative corneal endothelial cell density (1718.33 ± 267.19 cells/mm^2) was not significantly different from that after surgery (1434.67 ± 321.29 cells/mm^2 ($p = 0.242$) with a mean endothelial loss of 283.66 ± 681.71 cells/mm^2. The percentage of endothelial loss was 14%, which is similar to that reported (8 to 14%) after phacoemulsification in normal corneas [22, 23]. However, due to poor corneal transparency, the preoperative endothelial cell density was only accessible in seven eyes and eleven eyes postoperatively. Therefore, we used changes in corneal thickness as a surrogate for corneal endothelium dysfunction [16]. Complete corneal thickness data were obtained in nine eyes, and the mean preoperative corneal thickness was 497.56 ± 79.08 um and 509.22 ± 79.06 um postoperatively. There was no statistically significant perioperative difference ($P = 0.055$), indicating that the endothelium was not compromised after surgery.

Association of the severity of corneal opacity and surgical outcomes

Figure 4 demonstrates corneal haze grading increase with their OCT grading for opacity severity. Also, we found significant correlation of OCT grading with corneal densitometry within central 2 mm and 2 to 6 mm diameter (Spearman correlation $r = 0.794$, $P = .006$ and $r = 0.790$, $P = .007$ respectively) (Fig. 5). Regarding visual outcome, there is no significant correlation between logMAR BCVA and corneal densitometry (2 mm, $r = -0.224$, $P = .507$; 2 to 6 mm, $r = -0.309$, $P = .355$) and also OCT grading ($r = -0.223$, $P = .510$) (Fig. 6). We performed Pearson correlation analysis to investigate the association between postoperative visual outcomes improvement and the OCT grading method. Among the 14 eyes available for anterior segment OCT examinations, there was only a weak but insignificant correlation with improvements in UCVA postoperatively ($r = -0.118$, $P = 0.688$, Fig. 2c); in the other hand, the opacity grading value was negatively correlated with postoperative improvements in BCVA

Table 1 Demographics and corneal opacity severity of the patients

Case No.	Gender	Laterality	Etiology of corneal opacity	Location of corneal opacity	Percentage of opacity area involving central ellipse (%)	Average density of corneal opacity	Corneal opacity severity*	Associated ocular pathology	Cataract grading
1	F	OS	Traumatic scar	Superotemporal scar involving central cornea	NA	NA	NA		NS3+ CO2+
2	M	OD	Bullous keratopathy	Diffusive opacity sparing temporal side	68.9	70.9	4882	PPA	NS2+
	M	OS	Bullous keratopathty	Inferior focal scar involving central cornea	79.6	67.7	5389	PPA	NS2+ PSCO1+
3	M	OD	Herpetic keratitis	Central scar	41.4	87.1	3602	CR degeneration	NS3+
	M	OS	Herpetic keratitis	Paracentral scar	53.1	73.1	3877	CR degeneration	NS3+
4	M	OS	Herpetic keratitis	Central scar	62.7	101.2	6340		NS2+
5	M	OD	Herpetic keratitis	Central scar	31.1	43.9	1365		NS4+ PSCO3+
6	M	OD	OCP	Diffusive faint scar	NA	NA	NA		NS2+ CO2+ PSCO1+
	M	OS	OCP	Diffusive faint scar	NA	NA	NA		NS2+ CO2+ PSCO1+
7	M	OS	Traumatic scar	Diffusive dense scar	66.5	93.9	6246	CR degeneration	NS1+ CO1+ PSCO1+
8	F	OD	Idiopathic	Central focal scar	59.1	94.7	5592		NS2+
9	F	OS	Herpetic keratitis	Paracentral focal scar	40.0	119	4757	Macular degeneration	NS4+
10	M	OS	Traumatic scar	Central focal scar	NA	NA	NA		Traumatic cataract
11	F	OS	Idiopathic	Paracentral focal scar	NA	NA	NA		NS2+ CO2+
12	M	OS	Idiopathic	Paracentral dense scar	80	97.2	7780	Ambylopia	NS1+
13	F	OD	Herpetic keratitis	Central focal scar	93.8	89	8344		NS2+ CO1+
14	F	OD	SJS	Central scar	14.5	101.3	1470		NS4+
15	F	OS	Idiopathic	Paracentral scar	NA	NA	NA	Ambylopia	Total opacity
16	F	OD	Idiopathic	Diffusive scar	NA	NA	NA	CR degeneration	NS2+ CO2+
	F	OS	Herpetic keratitis	Diffusive scar	NA	NA	NA	CR degeneration	NS2+ CO2+
17	F	OS	Herpetic keratitis	Central scar	76.1	86	6548		NS3+ CO2+
18	F	OD	Neurotrophic keratitis	Diffusive faint scar	30.2	40	1207	Pale disc	NS4+ CO3+
19	M	OD	Fungal ulcer	Central focal scar	NA	NA	NA		NS2+ CO2+

M male, *F* female, *OD* right eye, *OS* left eye, *OCP* ocular cicatricial pemphigoid, *SJS* Stevens Johnson syndrome, *PPA* peripapillary atrophy, *CR degeneration* chorioretinal degeneration, *NS* nuclear sclerosis, *CO* cortical opacity, *PSCO* posterior subcapsular opacity, *NA* not accessible
*area percentage of central ellipse x average density

($r = -0.78$, $P < 0.05$, Fig. 2d). Our results suggest that the more severe the corneal opacity, the lesser the improvements in BCVA after cataract surgery.

Discussion

The presence of corneal opacities can be challenging for surgeons during cataract surgery and combined corneal

Table 2 Postoperative visual outcomes and complications

Case No.	Laterality	ECD (Pre- / post-op)	Corneal thickness (Pre- / post-op) (μm)	Pre-op UCVA	Post-op UCVA	Pre-op BCVA	Post-op BCVA	Early Complications (≤ 1 month)	Late Complications (> 1 month)	Secondary procedure	Follow-up period (months)
1	OS	NA/NA	484/481	20/200	20/100	20/200	20/100			PKP	24
2	OD	893/782	484/517	20/320	20/50	20/320	20/50				15
	OS	1318/1052	403/426	20/100	20/50	20/66	20/50				6
3	OD	NA/3106	NA/610	20/200	20/66	20/200	20/66				15
	OS	NA/2688	NA/555	20/2000	20/500	20/2000	20/500				14
4	OS	NA/NA	NA/601	20/1000	20/320	20/1000	20/320		Recurrent HSV keratitis		15
5	OD	NA/962	NA/569	20/2000	20/400	20/2000	20/400				19
6	OD	NA/NA	NA/NA	20/2000	20/2000	20/2000	20/2000		OCP progression		27
	OS	NA/NA	NA/NA	20/285	20/2000	20/300	20/2000		OCP progression		26
7	OS	2809/2488	596/615	20/2000	20/100	20/200	20/100				54
8	OD	NA/NA	418/406	20/500	20/50	20/100	20/50				26
9	OS	NA/NA	400/428	20/2000	20/2000	20/2000	20/2000				12
10	OS	NA/NA	NA/735	20/2000	20/100	20/2000	20/66			PKP	10
11	OS	NA/NA	NA/552	20/200	20/100	20/200	20/100				19
12	OS	1727/1664	567/581	20/100	20/66	20/66	20/66				10
13	OD	NA/2364	NA/592	20/200	20/100	20/66	20/66	MCE	Recurrent HSV keratitis		65
14	OD	NA/NA	NA/600	20/2000	20/100	20/2000	20/100	Diffusive SPK			13
15	OS	2008/495	593/622	20/20000	20/1000	20/20000	20/800				2
16	OD	NA/1969	NA/519	20/2000	20/200	20/2000	20/200				3
	OS	NA/NA	NA/412	20/1000	20/400	20/1000	20/400				2
17	OS	1555/2127	NA/471	20/2000	20/100	20/400	20/100	MCE	Recurrent HSV keratitis		12
18	OD	NA/NA	NA/453	20/2000	20/1000	20/2000	20/66				38
19	OD	1007/NA	533/529	20/500	20/100	20/200	20/66				6

OD right eye, *OS* left eye, *NA* not accessible, *ECD* corneal endothelial cell density, *OCP* ocular cicatricial pemphigoid, *SPK* superficial punctate keratitis, *HSV* herpetic simplex keratitis, *MCE* microcystic edema, *CF* counting fingers, *HM* hand motion, *UCVA* uncorrected visual acuity, *BCVA* best corrected visual acuity, *Pre-op* preoperative, *Post-op* postoperative, *PKP* penetrating keratoplasty

transplantation may be preferred. However, patients may hesitate to receive PKP for only mild-to-moderate nebulae. For one-eyed patients whose corneal opacities are accompanied by deep stromal vascularization, it may not be appropriate to perform corneal transplantation due to high-risk of graft rejection [8]. Therefore, cataract surgery may be an alternative in these patients [12].

Panda et al. reported that phacoemulsification with IOL implantation with 0.06% trypan blue improved BCVA from less than 40/200 to 20/60 [12]. A similar study reported that 64.7% of patients improved visual acuity, and that 47.1% of those with advanced cataracts achieved 20/100 or better [11]. In this study, 78% improved BCVA, with 60.8% achieving better than 20/100 postoperatively. Although final visual acuity was suboptimal, the patients had improvements of at least two lines except for one eye

with worse BCVA. Cataract surgery alone can also be an interim procedure for patients awaiting donor corneas. Two cases suffered from corneal lacerations and traumatic cataracts had improved vision after cataract surgery with a final BCVA of 20/22 after corneal transplantation (Fig. 3).

Corneal haze impedes visibility even with adequate fundus glow. Various techniques were used to improve visualization through opaque corneas during surgery [24]. To optimize visualization, attempts were made to adjust light setting and the following maneuvers resulted in high success rate. First, avoid the corneal opaque area and look for a transparent window to initiate continuous curvilinear capsulorhexis. Visualization during phacoemulsification in eyes with corneal opacity superimposed with mature cataracts can be extremely difficult and technically demanding, therefore we suggest that this procedure be

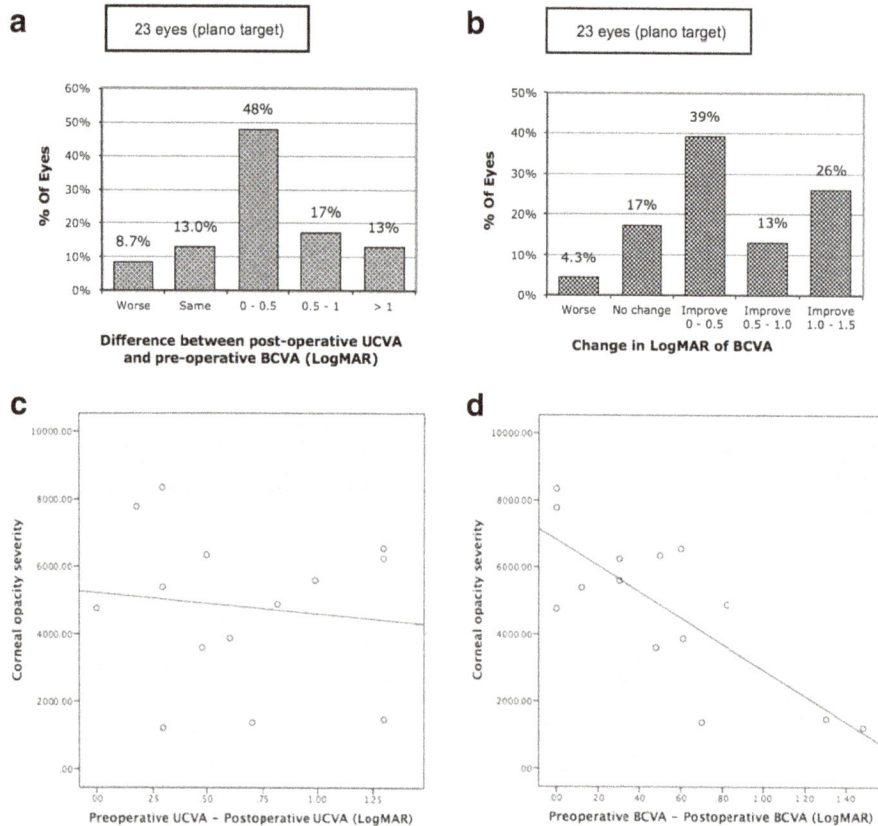

Fig. 2 Visual outcomes and the correlation with severity of corneal opacity after cataract surgery in eyes with visually debilitating cataracts and coexisting corneal opacities. **a** Comparison of pre-operative BCVA and post-operative UCVA in logMAR, histogram representing efficacy of cataract surgeries. **b** Comparison of pre-operative BCVA and post-operative BCVA in logMAR, histogram demonstrating safety of surgeries in our cases; only one case (4.3%) become worse in visual performance. **c** There was a statistically significantly negative linear relationship and strong correlation in terms of BCVA ($r = -0.782$, $P = 0.001$); **d** there was a mildly significantly negative linear relationship and weak correlation regarding UCVA ($r = -0.118$, $P = 0.688$). (BCVA = best corrected visual acuity; UCVA = uncorrected visual acuity)

reserved for experienced surgeons. Second, obtain favorable contrast in the surgical field by adjusting the illumination to low or medium intensity, as coaxial lighting of most operating microscopes may interfere with the surgical field due to backscatter and reflection of light from the cornea [25]. Finally, perform "continuous" capsulorhexis with a constant tethered force under the opaque area. Non-continuous capsulorhexis is likely to cause radial tearing and intraoperative complications are even harder to manage in eyes with poor corneal clarity. Therefore, patients must be aware of alternative surgical options and secondary surgeries during preoperative consultation.

Ocular surface diseases such as OCP and viral keratitis can be exacerbated by uneventful cataract surgery and limit surgical outcomes. Preoperative recognition and effective management can prevent devastating complications [26]. The safety and efficacy of cataract surgery has been reported in patients with OCP; however, reactivation of

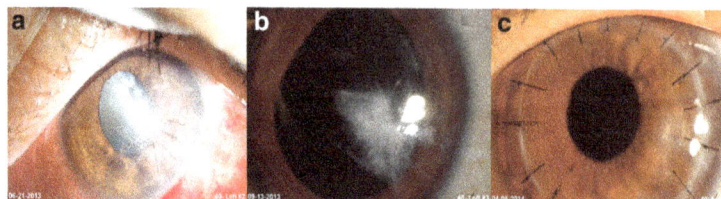

Fig. 3 Two stage surgery in case 10 suffering from traumatic corneal perforation and cataract. **a** Initial ocular penetrating trauma with coexisting traumatic cataract, BCVA was counting finger at 10 cm after primary eyeball repair. **b** BCVA achieved 20/66 after cataract surgery. **c** Penetrating keratoplasty was performed 6 months later. BCVA further improved to 20/22. (BCVA = best corrected visual acuity)

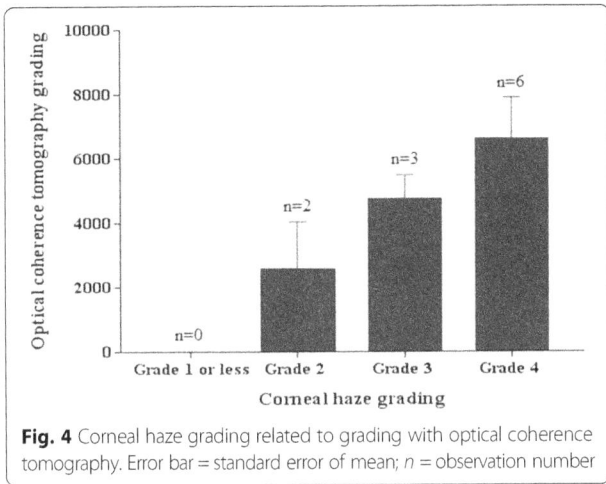

Fig. 4 Corneal haze grading related to grading with optical coherence tomography. Error bar = standard error of mean; *n* = observation number

OCP is possible and results in poor outcomes [27]. In a previous study, postoperative visual acuity was worse in eight of 15 eyes by about 2 years due to progressive cicatricial disease [28]. Similar to their findings, case 6 with OCP had a temporary visual improvement in early postoperative period, but visual acuity deteriorated 2 years later because of missed follow-up and uncontrolled disease. In contrast, Puranik et al. argued that surgeries were not associated with exacerbations of inflammation, and that stable visual outcomes could be anticipated in spite of ongoing disease [29]. However, we strongly recommend adequate preoperative immunosuppression therapy and the use of small corneal incisions in cases with OCP scheduled for cataract surgery in order to ensure better outcomes.

The onset of new and recurrent herpetic simplex virus (HSV) keratitis has been reported after uncomplicated cataract surgery [24]. Triggers for HSV keratitis such as surgical trauma and use of steroids have been proposed. Barequet et al. reported that new HSV keratitis may develop after uneventful surgery within 1–5 months

under corticosteroid treatment [30]. In this series, three eyes with preexisting herpetic keratitis had signs of reactivation with a mean inactive period of 14.8 weeks. All patients were under topical steroids for at least 4 weeks, and the mean flare-up time of HSV keratitis was 10 months. All eyes were treated with oral acyclovir or topical acyclovir ointment, and the lesions resolved over a mean period of 4 weeks. Unfortunately, two eyes developed further recurrence, and the final visual outcomes were not favorable due to exacerbation of HSV keratitis. Although herpetic eye disease study suggested that prophylactic oral antivirals for 1 year could be effective in preventing half of ocular and non-ocular cases of recurrence in patients with previous HSV keratitis (Herpetic Eye Disease Study Group 1998), no guidelines for antiviral prophylaxis currently exist for cataract surgery [26]. To prevent HSV exacerbations compromising well-tolerated cataract surgery, we suggest that oral antiviral prophylaxis in cases of suspected reactivation of HSV keratitis.

Recently, OCT has been shown a valuable tool to detect and analyze corneal opacities in different clinical situations [13, 31]. Accumulating evidence has demonstrated that cross-sectional images of the cornea in anterior segment OCT correlate well with the morphology in light microscopy [13]. Wirbelauer and Pham (2004) reported the quantitative assessment of calcified corneal lesions using anterior segment OCT. They found that reflectivity in OCT could be used to represent the severity of opacities, and concluded that OCT was helpful in quantifying the corneal opacity and in guiding the treatment plan. However, the parameters in their study included only depth of the calcified lesions and thickness of the corneas [16]. Normative corneal densitometry in healthy subjects using Oculus Pentacam system and its relation with refractive parameter were published before [32]. Effect of backscatters from corneal pathology on visual

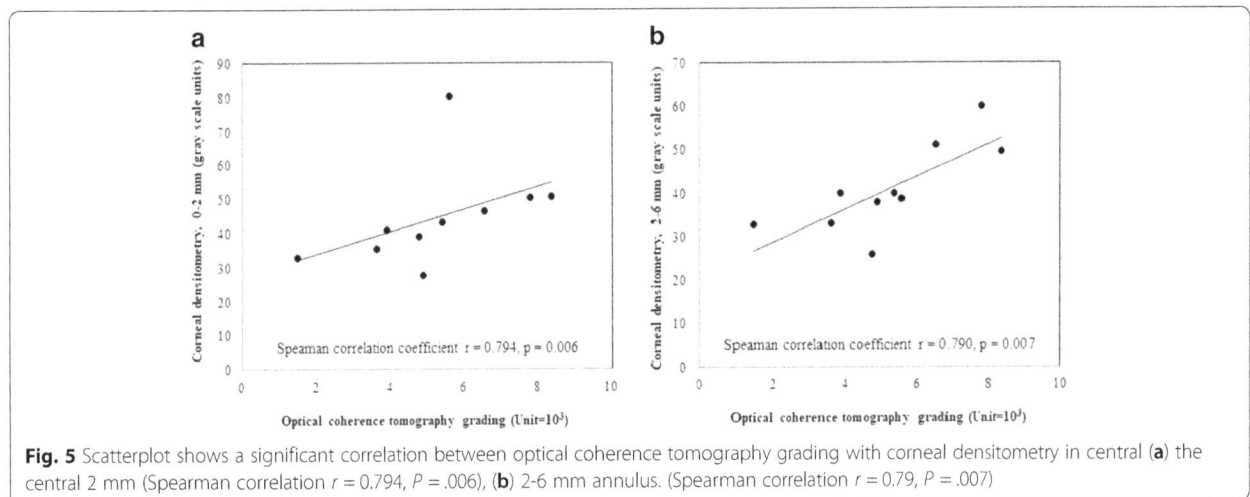

Fig. 5 Scatterplot shows a significant correlation between optical coherence tomography grading with corneal densitometry in central (**a**) the central 2 mm (Spearman correlation *r* = 0.794, *P* = .006), (**b**) 2-6 mm annulus. (Spearman correlation *r* = 0.79, *P* = .007)

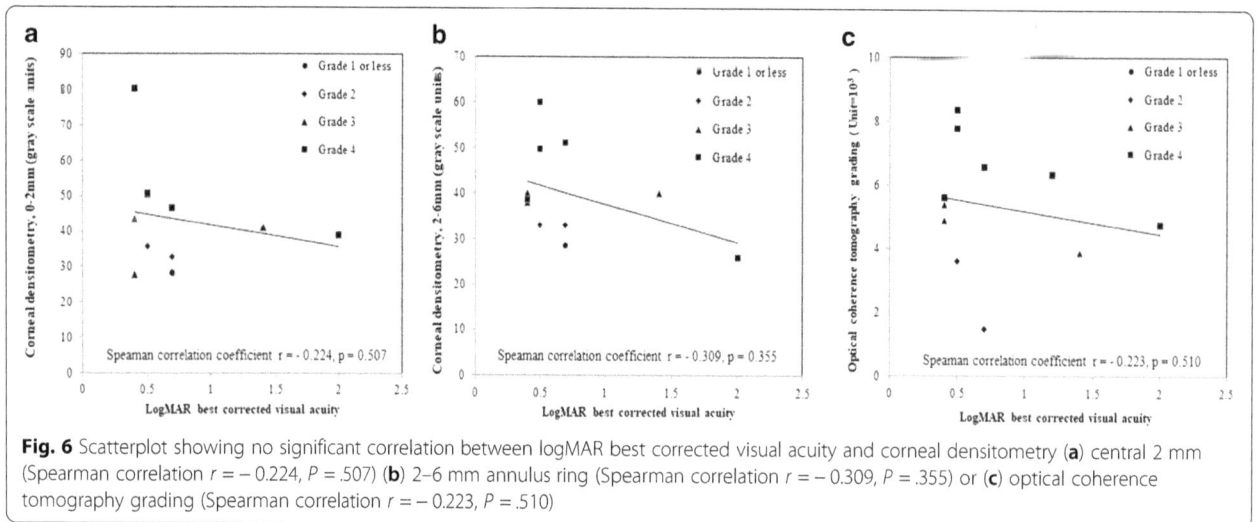

Fig. 6 Scatterplot showing no significant correlation between logMAR best corrected visual acuity and corneal densitometry (**a**) central 2 mm (Spearman correlation $r = -0.224$, $P = .507$) (**b**) 2–6 mm annulus ring (Spearman correlation $r = -0.309$, $P = .355$) or (**c**) optical coherence tomography grading (Spearman correlation $r = -0.223$, $P = .510$)

performance had also been proven by Kamiya et al. [17, 18]. However, no quantitative analysis using ASOCT and its relations with corneal densitometry and visual outcome has been so far elucidated.

Current study took into consideration the area and density of the corneal opacity involving the pupillary axis, and found that the more severe the opacity index according to the reflectivity signal, the less likely BCVA improvements would be achieved after surgery (Fig. 2d). The similar interfering effect of backward scattering has also been studied but no definite association was proved with corneal densitometry [17, 18]. This is might due to the similar conditions that we found in our study, Pentacam performed poorly to analyzed corneal opacity in moderate-to-high density, location closed to pupil center and pathology concentrated at superficial cornea. Also, the circle or annuli area Pentacam system analyzed is not useful if the opacity area is irregular in shape. In contrasts, one can delineate along contour of opacity area and quantified with the depth detected by ASOCT.

Confounding parameters such as the thickness of the cornea, irregularities of the corneal surface and refractive index in the opacified area were controlled for by comparing preoperative and postoperative visual acuity in the same individual. Because of the simplicity and reproducibility of OCT measurements, surgeons may adopt our proposed grading system as a useful guide to predict visual outcomes in patients who are not candidates or hesitate for combined PKP and cataract surgery.

Although anterior segment OCT allows for non-invasive and objective analysis of corneal structural abnormalities and has good predictability for postoperative BCVA, some limitations still exist. For example, simply averaging vertical and horizontal cross-sectional lines is inadequate to represent the size and shape of corneal opacities due to their non-homogenous properties. Severity of cataract also

contributes to the improvement of visual acuity. Above two factors may be reason why we did not find an association between corneal opacity severity and improvements in UCVA. Furthermore, corneal surface irregularities and tearing that may contribute to visual disturbance were not addressed. Finally, due to the retrospective nature, the effects of underlying posterior segment pathologies on visual outcomes were not excluded. Therefore, future prospective studies with well-designed anterior segment OCT software and strict criteria to exclude the confounding factors are warranted to investigate the effects of corneal opacity on visual outcomes after cataract surgery.

Conclusions

In conclusion, phacoemulsification is not an alternative to PKP, however it is a safe and feasible method for patients who are poor candidates for transplantation, especially for those with vision in only one eye and who are unable to comply with follow-up protocols after keratoplasty. Moreover, phacoemulsification can also serve as an interim procedure to allow patients to become ambulatory while they are waiting for PKP, especially in developing countries with a lack of good quality donor corneas.

Abbreviations
BCVA: Best corrected visual acuity; CF: Counting finger; HSV: Herpetic simplex virus; IOL: Intraocular lens; OCP: Ocular cicatricial pemphigoid; OCT: Optical coherence tomography; PKP: Penetrating keratoplasty; UCVA: Uncorrected visual acuity

Acknowledgements
There are no acknowledgements to note.

Funding
There is no financial and material support from any sponsor or funder for this study.

Authors' contributions
YJH was involved in analysis and interpretation of data and drafting the manuscript. CCS contributed to conception and design, analysis and interpretation of data, drafting and revising the manuscript. HCC made contribution to acquisition of data and drafting. All authors read and approved the final manuscript.

Competing interests
There were no financial or non-financial competing interests regarding to this study.

Author details
[1]Department of Ophthalmology, Chang Gung Memorial Hospital, Linkou, Taiwan. [2]Department of Ophthalmology, Chang Gung Memorial Hospital, 6F, Mai-Jing Road, An-Leh District, Keelung, Taiwan, Republic of China. [3]Department of Chinese Medicine, College of Medicine, Chang Gung University, Taoyuan, Taiwan.

References
1. Al Salem M, Ismail L. Factors influencing visual outcome after cataract extraction among Arabs in Kuwait. Br J Ophthalmol. 1987;71(6):458–61.
2. Javadi MA, Feizi S, Moein HR. Simultaneous penetrating keratoplasty and cataract surgery. J Ophthalmic Vis Res. 2013;8(1):39–46.
3. Davis EA, et al. Refractive and keratometric results after the triple procedure: experience with early and late suture removal. Ophthalmology. 1998;105(4):624–30.
4. Shimmura S, et al. Corneal opacity and cataract: triple procedure versus secondary approach. Cornea. 2003;22(3):234–8.
5. Moore JE, Herath GD, Sharma A. Continuous curvilinear capsulorhexis with use of an endoscope. J Cataract Refract Surg. 2004;30(5):960–3.
6. Chylack LT Jr, et al. The Lens opacities classification system III. The longitudinal study of cataract study group. Arch Ophthalmol. 1993;111(6):831–6.
7. Farjo AA, Meyer RF, Farjo QA. Phacoemulsification in eyes with corneal opacification. J Cataract Refract Surg. 2003;29(2):242–5.
8. Titiyal JS, et al. Dye-assisted small incision cataract surgery in eyes with cataract and coexisting corneal opacity. Eye (Lond). 2006;20(3):386–8.
9. Chowdhury PK, Raj SM, Vasavada AR. Inadvertent staining of the vitreous with trypan blue. J Cataract Refract Surg. 2004;30(1):274–6.
10. Al Sabti K, Raizada S, Al Abduljalil T. Cataract surgery assisted by anterior endoscopy. Br J Ophthalmol. 2009;93(4):531–4.
11. Chang YS, et al. Indocyanine green-assisted phacoemulsification in cases of complicated or simple advanced cataracts. J Formos Med Assoc. 2008;107(9):710–9.
12. Panda A, Krishna SN, Dada T. Outcome of phacoemulsification in eyes with cataract and cornea opacity partially obscuring the pupillary area. Nepal J Ophthalmol. 2012;4(2):217–23.
13. Wirbelauer C, et al. Histopathological correlation of corneal diseases with optical coherence tomography. Graefes Arch Clin Exp Ophthalmol. 2002;240(9):727–34.
14. Campos M, et al. Clinical follow-up of phototherapeutic keratectomy for treatment of corneal opacities. Am J Ophthalmol. 1993;115(4):433–40.
15. Wang J, Simpson TL, Fonn D. Objective measurements of corneal light-backscatter during corneal swelling, by optical coherence tomography. Invest Ophthalmol Vis Sci. 2004;45(10):3493–8.
16. Wirbelauer C, Pham DT. Imaging and quantification of calcified corneal lesions with optical coherence tomography. Cornea. 2004;23(5):439–42.
17. Kamiya K, et al. Effect of light scattering and higher-order aberrations on visual performance in eyes with granular corneal dystrophy. Sci Rep. 2016;6:24677.
18. Kamiya K, et al. Effect of scattering and aberrations on visual acuity for band keratopathy. Optom Vis Sci. 2017;94(11):1009–14.
19. Ni Dhubhghaill S, et al. Normative values for corneal densitometry analysis by Scheimpflug optical assessment. Invest Ophthalmol Vis Sci. 2014;55(1):162–8.
20. Kim TI, et al. Determination of treatment strategies for granular corneal dystrophy type 2 using Fourier-domain optical coherence tomography. Br J Ophthalmol. 2010;94(3):341–5.
21. Mori H, et al. Three-dimensional optical coherence tomography-guided phototherapeutic keratectomy for granular corneal dystrophy. Cornea. 2009;28(8):944–7.
22. Dick HB, et al. Long-term endothelial cell loss following phacoemulsification through a temporal clear corneal incision. J Cataract Refract Surg. 1996;22(1):63–71.
23. Kim EC, Kim MS. A comparison of endothelial cell loss after phacoemulsification in penetrating keratoplasty patients and normal patients. Cornea. 2010;29(5):510–5.
24. Muraine MC, Collet A, Brasseur G. Deep lamellar keratoplasty combined with cataract surgery. Arch Ophthalmol. 2002;120(6):812–5.
25. Srinivasan S, Kiire C, Lyall D. Chandelier anterior chamber endoillumination-assisted phacoemulsification in eyes with corneal opacities. Clin Exp Ophthalmol. 2013;41(5):515–7.
26. Greene JB, Mian SI. Cataract surgery in patients with corneal disease. Curr Opin Ophthalmol. 2013;24(1):9–14.
27. Sainz de la Maza M, Tauber J, Foster CS. Cataract surgery in ocular cicatricial pemphigoid. Ophthalmology. 1988;95(4):481–6.
28. Geerling G, Dart JK. Management and outcome of cataract surgery in ocular cicatricial pemphigoid. Graefes Arch Clin Exp Ophthalmol. 2000;238(2):112–8.
29. Puranik CJ, et al. Outcomes of cataract surgery in ocular cicatricial pemphigoid. Ocul Immunol Inflamm. 2013;21(6):449–54.
30. Barequet IS, Wasserzug Y. Herpes simplex keratitis after cataract surgery. Cornea. 2007;26(5):615–7.
31. Majander AS, et al. Anterior segment optical coherence tomography in congenital corneal opacities. Ophthalmology. 2012;119(12):2450–7.
32. Garzon N, et al. Corneal densitometry and its correlation with age, pachymetry, corneal curvature, and refraction. Int Ophthalmol. 2017;37(6):1263–8.

20

Surgical peripheral iridectomy via a clear-cornea phacoemulsification incision for pupillary block following cataract surgery in acute angle closure

Aiwu Fang, Peijuan Wang, Rui He and Jia Qu*

Abstract

Background: To describe a technique of surgical peripheral iridectomy via a clear-cornea tunnel incision to prevent or treat pupillary block following phacoemulsification.

Methods: Description of technique and retrospective description results in 20 eyes of 20 patients with acute angle closure with coexisting visually significant cataract undergoing phacoemulsification considered at risk of postoperative papillary block as well as two pseudo-phakic eyes with acute postoperative pupillary-block. Following phacoemulsification and insertion of an intraocular lens, a needle with a bent tip was inserted behind the iris through the corneal tunnel incision. A blunt iris repositor was introduced through the paracentesis and placed above the iris to exert posterior pressure and create a puncture. The size of the puncture was enlarged using scissors. For postoperative pupillary block the same technique was carried out through the existing incisions created for phacoemulsification.

Results: Peripheral iridectomy was successfully created in all 22 eyes. At a mean follow-up of 18.77 ± 9.72 months, none of the iridectomies closed or required enlargement. Two eyes had mild intraoperative bleeding and one eye a small Descemet's detachment that did not require intervention. No clinically significant complications were observed. Visual acuity and IOP improved or was maintained in all patients. The incidence of pupillary block in our hospital was 0.09% overall, 0.6% in diabetics and 3.5% in those with diabetic retinopathy.

Conclusions: This technique of peripheral iridectomy via the cornea tunnel incision can be safely used during phacoemulsification in eyes at high risk of pupillary block or in the treatment of acute postoperative pupillary-block after cataract surgery. The technique is likely to be especially useful in brown iris, or if a laser is not available.

Keywords: Surgical peripheral iridectomy, Phacoemulsification, Pupillary block, Acute angle closure

Background

Pupillary block is a rare complication in cataract surgery wit IOL in lens bag [1]. Accordingly peripheral iridectomy (PI) is not performed during routine phacoemulsification but may be indicated in special situations such as implantation of an anterior chamber (or iris-fixated) lens and perhaps in patients prone to inflammation and pupillary block [1, 2].

Phacoemulsification is increasingly being used for the primary management of acute angle closure (AAC) [1, 3–7], where, theoretically the shorter axial length and higher risk of post-operative inflammation may increase the risk of postoperative pupillary block, especially if other risk factors like diabetes are present [1, 6, 8]. An elective intra-operative iridectomy is difficult to execute through the length of the corneal tunnel incision. The alternatives are to create an additional limbal incision for this purpose, or perform a laser peripheral iridotomy (LPI) either prior to or after surgery if required. In the setting of inflammatory post-operative pupillary block, LPI is more difficult to perform and is prone to occlusion. In this situation, it is even more difficult to perform LPI on Chinese people due to the brown irises, which are thicker than blue irises. Furthermore, a Neodymium-YAG laser is not universally available,

* Correspondence: wzjiaqu@126.com
Wenzhou Medical University Eye Hospital, Wenzhou 325027, China

especially in poorly resourced countries. We describe a surgical technique and retrospectively describe the results of performing a surgical iridectomy through the cornea tunnel incision used for phacoemulsification.

Methods

This was a retrospective case series. The technique was used on a series of patients with AAC seen between September 2009 and January 2013 at the glaucoma unit of the eye hospital, Wenzhou Medical University. Patients were included if they had concomitant visually significant cataract where the surgeon considered the risk of pupillary block (AAC concomitant diabetic retinopathy, uveitis and short axial length) following phacoemulsification for AAC warranted an intra-operative iridectomy. The institutional review board approved the study and informed consent was obtained from all patients.

The inclusion criteria were: (1) AAC concomitant diabetic retinopathy, uveitis and short axial length (<22 mm); (2) visually significant cataract or pseudophakic eye following phacoemulsification recently; (3) IOP and inflammation was under control prior to surgery. Exclusion criteria were: (1) AAC was not caused by non-pupillary block glaucoma such as neovascular glaucoma, trauma; (2) corneal opacity prevent to perform a surgical iridectomy; (3) AAC with clear opening of laser peripheral iridotomy.

Surgical procedure

Surgery was performed by a single surgeon under topical or peribulbar anesthesia. A standard clear-cornea phacoemulsification was performed with implantation of a foldable post chamber intraocular lens (IOL). The position of the clear-cornea tunnel was located in the nasal superior quadrant. Following insertion of the IOL in the capsular bag, a viscoelastic agent was injected into the anterior chamber and the posterior chamber at the site of the intended surgical iridectomy. A 26G needle with its tip bent to approximately 45 degrees about 1 mm from the tip was inserted into the corneal tunnel and advanced behind the iris, anterior to capsule and IOL to the selected site. The tip was kept horizontal to avoid snagging the iris. A blunt iris repositor was introduced into the eye through the paracentesis and placed above the iris adjacent to the needle. The needle tip was then turned anteriorly towards the iris and posterior pressure exerted with the repository to create a temperal inferior puncture. The size of the puncture was enlarged using fine long bladed microsurgical scissors to excise a small piece of iris tissue and the excised iris tissue removed with microsurgery forceps. The surgical technique can also create a nasal iridectomy through a temporal corneal tunnel. In the first three cases intra-cameral Carbamylcholine Chloride (0.01%) was administered to constrict the pupil following intraocular lens implantation. The surgical steps are illustrated in Fig. 1 and a typical post-operative result is

shown in Fig. 2. Viscoelastic material was evacuated as is routine at the end of surgery.

The technique was used in twenty eyes of 20 patients with AAC and coexisting visually significant cataract considered to be at high risk of postoperative pupillary block due to the presence of factors such as poorly controlled diabetes, uveitis and short axial length. Two pseudophakic eyes that developed acute postoperative pupillary-block following phacoemusificatoin for AAC (in whom intraoperative iridectomy was not performed) also underwent this procedure.

Clinical observations

Preoperative examination included decimal visual acuity (VA), applanation tonometry, biomicroscopy, ophthalmoscopy, gonioscopy, specular microscopy, and ultrasound biomicroscopy (UBM, OTI, Inc. CA). Anterior chamber depth was measured with UBM, Keratometry, and axial length were measured with an IOL Master (Carl Zeiss Meditec, Inc. Dublin, CA).

In all patients the acute attack was controlled with medications and/or paracentesis prior to surgery. Phacoemusification was undertaken as soon as the IOP decreased and the inflammation was under control. The time to surgery was 2 to 30 days.

Postoperative care included topical steroids and antibiotics, as is routine following phacoemulsification. Systemic steroids were administered if a fibrin reaction was seen in the anterior chamber. Patients were followed up on day 1 and 2, week 1 and 2, months 1, 2, 3, 6, 9, and 12 and then every 6 months thereafter. VA, intraocular pressure (IOP), disc assessment and postoperative complications were recorded.

Statistical analysis

Statistical analysis was performed using the SPSS 20 software package (SPSS Inc., Munich, Germany). Results are reported as the mean ± standard deviation. A paired t test was used to evaluate changes in IOP and VA before and after surgery. VA was analyzed after conversion to the logarithm of the minimal angle resolution (logMAR) score. Hand-motion VA and counting fingers were assigned decimal equivalents of 0.001(+ 3.0 logMAR) and 0.01 (+ 2.0 logMAR). A p value less than 0.05 was considered statistically significant.

Results

A patent surgical peripheral iridectomy was successfully achieved in the twenty eyes that underwent phacoemulsification for AAC and the two pseudophakic eyes with pupillary block that followed phacoemulsification.

Three patients were male and 19 were females. Mean patient age was 56.86 ± 12.90 years (range: 27 to 75). The table details demographics, eye characteristics and results. There were no complications during phacoemulsification

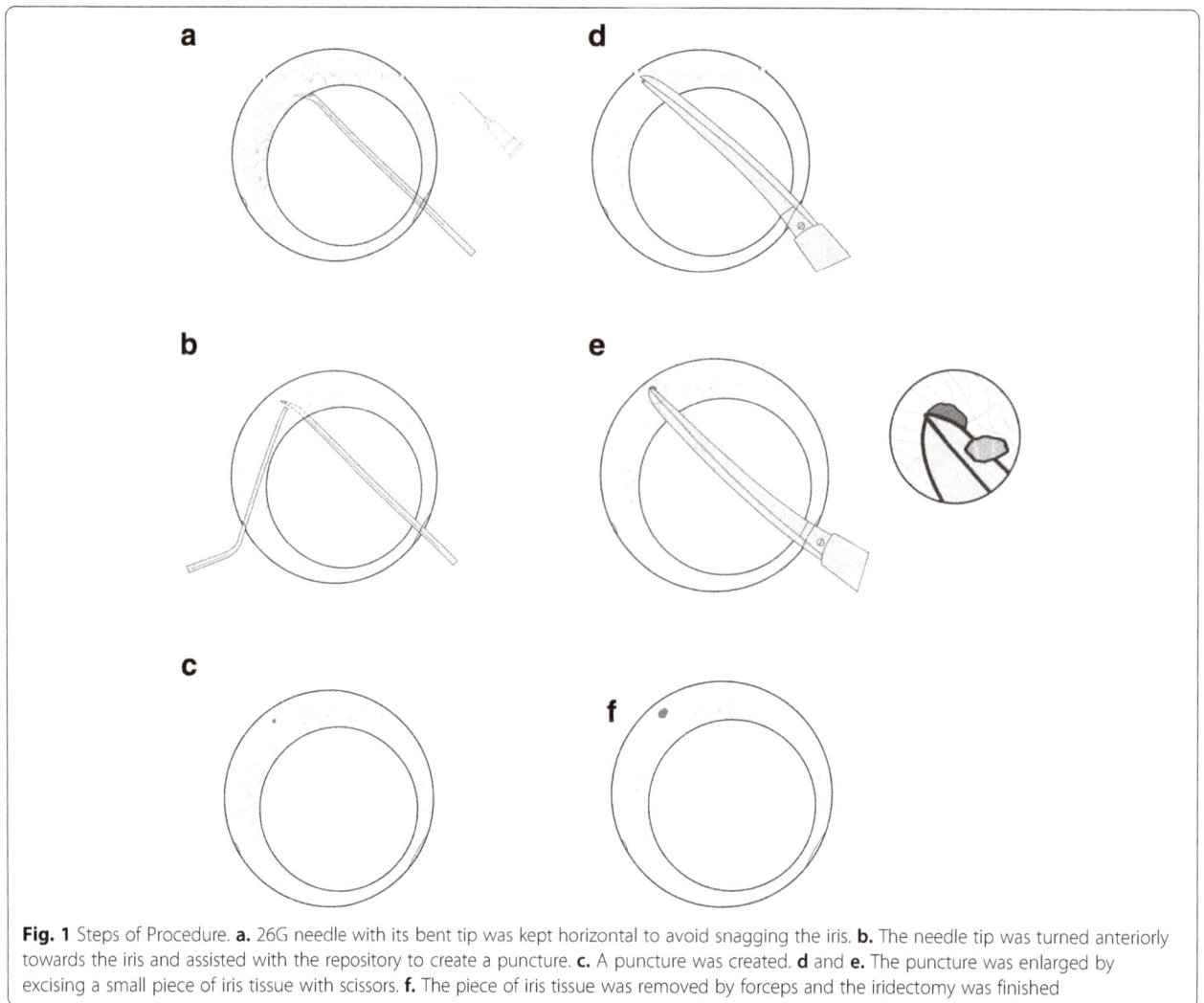

Fig. 1 Steps of Procedure. **a.** 26G needle with its bent tip was kept horizontal to avoid snagging the iris. **b.** The needle tip was turned anteriorly towards the iris and assisted with the repository to create a puncture. **c.** A puncture was created. **d** and **e.** The puncture was enlarged by excising a small piece of iris tissue with scissors. **f.** The piece of iris tissue was removed by forceps and the iridectomy was finished

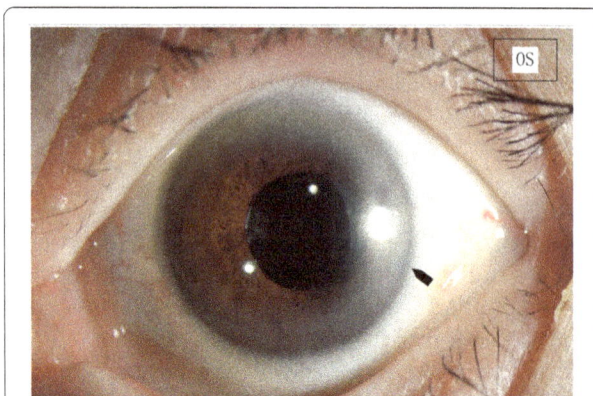

Fig. 2 Patent Surgical Iridectomy. The iridectomy remained patent over a follow up of 12 months

and the IOL was implanted in capsular bag in all 20 eyes. During surgical peripheral iridectomy, two eyes had intraoperative bleeding resulting in a 1–2 mm hypaema that resolved spontaneously within a week. One eye had a small (approximately 1 mm^2) Descemet's detachment caused by the needle tip, but did not require any intervention. Two eyes that underwent phacoemulsification within two weeks of the acute attack developed intraoperative corneal edema that did not preclude completion of iridectomy. Complications such as iridodialysis/cyclodialysis were not observed and none of the patients reported dysphotopsia. All iridectomies remained patent through the mean follow-up of 18.8 ± 9.7 months (range 12–48 months).

Two patients had an IOP elevation on the first postoperative day. The IOP was lowered by pressure on the posterior lip of the paracentesis with a 26G needle at the slit lamp to allow egress of aqueous and any residual viscoelastic. None of the patients required long term anti-glaucoma medications.

Significant postoperative inflammation and corneal edema were the most common complications. Four eyes that developed a fibrin aqueous reaction and/or corneal edema had undergone surgery within 2 weeks of the acute attack. Three of the eyes had received intracameral Carbamylcholine Chloride; two eyes developed the fibrin reaction immediately after injection of this miotic. Four eyes developed significant stromal edema of the cornea, which subsided within 4 weeks.

Postoperative visual acuities improved or remained unchanged (Table 1). Visual acuity improved from 0.96 ± 1.03logMAR preoperatively to 0.18 ± 0.21 logMAR after surgery ($p = 0.01$).

The mean preoperative IOP at presentation was 50.81 ± 6.0 mmHg (range, 41–60 mmHg) (Table 1). At the final examination for IOP was 12.95 ± 3.36 mmHg (range, 8–20 mmHg) without medication (Table 1). The difference in pre and post-operative IOP was statistically significant ($p = 0.000$).

Discussion

Postoperative pupillary block is a rare complication following phacoemulsification [1]. A surgical iridectomy may be indicated in high risk situations such as implantation of an anterior chamber (AC) or iris-fixed intraocular lens, perhaps in patients who are more prone to inflammation such as diabetics and those with current and past inflammation, especially where a YAG laser is not available [1, 2, 8]. In eyes with posterior chamber IOL, papillary block may be related to excessive postoperative inflammation, with the formation of posterior synechiae [9, 10]. This risk is higher in diabetics [1, 8], and in angle closure glaucoma [11].

Phacoemulsification is increasingly being used for the primary management of AAC [1, 3–7]. Two randomized trials have investigated phacoemulsification as a primary treatment for AAC [3, 6]. None of the patients undergoing phacoemulsification in those studies developed pupillary block; as numbers were small the upper end of the confidence interval is actually compatible with a true rate of 10–22% [3, 6].

A short axial length and higher risk of post-operative inflammation may increase the risk of pupillary block [1, 2]. Gaton's series of pupillary block following posterior IOL implantation included two patients (2/6) with known diabetic retinopathy and four (4/6) with glaucoma [1]. Diabetes was also present in 3 of 4 patients who developed acute postoperative pupillary-block following phacoemulsification [12]. Acute postoperative pupillary block occurred in 11 eyes (11 patients) of 12,016 phacoemulsifications (0.09%) performed by one unit in our hospital between 2011 and 2014 (unpublished data). 10 of the 11 patients that developed pupillary block were diabetic while one had uveitis. Pupillary block occurred in 10 of 1704 (0.6%) diabetics undergoing phacoemulsification; all had diabetic retinopathy. The incidence of pupillary block in those with diabetic retinopathy was 3.5% (10 of 290).

Table 1 The demographics, eye characteristics and results of this study

Patient characteristics	Mean ± SD (range)	
Number of patients	22	
Female/male ratio	19/3	
Age	56.86 ± 12.90 (27–75)	
Follow-up range (months)	18.9 ± 9.72 (12–48)	
Diagnosis		
a. AAC with cataract ($n = 20$)		
PAS (clock hours)	6.95 ± 3.15 (0–12)	
ACD (mm)	1.59 ± 0.20 (1.22–1.90)	
AL (mm)	21.44 ± 0.58 (19.65–21.97)	
b. Postoperative pupillary block after phacoemulsification ($n = 2$)	Case 1	Case 2
PAS (clock hours)	9	11
ACD (mm)	3.75	3.15
AL (mm)	22.86	23.26
Preoperative data		
IOP at presentation (mmHg)	50.81 ± 6.01 (41–60)	
LogMAR BCVA	0.96 ± 1.03 (0.1–3)	
Postoperative data		
IOP at last follow up (mmHg)	12.95 ± 3.36 (8–20)	
LogMAR BCVA	0.18 ± 0.21 (0–0.8)	

PAS Periphery anterior aynechia, *ACD* Anterior chamber depth, *AL* Axial lenth, *IOP* Intraocular pressure, *BCVA* Best corrected visual acuity, *SD* Standard deviation

A surgical iridectomy may be warranted in cases considered high risk for postoperative pupillary block. Performing LPI postoperatively only if papillary block occurs is certainly an option. However LPI in the situation of postoperative pupillary block, especially in the presence of inflammation that follows an acute attack is more difficult and associated with more complications [13–16]. Moreover it is also more difficult to perform LPI in brown irises in this situation, and in many locations a YAG laser may not be available. If YAG laser is not available, the described technique can also be used for the pupillary block that may follow AC or iris fixated IOL's.

Performing a surgical iridectomy through a tunnel incision can be technically challenging. An elegant technique that creates a small incision in the bed of a 4–5 mm scleral tunnel during the course of manual small incision cataract surgery has been described and can be used if a scleral tunnel is employed for phacoemulsification [17, 18]. This method can also be used with a corneal tunnel, but is easier with a longer incisional length and width. Also, an incision in the bed of a corneal tunnel has the potential to distort the wound and cause leakage; a watertight closure in this situation needs a larger tunnel length which can make phacoemulsification more difficult.

Other alternatives include an additional limbal incision for the iridectomy or the use of a vitrector. An extra limbal incision that requires a suture will be unattractive to most surgeons. We tend to avoid a vitrector primarily because it adds considerable expense to the procedure but also because it is more difficult and traumatic in a dilated pupil [19, 20].

Proper positioning of the iridectomy when performed through the tunnel is difficult in patients with the dilated pupils encountered in AAC. While miochol can be used to constrict the pupil, some pupils are unreactive, and, in our experience, inflammation in eyes that have recently suffered AAC is aggravated by Miochol [3, 6].

Potential complications of this method include complications related to introduction of a sharp needle behind the iris. While damage to the posterior capsule is conceivable, the needle is introduced under viscoelastic with the tip oriented horizontally and the maneuvers are undertaken following intraocular lens implantation. Introducing a scissor into the AC can cause damage to tissues. While an iridotomy alone might suffice, we elected to excise tissue, as the larger opening is less likely to occlude in the presence of inflammation. Bleeding from the iris and damage to Descemets membrane (as occurred in one case) and to the corneal endothelium is also possible. In order to avoid the immediate postoperative pressure spike, residual viscoelastic agent should be removed completely at the end of the surgery.

We acknowledge that an iridectomy adds an extra step to surgery and as there is potential for complications, it is only indicated in cases at higher risk of pupillary block. We also acknowledge that it is difficult to accurately predict post-operative pupillary block and that our own data suggests that some of the iridectomies were probably unnecessary. A risk of 3.5% has a number needed to treat of 29 and may help the decisions in specific situations/locations [21].

To conclude, this surgical technique for iridectomy can be safely and conveniently used for cases with or at high risk of postoperative pupillary block following cataract surgery, especially in settings where a YAG laser is not available.

Abbreviations

AAC: Acute angle closure; AC: Anterior chamber; IOL: Intraocular lens; IOP: Intraocular pressure; logMAR: Logarithm of the minimal angle resolution; LPI: Laser peripheral iridotomy; PI: Peripheral iridectomy; UBM: Ultrasound biomicroscopy; VA: Visual acuity

Acknowledgments

We appreciate the generous help and contributions made by professor Ravi Thomas to this manuscript.

Authors' contributions

AWF performed the surgery, participated in the design of the study, and drafted the manuscript; PJW analyzed the data and revised the manuscript; RH collected and analyzed the data; JQ participated in the design of the study and gave final approval of the version to be published. All authors read and approved the final manuscript.

Competing interests

The authors declare that they have no competing interests.

References

1. Gaton DD, Mimouni K, Lusky M, Ehrlich R, Weinberger D. Pupillary block following posterior chamber intraocular lens implantation in adults. Br J Ophthalmol. 2003;87(9):1109–11.
2. Stamper RL, Lieberman MF, Drake MV. Becker-Shaffer's diagnosis and therapy of the glaucomas. 7th ed. San Diego: Harcourt Publishers Limited; 2001.
3. Husain R, Gazzard G, Aung T, Chen Y, Padmanabhan V, Oen FT, Seah SK, Hoh ST. Initial management of acute primary angle closure: a randomized trial comparing phacoemulsification with laser peripheral iridotomy. Ophthalmology. 2012;119(11):2274–81.
4. Imaizumi M, Takaki Y, Yamashita H. Phacoemulsification and intraocular lens implantation for acute angle closure not treated or previously treated by laser iridotomy. J Cataract Refract Surg. 2006;32(1):85–90.
5. Hwang JU, Yoon YH, Kim DS, Kim JG. Combined phacoemulsification foldable intraocular lens implantation, and 25-gauge transconjunctival sutureless vitrectomy. J Cataract Refract Surg. 2006;32(5):727–31.
6. Lam DS, Leung DY, Tham CC, Li FC, Kwong YY, Chiu TY, Fan DS. Randomized trial of early phacoemulsification versus peripheral Iridotomy to

prevent intraocular pressure rise after acute primary angle closure. Ophthalmology. 2008;115(7):1134–40.

7.   Teekhasaenee C, Ritch R. Combined phacoemulsification and goniosynechialysis for uncontrolled chronic angle-closure glaucoma after acute angle-closure glaucoma. Ophthalmology. 1999;106(4):669–74. discussion 674-5

8.   Naveh N, Wysenbeek Y, Solomon A, Melamed S, Blumenthal M. Anterior capsule adherence to iris leading to pseudophakic pupillary block. Ophthalmic Surg. 1991;22(6):350–2.

9.   Ferris FL 3rd, Kassoff A, Bresnick GH, Bailey I. New visual acuity charts for clinical research. Am J Ophthaloml. 1982;94(1):91–6.

10.   Vajpayee RB, Angra SK, Titiyal JS, Sharma YR, Chabbra VK. Pseudophakic pupillary-block glaucoma in children. Am J Ophthalmol. 1991;111(6):715–8.

11.   Weinreb RN, Wasserstrom JP, Forman JS, Ritch R. Pseudophakic papillary block with angle-closure glaucoma in diabetic patients. Am J Ophthalmol. 1986;102(3):325–8.

12.   Khor WB, Perera S, Jap A, Ho CL, Hoh ST. Anterior segment imaging in the management of postoperative fibrin pupillary-block glaucoma. J Cataract Refract Surg. 2009;35(7):1307–12.

13.   Sihota R, Lakshmaiah NC, Walia KB, Sharma S, Pailoor J, Agarwal HC. The trabecular meshwork in acute and chronic angle closure glaucoma. Indian J Ophthalmol. 2001;49(4):255–9.

14.   Saw SM, Gazzard G, Friedman DS. Interventions for angle-closure glaucoma: an evidence-based update. Ophthalmology. 2003;110(10):1869–78.

15.   Sakai H, Ishikawa H, Shinzato M, Nakamura Y, Sakai M, Sawaguchi S. Prevalence of ciliochoroidal effusion after prophylactic laser iridotomy. Am J Ophthalmol. 2003;136(3):537–8.

16.   Athanasiadis Y, de Wit DW, Nithyanandrajah GA, Patel A, Sharma A. Neodymium: YAG laser peripheral iridotomy as a possible cause of zonular dehiscence during phacoemulsification cataract surgery. Eye (Lond). 2010; 24(8):1424–5.

17.   Blumenthal M, Kahana M. Performing peripheral Iridectomy via a scleral tunnel incision: a new technique. Ophthalmic Surg and Lasers. 1997; 28(2):162–4.

18.   Thomas R, Parikh R, Muliyil J. Comparison between phacoemulsification and the Blumenthal technique of manual small-incision cataract surgery combined with trabeculectomy. J Glaucoma. 2003;12(4):333–9.

19.   Bitrian E, Caprioli J. Pars plana anterior vitrectomy, hyaloido-zonulectomy, and iridectomy for aqueous humor misdirection. Am J Ophthalmol. 2010; 150(1):82–7.

20.   Debrouwere V, Stalmans P, Van Calster J, Spileers W, Zeyen T, Stalmans I. Outcomes of different management options for malignant glaucoma: a retrospective study. Graefes Arch Clin Exp Ophthalmol. 2012;250(1):131–41.

21.   Thomas R, Padma P, Braganza A, Muliyil J. Assessment of clinical significance: the number needed to treat. Indian J Ophthalmol. 1996; 44(2):113–5.

21

Case report of secondary pigment dispersion glaucoma, recurrent uveitis and cystoid macular oedema following inadvertent implantation of an intraocular lens into the ciliary sulcus following cataract surgery

Alastair Porteous* and Laura Crawley

Abstract

Background: This case highlights the important sequelae that can occur following the inadvertent implantation of a single-piece intraocular lens into the ciliary sulcus during cataract surgery; secondary pigment dispersion glaucoma, recurrent anterior uveitis and macular oedema.

Case presentation: A 67-year-old lady underwent routine left cataract surgery in a separate unit but subsequently attended our eye casualty with recurrent hypertensive anterior uveitis. She was found to have secondary pigment dispersion glaucoma as the intraocular lens had been inadvertently placed into the ciliary sulcus. She underwent a trabeculectomy to control the intraocular pressure and initially settled well but 12 months later developed persistent anterior segment inflammation and macular oedema. She subsequently had the intraocular lens removed and the macular oedema was treated successfully with intravitreal Bevacizumab.

Conclusions: We provide a summary of the evidence and a discussion over the management options available in managing such a difficult case.

Keywords: Glaucoma, Intraocular-lens, Sulcus, Pigment dispersion

Background

The following case of a 67-year-old lady highlights some interesting and important learning points that would be of value to both trainee and practising ophthalmologists involved in the management of post-operative cataract patients and of patients presenting to eye casualty. The case details the important sequelae that can occur following the inadvertent implantation of a single-piece intraocular lens into the ciliary sulcus during cataract surgery; secondary pigment dispersion glaucoma, recurrent anterior uveitis and macular oedema. A timeline detailing the patient's management can be seen in Fig. 1.

Implantation of a single-piece intraocular lens into the ciliary sulcus has been shown to lead to secondary pigment dispersion [1–3], and for those cases where a foldable intraocular lens has been placed in the ciliary sulcus 60% experience a chronic recurrent iridocyclitis and 60% require a further surgical procedure, either intraocular lens exchange alone or combined with trabeculectomy [4]. Cystoid macular oedema has been shown to be a sequelae of both the implantation of an intraocular lens into the ciliary sulcus [3], and of uveitis [5]. We aim to provide a summary of the evidence and a discussion over the management options available in managing such a difficult case.

* Correspondence: alastair.porteous1@nhs.net
Western Eye Hospital, London, UK

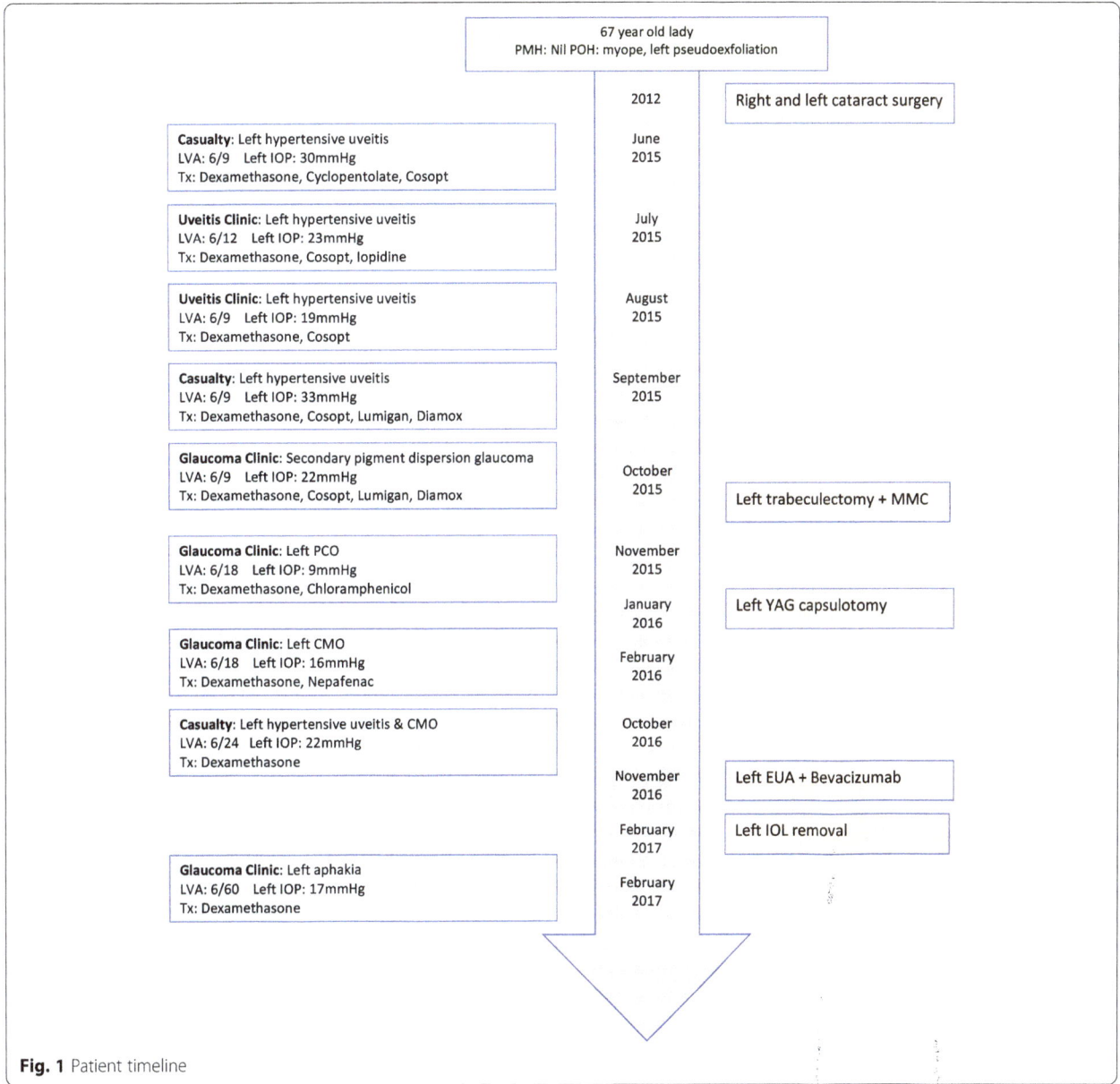

Fig. 1 Patient timeline

Case presentation

Our patient initially presented to our ophthalmic emergency department in June 2015 with pain, redness and a feeling of pressure in her left eye. She was found to have intraocular pressures (IOP) of 18 mmHg right 30 mmHg left, visual acuities (VA) of 6/4 right 6/9 left, clear corneas, deep anterior chambers, myopic optic discs and flat retinas in both eyes but with cells and flare in the left anterior segment. She was bilaterally pseudophakic having had both cataracts operated on at a different hospital 3 years prior, before which she was myopic with refractions of − 10.75/− 0.25 × 90 right and − 11.0/− 0.5 × 125 left. She was otherwise fit and healthy with no past medical history and was not on any topical medication at this point. She was diagnosed with a left hypertensive uveitis, started on a reducing course of Dexamethasone 0.1% along with Cyclopentolate 1% and Cosopt eye drops in the left eye and referred to the uveitis clinic.

On review in the uveitis clinic 6 weeks later her IOPs were 22 mmHg right 23 mmHg left with VAs of 6/5 right and 6/18 left (with glasses) improving to 6/12 left with pinhole, but with mild persistent anterior segment inflammation in the left eye; Iopidine 0.5% was added and a reducing course of Dexamethasone 0.1% was continued. On further review in August 2015 she had VAs of 6/5 right 6/9 left and IOPs of 17 mmHg right 19 mmHg but on Dexamethasone 0.1% every 2 h, Iopidine 0.5% and Cosopt to the left eye. She was referred to the glaucoma service where detailed anterior examination suggested that the inferior haptic of the intraocular lens was in fact in the sulcus. The findings included pigment on the inferior third of the corneal endothelium along with some transillumination iris defects inferiorly. As the intraocular pressures and inflammation were controlled on drops these were continued, but a diagnosis of secondary intraocular lens-induced pigment dispersion was made.

The pressure control was variable in the ensuing few months eventually requiring Diamox 250 mg slow-release (SR) twice daily and maximal topical treatment. She was reviewed in the glaucoma clinic in Oct 2015 with VAs of 6/5 right 6/9 left and IOPs of 12 mmHg right 22 mmHg left on oral Diamox 250 mg SR twice daily, Dexamethasone 0.1% two hourly, Cosopt, Iopidine 0.5% and Lumigan 0.01% to the left eye. Her optic discs were myopic and tilted but the left did appear suspicious for glaucomatous optic neuropathy [Fig. 2], although her visual fields did not show any overt glaucomatous defects [Fig. 3]. To get further information regarding her past ocular history a correspondence was sent to the consultant who performed her cataract operations. The surgeon replied stating that the left eye had pseudoexfoliation prior to surgery with IOPs of 19 mmHg right 23 mmHg left, both operations were uncomplicated but she did have previous episodes of left sided anterior hypertensive uveitis.

Following a discussion over further management, as her left IOP was only controlled on maximal therapy she was listed for a left trabeculectomy with Mitomycin-C. This operation was performed without complication on the 25th Oct 2015 with one fixed and two releasable sutures and an application of 0.4 mg/ml Mitomycin C for 3 min. Following the operation her left IOP was 9 mmHg on preservative free (PF) Dexamethasone 0.1% and PF Chloramphenicol 0.5% only. Although the IOP was subsequently controlled, the VA in the left eye started to reduce to 6/18 due to posterior capsular opacification and the decision was made to offer her a Nd:YAG (neodymium-doped yttrium aluminium garnet) laser

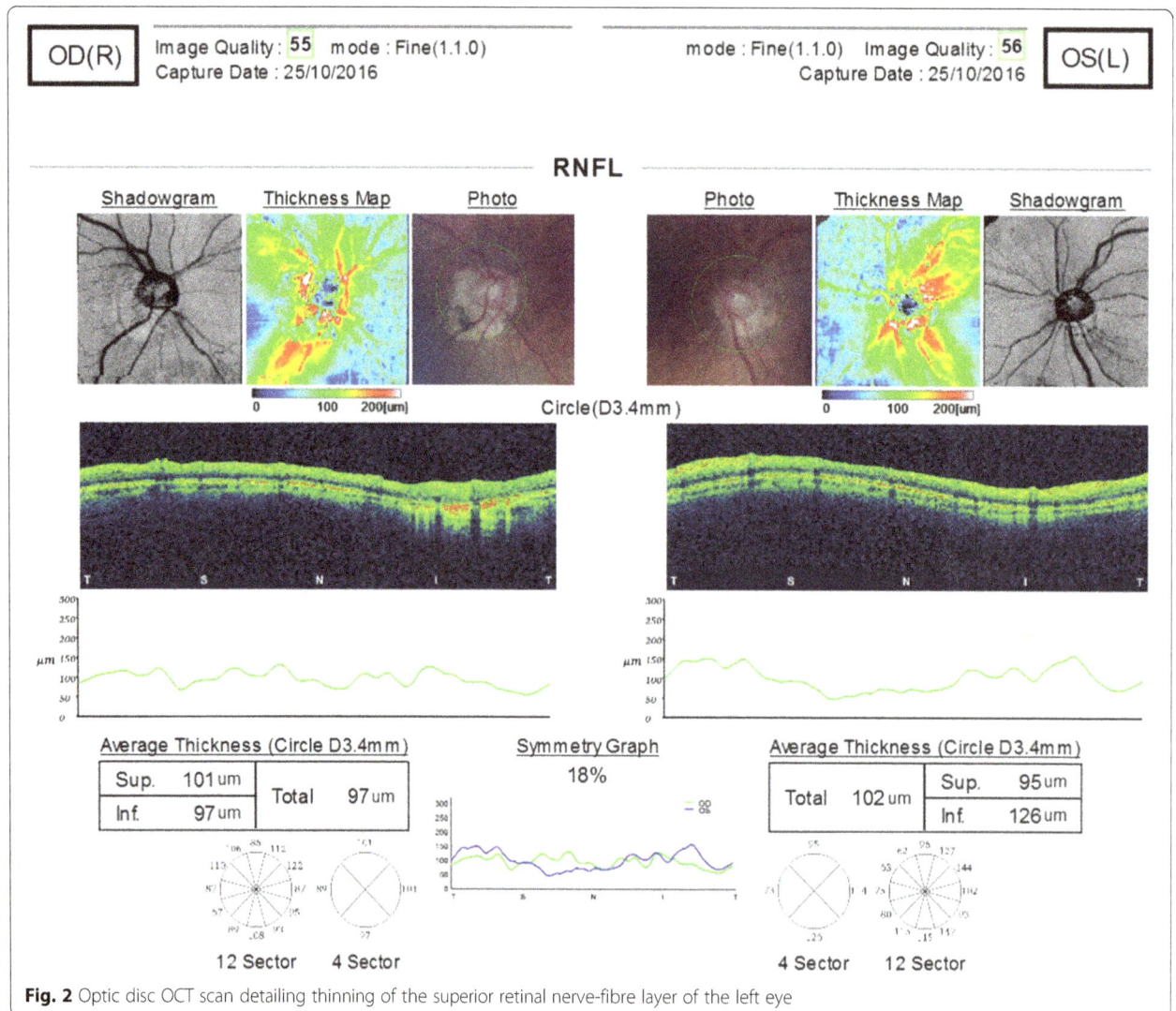

Fig. 2 Optic disc OCT scan detailing thinning of the superior retinal nerve-fibre layer of the left eye

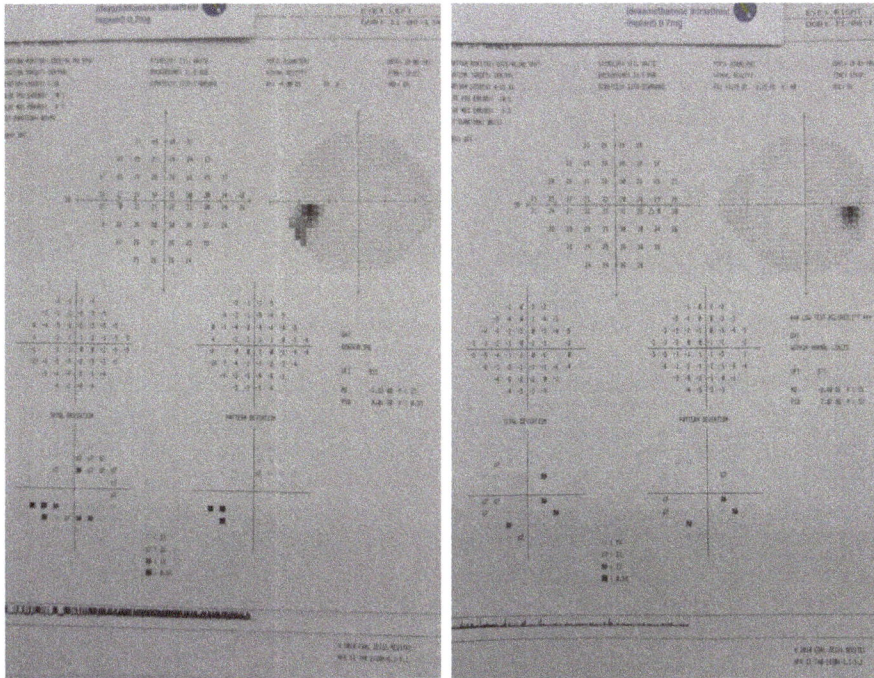

Fig. 3 24–2 Humphrey visual fields of the right and left eye

capsulotomy as there was currently enough anterior capsular support for the intraocular lens and she had not had any uveitis or raised IOP since the trabeculectomy. This was performed in January 2016 without complication but the vision following the laser remained at 6/18. On review in clinic the following month she was found to have some cystoid macular oedema of the left eye on macular OCT (ocular coherence tomography) [Fig. 4] and was started on topical Dexamethasone 0.1% and Nepafenac drops. This oedema slowly resolved and by July there was only a small epiretinal membrane visible on OCT with no oedema.

In Sept 2016 she was off all drops but was found to have some grumbling anterior segment inflammation in the left eye and was restarted on a long reducing course of topical Dexamethasone 0.1%. Unfortunately, she presented to casualty in Oct 2016 with a worsening of this inflammation, the left IOP increasing to 22 mmHg and the cystoid macular oedema starting to recur. The decision was therefore made to proceed with an EUA

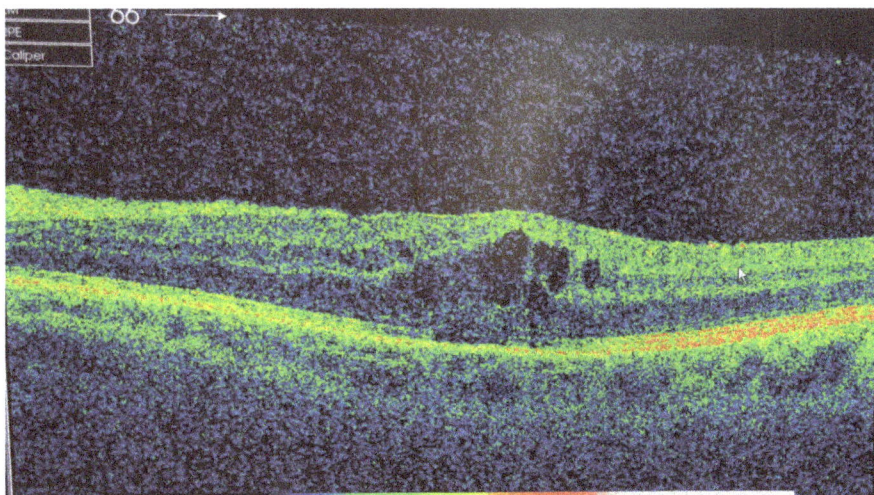

Fig. 4 Macular OCT scan of the left eye showing macular oedema

(examination under anaesthetic) of the left eye along with an intravitreal injection of Bevacizumab. This was performed in Nov 2016 and the intraocular lens was indeed found to be in the sulcus.

As the intraocular lens had now been confirmed to be in the sulcus and the patient was developing recurrent episodes of anterior uveitis due to the secondary pigment dispersion, complicated by macular oedema, a decision was made to proceed to removal of the lens [Fig. 5]. This was performed in Feb 2017, the upper haptic was found to be in the bag with the lower haptic in the sulcus. The intraocular lens was folded in the anterior chamber and removed, followed by a triamcinolone-assisted anterior vitrectomy with intracameral Dexamethasone and sub-conjunctival 5-FU (5-fluorouracil) injections given at the end of the procedure. She was left aphakic.

On review in clinic in Feb 2017 the left VA (aphakic) was CF (count fingers) unaided improving to 6/60 with pin-hole and 6/18 with aphakic correction. The IOP in the left eye was 17 mmHg on topical Dexamethasone 0.1% only, the trabeculectomy bleb was functioning well and the retina was flat with no macular oedema on OCT. The further management for this patient will involve a contact lens fitting in the first instance once the eye has settled following the recent surgery, and preservation of bleb function. With regards to secondary intraocular lens insertion this would be complicated by the

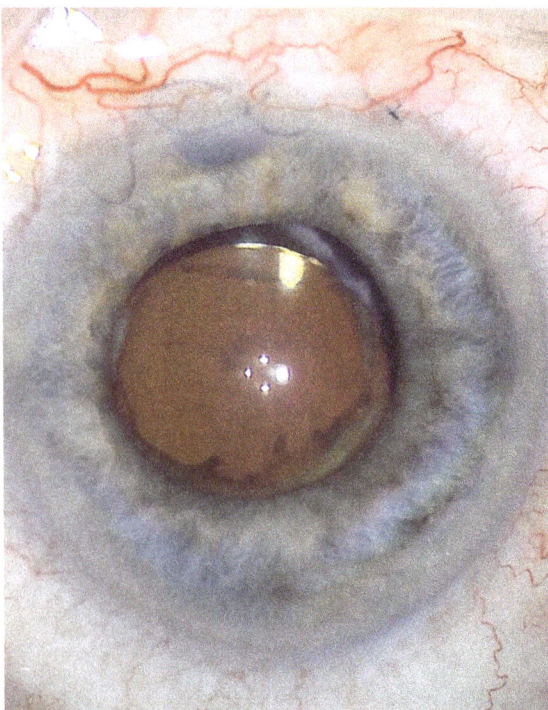

Fig. 5 Still taken during IOL removal

lack of capsular support, concerns about failure of the trabeculectomy bleb and, given her previous myopia, the risk of retinal detachment with repeated surgical intervention. A detailed discussion over the correct placement of an intraocular lens, if possible, would therefore need to be had with the patient before proceeding with any further surgery.

Discussion

This case highlights some very important learning points for any ophthalmologist involved in either the management of post-operative cataract surgery patients or managing patients presenting to eye casualty. The first point is to always consider the intraocular lens position in patients with persistent anterior segment inflammation following cataract surgery. Chronic post-operative uveitis (persistent inflammation more than 6 months after cataract surgery) has been quoted as occurring in 1 in 400 operations with a much higher incidence in those eyes that had an intraoperative complication [6]. In our case the important signs of endothelial pigment deposition and inferior iris transillumination defects made us very suspicious that the intraocular lens may have been in the sulcus rather than in the capsular bag, and was therefore leading to iris chaffe and pigment shedding causing the persistent inflammation and high intraocular pressure. The complicating factor in our case was that the surgeon who performed the operation was adamant that the intraocular lens was placed inside the capsular bag during the operation. On EUA, however, the intraocular lens was confirmed to be in the sulcus. This therefore highlights the importance of careful placement of the intraocular lens at the time of surgery to make sure it is inserted into the capsular bag. The fact that the intraocular lens in this case was a one-piece polymethylmethacrylate (PMMA) lens designed to be placed inside the capsular bag and not in the sulcus subsequently led to the pigment shedding.

Secondary pigment dispersion following implantation of a single-piece intraocular lens into the ciliary sulcus has been well described [1–3]. Patients may present with either pigment dispersion with a normal IOP or pigmentary glaucoma associated with elevated IOP, glaucomatous optic neuropathy and corresponding visual field loss. One study looking at the long-term outcomes of eyes with secondary pigmentary glaucoma associated with the implantation of foldable intraocular lenses in the ciliary sulcus [4] found that the average time to the onset of elevated IOP was 21.9 months, with 60% of the eyes experiencing chronic recurrent iridocyclitis. This study found 60% of the eyes required further surgical procedures, either intraocular lens exchange alone or combined with trabeculectomy. This current case highlights the fact that eyes where the intraocular lens was inadvertently placed into the sulcus can present both with acute episodes of inflammation leading to high IOP shortly after the surgery, which can be managed with drops, and delayed chronically elevated IOP that can be much more difficult to manage. Over time, as the intra-ocular lens continues to chafe the posterior iris leading to a continual shedding of pigment, there can be recurrent episodes of inflammation and elevated IOP which is likely to be related to an increase in pigment blocking the trabecular meshwork and reducing the outflow, therefore making this elevation in IOP more likely to be refractory to topical medications and more likely to require surgical intervention.

The second point is to highlight the incidence and management of CMO in a case such as this. The cause of the oedema in this case could be due to a number of factors; CMO has been shown to be a sequelae of the implantation of a single-piece intraocular lens into the ciliary sulcus [3], CMO is a well-documented complication following Nd:YAG laser posterior capsulotomy [7, 8] but in this case was most likely due to persistent uveitis. CMO is a well-recognised sequelae of uveitis [5] and CMO is also a well-recognised complication of cataract surgery alone, with one large study quoting an incidence of 1.17% in eyes of patients who did not have diabetes [9]. The initial treatment for CMO associated with uveitis is with topical steroid and topical non-steroidal anti-inflammatory drops [10] but the benefit of topical non-steroidals in treating CMO following cataract surgery alone has not been confirmed [11]. In the current case there was an initial good response to topical treatment with a resolution of the CMO but with continued inflammation this oedema started to return. In cases of CMO associated with uveitis that becomes refractory to topical treatment, both intravitreal Triamcinolone [12] and intravitreal Bevacizumab [13] have shown to be both safe and effective, with both treatments showing comparable efficacy [14]. In this case, as the CMO had re-occurred the decision was made to proceed with an injection of intravitreal Bevacizumab. Bevacizumab was chosen over Trimacinolone due to the possible risk of raised IOP associated with the use of intraocular steroids.

Conclusions

In summary, we believe this case highlights the importance of including the inadvertent placement of an intraocular lens into the sulcus during cataract surgery as an important differential diagnosis for persistent post-operative uveitis, but it also illustrates the possible sequelae that can occur including secondary pigmentary glaucoma and cystoid macular oedema, and the difficult decisions managing these complications can pose. In this case any further surgery has to balance visual rehabilitation with preserving the bleb for pressure control and minimising the risk of further cystoid macular oedema.

Abbreviations
5-FU: 5-fluorouracil; CF: Count fingers; CMO: Cystoid macular oedema; EUA: Examination under anaesthetic; IOP: Intraocular pressure; Nd:YAG: Neodymium-doped yttrium aluminium garnet; OCT: Ocular coherence tomography; PF: Preservative free; PMMA: Polymethylmethacrylate; SR: Slow release; VA: Visual acuity

Funding
This supplement and the meeting on which it was based were sponsored by Novartis (tracking number OPT17-C041). Novartis did not contribute to the content and all authors retained final control of the content and editorial decisions. Novartis have checked that the content was compliant with the Association of the British Pharmaceutical Industry Code of Practice.

Authors' contributions
AP wrote the manuscript. LC managed the patient clinically, performed the surgery and approved the final manuscript. Both authors read and approved the final manuscript.

Consent for publication
The patient discussed in this case report gave informed consent.

Competing interests
The authors declare that they have no competing interests.

References
1. Hadid O, Megaw R, Owen R, Fraser S. Secondary pigment dispersion syndrome with single-piece acrylic IOL. J Cataract Refract Surg. 2010;36: 1610–1.
2. Uy HS, Chan PS. Pigment release and secondary glaucoma after implantation of single-piece acrylic intraocular lenses in the ciliary sulcus. Am J Ophthalmol. 2006;142:330–2.
3. Chang DF, Masket S, Miller KM, et al. Complications of sulcus placement of single-piece acrylic intraocular lenses: recommendations for backup IOL implantation following posterior capsule rupture. J Cataract Refract Surg. 2009;35:1445–8.
4. Chang SHL, Wu W, Wu S. Late-onset secondary pigmentary glaucoma following foldable intraocular lenses implantation in the ciliary sulcus: a long-term follow-up study. BMC Ophthalmol. 2013;13:22.
5. Lardenoye CWTA, van Kooij B, Rothova A. Impact of macular edema on visual acuity in uveitis. Ophthalmology. 2006;113(8):1446–9.
6. Patel C, Kim SJ, Chomsky A, Saboori M. Incidence and risk factors for chronic uveitis following cataract surgery. Ocul Immunol Inflamm. 2013; 21(2):130–4.
7. Steinert RF, Puliafito CA, Kumar SR, Dudak SD, Patel S. Cystoid macular edema, retinal detachment, and glaucoma after Nd:YAG laser posterior capsulotomy. Am J Ophthalmol. 1991;112:373–80.

8.   Burq MA, Taqui AM. Frequency of retinal detachment and other complications after neodymium:Yag laser capsulotomy. J Pak Med Assoc. 2008;58(10):550–2.

9.   Chu CJ, Johnston RL, Buscombe C, Sallam AB, Mohamed Q, Yang YC. Risk factors and incidence of macular edema after cataract surgery: a database study of 81984 eyes. Ophthalmology. 2016;123(2):316–23.

10. Hariprasad SM, Callanan D, Gainey S, He Y, Warren K. Cystoid and diabetic macular edema treated with nepafenac 0.1%. J Ocul Pharmacol Ther. 2007; 23(6):585–9.

11. Sivaprasad S, Bunce C, Crosby-Nwaobi R. Non-steroidal anti-inflammatory agents for treating cystoid macular oedema following cataract surgery. Cochrane Database Syst Rev. 2012;15(2):CD004239.

12. Androudi S, Letko E, Meniconi M, Papadaki T, Ahmed M, Foster CS. Safety and efficacy of intravitreal triamcinolone acetonide for uveitic macular edema. Ocul Immunol Inflamm. 2005;13(2–3):205–12.

13. Al-Dhibi H, Hamade IH, Al-Halafi AA, Barry M, Chacra CB, Gupta V, et al. The effects of intravitreal Bevacizumab in infectious and noninfectious uveitis macular edema. J Ophthalmol. 2014; https://doi.org/10.1155/2014/729465.

14. Bae JH, Lee CS, Lee SC. Efficacy and safety of intravitreal Bevacizumab compared with intravitreal and posterior sub-tenon triamcinolone acetonide for treatment of uveitic cystoid macular edema. Retina. 2011; 31(1):111–8.

22

Budget impact model of Mydrane®, a new intracameral injectable used for intra-operative mydriasis

Keith Davey[1]*, Bernard Chang[2], Christine Purslow[3], Emilie Clay[4] and Anne-Lise Vataire[4]

Abstract

Background: During cataract surgery, maintaining an adequate degree of mydriasis throughout the entire operation is critical to allow for visualisation of the capsulorhexis and the crystalline lens. Good anaesthesia is also essential for safe intraocular surgery.

Mydrane® is a new injectable intracameral solution containing two mydriatics (tropicamide 0.02% and phenylephrine 0.31%) and one anaesthetic (lidocaine 1%) that was developed as an alternative to the conventional topical pre-operative mydriatics used in cataract surgery. This study aimed to estimate the budget impact across a one year time frame using Mydrane® instead of topical dilating eye drops, for a UK hospital performing 3,000 cataract operations a year.

Methods: A budget impact model (BIM) was developed to compare the economic outcomes associated with the use of Mydrane® versus topical drops (tropicamide 0.5% and phenylephrine 10%) in patients undergoing cataract surgery in a UK hospital. The outcomes of interest included costs and resource use (e.g. clinician time, mydriasis failures, operating room time, number of patients per vial of therapy etc.) associated with management of mydriasis in patients undergoing cataract surgery. All model inputs considered the UK hospital perspective without social or geographical variables. Deterministic sensitivity analyses were also performed to assess the model uncertainty.

Results: Introduction of Mydrane® is associated with a cost saving of £6,251 over 3,000 cataract surgeries in one year. The acquisition costs of the Mydrane® (£18,000 by year vs. £3,330 for eye drops) were balanced by substantial reductions in mainly nurses' costs and time, plus a smaller contribution from savings in surgeons' costs (£20,511) and lower costs associated with auxiliary dilation (£410 due to avoidance of additional dilation methods). Results of the sensitivity analyses confirmed the robustness of the model to the variation of inputs. Except for the duration of one session of eye drop instillation and the cost of Mydrane®, Mydrane® achieved an incremental cost gain compared to tropicamide/phenylephrine eye drops.

Conclusions: Despite a higher acquisition cost of Mydrane®, the budget impact of Mydrane® on hospital budgets is neutral. Mydrane® offers a promising alternative to traditional regimes using eye drops, allowing for a better patient flow and optimisation of the surgery schedule with neutral budget impact.

Keywords: Cataract surgery, Mydriasis, Mydriatics, Anaesthesia, Budget impact model

* Correspondence: keithgdavey@gmail.com
[1]Calderdale and Huddersfield NHS Foundation Trust, Huddersfield, UK
Full list of author information is available at the end of the article

Background

Cataract surgery is a very common procedure that is anticipated to increase in the coming years with the expected aging of the population [1, 2]. In 2014–2015, there were a total of 396,000 cataract surgeries performed in England [3]. Phacoemulsification is the most common procedure; it is minimally invasive, and mostly completed in an outpatient setting involving an expedited post-operative recovery [4].

During this procedure, induction of pupil mydriasis and maintenance of an adequate degree of mydriasis throughout the entire operation are critical for successful lens removal and replacement [5, 6]. Additionally, good anaesthesia is essential for the performance of safe intraocular surgery, creating a comfortable environment for the patient and the surgeon during surgery. Insufficient mydriasis or pupillary constriction due to surgical trauma can lead to several risks in the course of surgery, including incomplete cortex removal, posterior capsule rupture, vitreous loss and dislocation of lens material [7]. Insufficient mydriasis is also a source of discomfort for the surgeon as it makes instrument manoeuvring within the eye difficult. If mydriasis fails during the surgical process, surgeons might utilise rescue mydriatic therapies and procedures (e.g. ophthalmic injections and iris hooks) to re-dilate the pupils and maintain iris retraction and/or control iris floppiness [5, 6].

The standard combination of two topical mydriatic drugs (parasympatholytic and sympathomimetic, typically tropicamide or cyclopentolate, and phenylephrine) to achieve appropriate pre-operative mydriasis presents several disadvantages. From the nurse's perspective, mydriatic eye drop application is time-consuming and stressful associated with a risk of mistakes, leading to delay of the surgery or risks of overdosing. From the patient's perspective, mydriasis with drops involves a long waiting time, which may increase his/her anxiety and stress before cataract surgery. Moreover, the unpredictable time to mydriasis can make it difficult to control the flow of patients ready to be operated and to optimize the surgical schedule. The use of rescue mydriatics by the surgeon occurs in 15 to 18% of the operations and may lead to delays in theatre [8]. Specifically, the time taken to achieve maximal mydriasis can be much longer than the surgical procedure itself.

Mydrane® was developed as an alternative to the conventional topical pre-operative mydriatics for cataract surgery. It is an intracameral (IC) injectable solution containing a combination of two mydriatics (tropicamide 0.02% and phenylephrine 0.31%) and one anaesthetic (lidocaine 1%). It is injected intracamerally under topical anaesthesia by the surgeon at the beginning of the surgery through the side or primary port. Due to the specific, localised therapy, Mydrane® was shown to achieve fast onset of mydriasis and low systemic absorption [7]. Additionally, Mydrane's administration route alleviates the limitations of the topical mydriatics [9].

Since the number of cataract procedures is increasing due to the combined effects of population ageing and higher life expectancy, innovative treatments are essential to improve cataract surgery efficiency with the aim to regulate patient's flow with moderate health care expenditure. For this purpose, we developed an economic model to estimate the budget impact for a UK hospital performing cataract surgeries of Mydrane® for injection use instead of topical dilating eye drops over a one year time-frame.

Methods

A budget impact model (BIM) was developed using Microsoft Excel 2010 (Microsoft Corp., Redmond, WA, USA) to compare the economic outcomes associated with utilisation of Mydrane® versus topical eye drops (tropicamide 0.5% and phenylephrine 10%) in adult patients undergoing phacoemulsification cataract surgery in a UK hospital. The outcomes of interest include cost and resource use (e.g. clinician time, mydriasis failures, operating room time, number of patients per vial of therapy etc.) associated with management of mydriasis in patients undergoing cataract surgery. All model inputs considered the UK hospital perspective without social or geographical variables.

Model settings

The budget impact model predicted health care costs of one year for cohorts of adult patients with cataract to be operated by phacoemulsification, in a given hospital, in the UK in two situations: the use of Mydrane® (intervention group) and the use of topical eye drops (tropicamide (0.5%) and phenylephrine (10%)) for mydriasis (reference group). It was assumed that 3,000 patients a year could be operated for cataract.

A decision tree was chosen to represent the patient's pathway (Fig. 1). The model was divided into three time phases: pre-surgery (pre-operative), surgery (intra-operative) and post-surgery (post-operative). At each state of the decision tree, resource use and costs were calculated and summed together to obtain total costs with respect to each treatment strategy. 1) The pre-surgery period included all administered interventions and outcomes achieved between the time of the patient's arrival at the hospital and the time of the ophthalmologist initial surgical methods. The nurse is typically the key person during the pre-operative phase of the cataract surgery procedure. She/he takes care of the patient before his/her arrival at the operating room and undertakes most of the care before the surgical procedure, including checking the condition of the eye and dilating the pupil

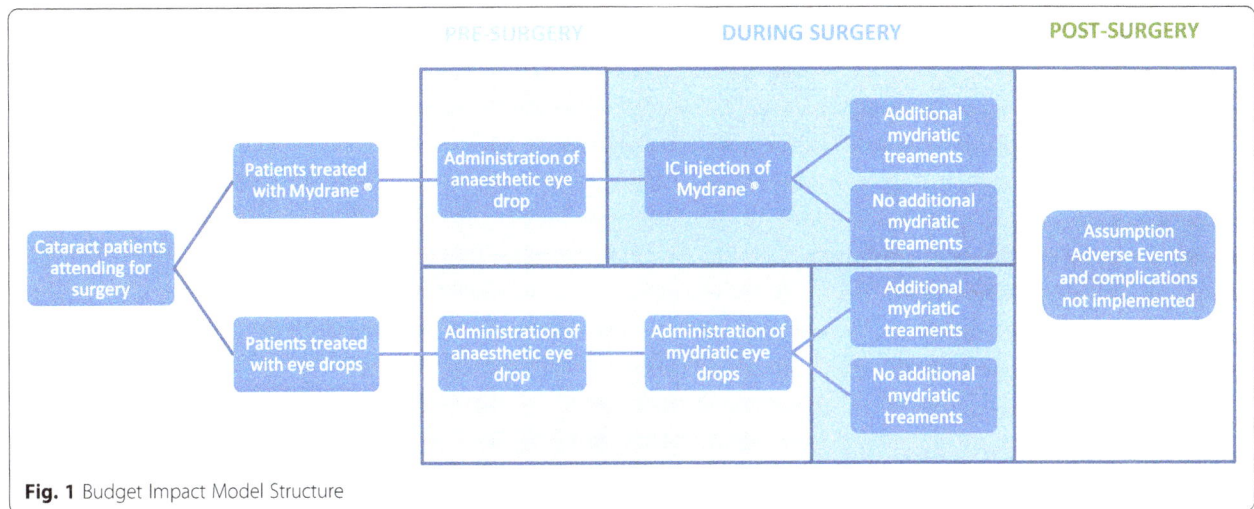

Fig. 1 Budget Impact Model Structure

with mydriatic eye drops. Anaesthesia costs were not taken into account as it is similar for the two strategies. 2) The surgery period was defined as the complete time of cataract surgery and included all methods, resources, and outcomes achieved through completion of the procedure. The surgical procedure can be divided into 2 main phases, a first phase of preparation involving the ocular surface and a second phase involving tissue manipulations inside the anterior chamber. 3) Finally, the post-surgery period was defined as the time period following all surgical activities by the ophthalmologist, which may include patients receiving medication for the prevention of post-operative infections and alleviation of ocular inflammation and pain [10, 11].

Clinical treatment protocol used in the model

Patient treatment groups differed in frequency and timing of drugs administered during the pre-surgery and surgery phases. For cataract patients treated with standard care (topical eye drops), the administration schedule included instillation of one drop of tropicamide 0.5% and one drop of phenylephrine 10% instilled by nurses in three instances; at 30, 20, and 10 min prior to surgery. In the Mydrane® group, the surgeon injected Mydrane® 200 μL IC at the beginning of surgery. Both patient groups also received topical anaesthetics 5 min and 1 min prior to surgery. Based on the phase III LT2380-PIII-05/10 clinical trial data [9], these treatment strategies were well tolerated and did not differ in their short-term adverse events profiles, hence these variables were not incorporated in the model.

Following appropriate administration of mydriatic and local anaesthetic, the surgeon proceeded with phacoemulsification. If adequate dilation was not achieved, additional therapy or mechanical methods were used. When such steps were taken, the model

took account of this (e.g. increased waiting time during surgical procedures).

Model inputs and outcomes

All model inputs (with associated sources) are presented in Table 1. Pre-surgery inputs included proportion of mydriasis failures, quantity of eye drop instillations, number of patients per vial of therapy, and nursing time costs. During the surgery phase, many of the pre-surgery inputs carried over, with additional inputs for operating room occupancy time, cost of treatments, time for mydriasis failure, surgeon cost and procedure time. The number of annual procedures was calculated by dividing the total surgeon working time gained by the time needed for a cataract surgery. Additionally, hospital revenue was calculated based on the number of operations performed by each surgeon. The structure of the model and its conformity with UK clinical practice was validated by the co-authors with clinical expertise.

Costs of treatment strategies

The reference treatment group was composed of patients treated with one drop of tropicamide 0.5% and one drop of phenylephrine 10% instilled by nurses in three instances at 30, 20 and 10 min prior to surgery. Comprehensive clinical information, resource use and unit cost are presented in Table 3. Costs were expressed in British pounds (£, January 2015).

Sensitivity analysis

Deterministic sensitivity analyses were performed to assess the model uncertainty. All input parameters are varied one by one according to bounds defining the possible range of variation of the considered parameter. These analyses ran the model while simultaneously varying one specific variable and holding all others constant.

Table 1 Model inputs

Variable		Base case	Low value	High value	Source
Pre-surgery					
Mydrane®: Percentage of mydriasis failure during surgery needing additional mydriatic treatments					
Mydrane®		1.1%	0.2%	3.2%	Phase III clinical trial results, Confidence Interval 95% [9]
Eye drops		5.3%	3.0%	8.7%	
Number of eye drop instillation sessions by nurses		3	2	4	Assumption
Duration of one session of eye drop (min)		3	1.5	5	Assumption, Mydriasert report, Office for National Statistics [15]
Number of patients per vial of eye drops		1	1	5	Assumption, Mydriasert report, Office for National Statistics [15]
Patient waiting time before surgery (min)					
Mydrane®		8.70	8.19	9.21	Phase III clinical trial results, Confidence Interval 95% [9]
Eye drops		37.90	36.73	39.07	
Nurse cost/h in £		43.12	35.76	59.95	PSSRU 2012–2013, Lower: nurse day ward without qualification costs, Higher: nurse team manager [16]
During surgery					
Mydrane®: Surgeon working time (no mydriasis failure) (min)		12.03	11.51	12.52	Phase III clinical trial results [9], Phase II clinical trial results, Confidence Interval 95%
Eye drops: Surgeon working time (no mydriasis failure) (min)		11.34	10.64	12.04	Phase III clinical trial results, Confidence Interval 95% [9]
Mydrane®: Operation room occupancy time (min)		12.03	11.51	12.52	Phase III clinical trial results [9], Phase II clinical trial results, Confidence Interval 95%
Eye drops: Operation room occupancy time (min)		11.34	10.64	12.04	Phase III clinical trial results [9], Confidence Interval 95%
Mydrane®: Additional time needed if mydriasis failure (min)		10.00	2.50	7.50	UK, 2013, Molecule used for additional mydriasis, European Observatory for Cataract Surgery 2014 [7]
Eye drops: Additional time needed if mydriasis failure (min)		10.00	2.50	7.50	UK, 2013, Molecule used for additional mydriasis, European Observatory for Cataract Surgery 2014 [7]
Mydrane®: Surgeon time loss between operations caused by mydriasis failure (min)		10.00	5.00	20.00	Assumption
Eye drops: Surgeon time loss between operations caused by mydriasis failure (min)		10.00	5.00	20.00	Assumption
Additional mydriatic treatments distribution (more than 1 possible)	Adrenaline	4%	39%	4%	UK, 2013, Molecule used for additional mydriasis, European Observatory for Cataract Surgery 2014 [7]
	Phenylephrine	93%	57%	93%	
	Tropicamide	14%	0%	14%	
	Mechanical tools	4%	5%	4%	
	Cyclopentolate	32%	1%	32%	
	Others	0%	0%	0%	
Cost Mydrane® in £		6.00	3.00	9.00	Assumption
Cost Adrenaline in £		4.95	0.39	8.31	British National Formulary 2015 [17]
Cost Phenylephrine in £		0.57	0.57	0.57	British National Formulary 2015 [17]
Cost Tropicamide in £		0.54	0.50	1.60	British National Formulary 2015 [17]
Cost Mechanical tools in £		56.80	28.40	85.20	Mydriasert pupillary dilation for cataract surgery.
Costs Cyclopentolate in £		0.56	0.50	12.96	British National Formulary 2014
Surgeon cost/h in £		147.26	105.18	189.33	Lower: consultant surgery without costs including qualifications, Upper: assumption

This process tests the model assumptions and parameter estimates validity, given their uncertainty. Parameters of the model were varied using data from alternative publications or confidence intervals obtained from clinical trials. In case of no available relevant information on uncertainty, the base case value was between 50 to 150%. The list of inputs used in the deterministic sensitivity analysis is described in Table 1. All deterministic and

Table 2 Base case results - Resource use

	Mydrane®	Eye drops	Difference Mydrane® - Eye drop
Occupation of rooms			
Total time spent in waiting room (hours)	435.00	1895.00	-1460.00
Total time spent in operation room (hours)	612.25	619.75	−7.50
Surgeon time			
Number of unexpected delays due to insufficient mydriasis during surgery	33.00	159.00	−126.00
Total surgeon time in operation (hours)	601.25	566.75	34.50
Total delay for surgeons due to insufficient mydriasis (hours)	11.00	53.00	−42.00
Total surgeon time (hours)	612.25	619.75	−7.50
Nurse time			
Total nurse time (hours)	0.00	450.00	−450.00

sensitivity analyses were then compared between groups based on incremental costs calculated according to the various inputs.

Results

Resource outcomes

Overall, Mydrane® was found to be a beneficial treatment reducing costs from the hospital, surgeon, and nurse perspectives (Table 2 and Fig. 2). With respect to hospital outcomes, Mydrane® decreased the time spent in the waiting rooms. Specifically, during the pre-surgery phase, patients' total time in the waiting room was lower compared to the reference group (435 vs. 1895 h, respectively; incremental difference 1460 h).

The number of unexpected delays caused by mydriasis failure was significantly reduced between treatment groups [33 (Mydrane®) vs. 159 (tropicamide/phenylephrine) delay cases; difference – 126]. Throughout the year, surgeon time delay was reduced of 42 h, decreasing from 53 h for the reference group to 11 h for the Mydrane® group. However, patients in the Mydrane® group

experienced more "working time" in surgery (601 h vs. 567 h; difference 35 h); subsequently, considering the pre-operative mydriasis time savings, the total procedure time was lower for the Mydrane® group (7 h saved over one year). Lastly, in terms of nursing time, Mydrane® patients did not need additional topical eye drop instillations to achieve mydriasis and this time was freed up (450 h over one year).

Economic outcomes

In the two treatment groups, the predicted total costs over one year were £108,264 (Mydrane®) and £114,515 (tropicamide/phenylephrine) (Table 3 and Fig. 3). We assumed that one vial of each eye drop per patient was used in line with good clinical practice and product licence. Therefore, the Mydrane® strategy realised an annual cost saving of £6,251 and supported budget impact savings from a hospital perspective. Mydrane® also decreased hospital staff costs compared to traditional topical tropicamide/phenylephrine drops. Specifically, significant cost savings were obtained in nursing

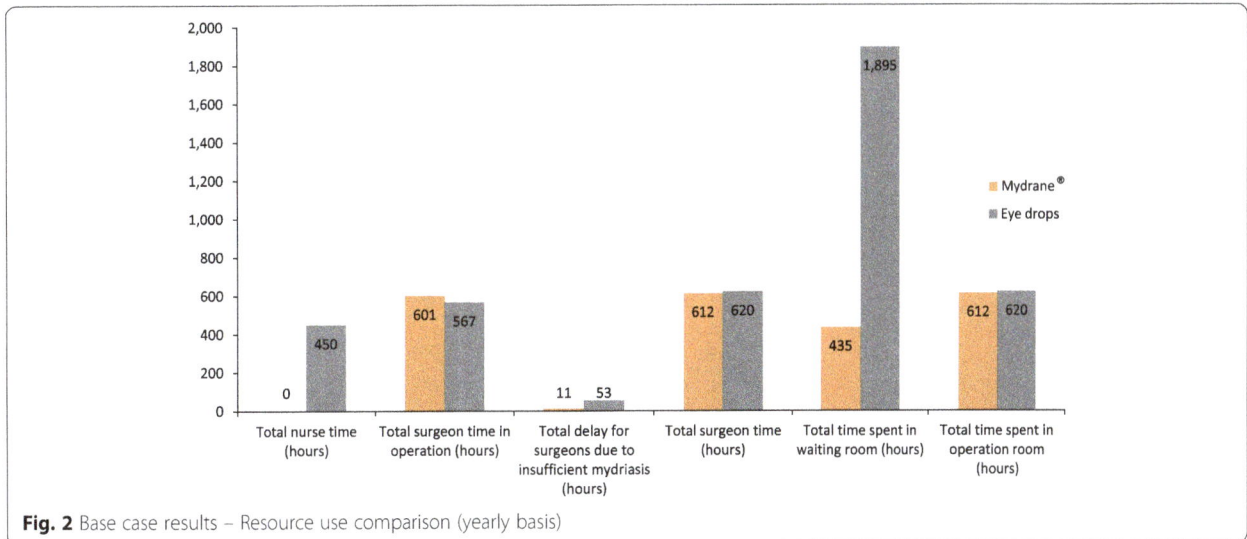

Fig. 2 Base case results – Resource use comparison (yearly basis)

Table 3 Base case results – Costs

	Mydrane®	Eye drops	Difference Mydrane® - Eye drop
Total nurse costs (£)	0	19,406	−19,406
Total surgeon costs (£)	90,157	91,261	− 1104
Total work-related costs (£)	90,157	110,668	−20,511
Mydrane® costs (£)	18,000	0	18,000
Eye drop costs (£)	0	3330	−3330
Additive mydriatic treatment costs (£)	107	518	−410
Total treatment-related costs (£)	18,107	3848	14,260
Total costs (£)	108,264	114,515	−6251
Costs per patient (£)	36.09	38.17	−2.08

time to instil drops in the pre-operative period. Over one year, cost savings amounted to £19,406.

The predicted annual work-related costs were similar in the Mydrane® and the topical eye drops arms (£90,157 vs. £91,261, respectively). The Mydrane® strategy gave the surgeon additional working time. Overall, using Mydrane® provided a total net cost saving as a consequence of the reduction of cases with insufficient mydriasis. Furthermore, compared to the Mydrane® group, the topical eye drops group had higher predicted treatment costs due to additional mydriatic therapies required for patients who initially failed mydriasis (£518 vs. £107, respectively; Table 3). Overall, the predicted treatment related costs were lower among patients in topical eye drops group compared to the Mydrane® group (£3848 vs. £18,107, respectively).

Surgeons experienced reduced working time for patients treated with Mydrane®; thus, allowing for more efficient clinical throughput and providing opportunities for resource optimisation. More specifically, considering the increased time to perform additional operations, the model indicated that changing to Mydrane® could potentially free up sufficient time to allow approximately 36. 81 more cataract procedures per year, bringing in an additional £27,412 in revenue (Table 4).

Sensitivity analysis
The tornado diagram presented in Fig. 4 illustrates the results of the deterministic sensitivity analyses. Results of the sensitivity analyses confirmed the robustness of the model to the variation of inputs. Except for the duration of one session of eye drop instillation and the cost of Mydrane®, Mydrane® achieved an incremental cost gain compared to topical eye drops. The model results were most sensitive to the following parameters: duration of one session of eye drop instillation, cost of Mydrane®, number of eye drop instillations sessions by nurses, and nursing costs.

Discussion
A budget impact model was developed for the introduction of Mydrane® in the UK over a 1-year time horizon. The model showed that the introduction of Mydrane® is associated with cost savings of £6398 by year for the hospital. The acquisition costs of Mydrane® compared to topical eye drops (£18,000/year vs. £3,330/year, respectively) were balanced by substantial reductions in nurses and surgeons costs (£20,658) and lower costs associated with distant recurrence (£410 due to additive mydriatic treatment avoided).

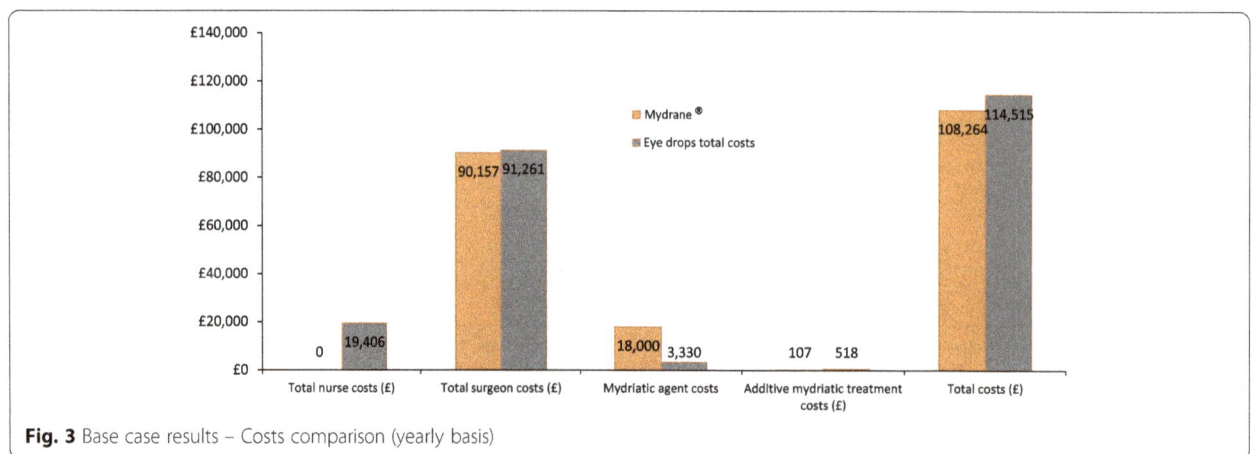

Fig. 3 Base case results – Costs comparison (yearly basis)

Table 4 Results: Benefits for the hospital

	Consequences of Mydrane® introduction
Total number of operations gained	36.81
Total additional revenue (£)	27,412
Total expected net benefit (£)	11,733

The BIM calculated similar costs between each treatment strategy and demonstrated the economic benefits of Mydrane® as an efficient treatment for mydriasis in cataract procedures. By producing a stable and fast mydriasis, it leads to less unexpected events, reduced lost time, freed up nursing time, optimised theatre time, and potentially reduces costs. Specifically, the time savings were achieved by decreasing the number of topical drop instillations and reduced mydriasis failure. The saved time potentially allows increased throughput with associated increased revenue. Our findings show that using Mydrane® instead of topical eye drops for cataract surgery patients should produce a net benefit for the hospital.

Additionally, Mydrane® treatment potentially provides a variety of indirect benefits to an adopting hospital. Amidst an aging population and capacity challenges, many patients face long waiting times for operations [12]. The savings achieved with respect to health care professionals' time and prospective increase in patients treated per day, positions Mydrane® to positively impact the waiting time before surgery. Secondly, patients in the pre-operative area may experience deteriorated

vision or increased anxiety as eye drops are applied; this may be alleviated by using an injectable treatment. Thirdly, patients treated with Mydrane® may be more likely to recover at a faster rate due to the lower risk of mydriatic failures and surgery complications. Overall, Mydrane® strategy offers reduced cost, improved health outcomes and minimised time losses from the institution, clinician, and patient's perspectives.

While every effort was made to obtain key model inputs from the best available evidence, assumptions about some parameters were necessary for the budget impact estimation and may impact the model output. Therefore, limitations of this study need to be acknowledged. The model included a simple design to reflect the available data and transparency of calculations, but did not include all the specific processes of an ophthalmic surgery unit. The number of operations (3,000) is typical of an average ophthalmology unit in a UK city, and it is assumed that human resources and patient flow are already optimised for the throughput of the surgical unit, but it is possible that savings due to nurse time might be further influenced by local organisation. A literature search was conducted to identify previously published

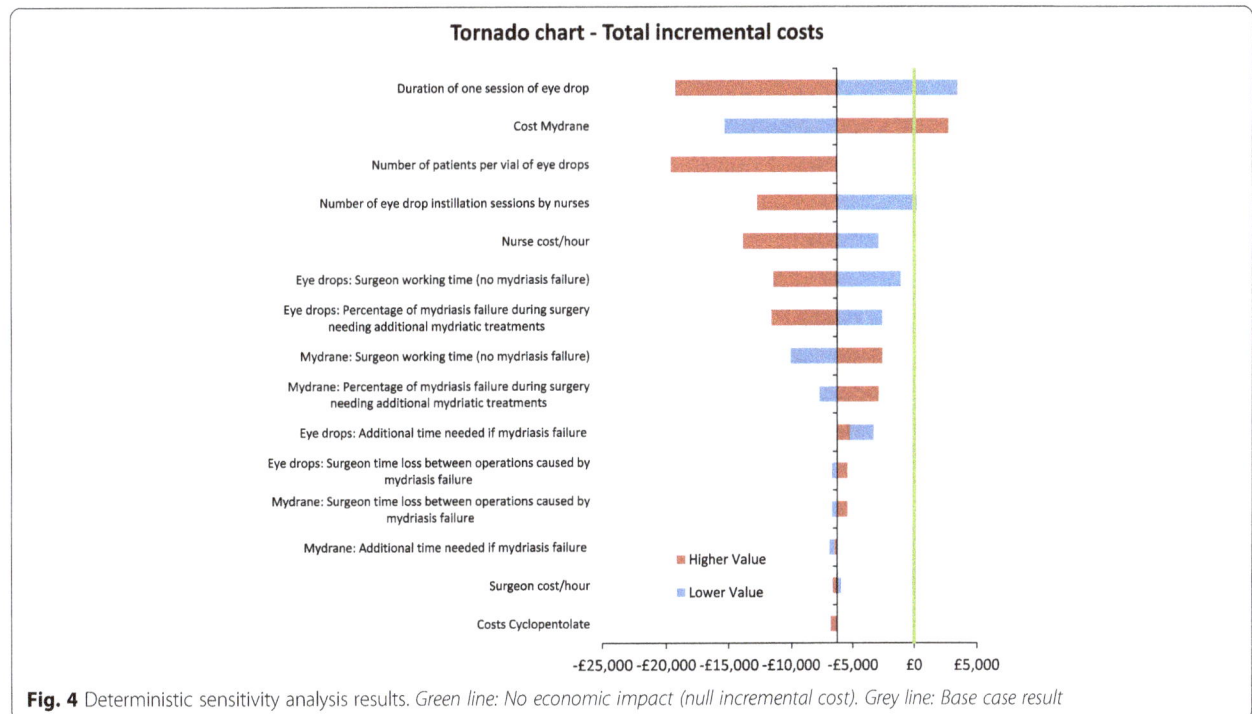

Fig. 4 Deterministic sensitivity analysis results. *Green line: No economic impact (null incremental cost). Grey line: Base case result*

models for cataract surgery. In 2001, Lundström described a model comparing performance of different cataract surgery management in an ophthalmology department [8]. An index approach was modelled to measure cataract surgery outcome. Moreover, one previously microsimulation model included a detailed depiction of the cataract procedure process [13] but extended beyond the framework in Mydrane® clinical trial and could not be used in this model. Also, the number of procedures gained due to time saving and financial benefits for the hospital is not part of the BIM. However, for the purposes of this analysis, the methodology deviates from classic BIM structure and guidelines. Additionally, hospital room costs were not included in the BIM due to lack of official data.

The structure and primary components of this BIM are derived from clinical trials data [9]. Two deviations from the clinical trial protocol versus daily practice have to be considered in the model. In the Mydrane® group, according to the trial protocol, if mydriasis was not achieved following one injection, a second (lower dose) injection was indicated before rescue therapy. However, to appropriately represent clinical practice, Mydrane® patients received only one injection in the BIM. The percentage of mydriasis failure in the model was established taking into account data from patients that received one or two injections (causing an underestimation of the percentage of mydriasis failure), while the duration of operations used in the model corresponded to patients who had only one injection. Furthermore, the trial protocol required the surgeon to wait 1.5 min to proceed with operation, even if mydriasis was obtained immediately, although this wait is not standard in clinical practice. The Phase II LT2380-PII-11/07 trial showed that 95% of the pupil dilation (6.9 mm before viscoelastic injection) was reached in less than 30 s following Mydrane® administration [14]. Thus, following Mydrane® injection, more accurate mydriasis time estimation (29 s) was applied from a phase II clinical trial study and substituted in the BIM.

The sensitivity analyses indicated that the BIM was sensitive to several nurse-specific variables (e.g. duration of eye drops applications, number of eye drops instillations); both values were obtained after consultation with experts. Also, the patient's (and any accompanying carer's) perspective was not considered; because Mydrane® reduces waiting time for patients, the group would waste less time arriving early for drops to be applied and being monitored during that time.

Conclusions

Despite a higher acquisition cost of Mydrane®, the economic impact is associated with benefits. Mydrane® represents a promising alternative to eye drops, permitting improved patient flow and optimization of the surgical schedule.

Abbreviations
BIM: Budget impact model; IC: Intracameral; min: minutes; UK: United Kingdom

Acknowledgments
Not applicable.

Funding
The study was funded by Thea Pharmaceuticals. Thea Pharmaceuticals contracted Creativ-Ceutical to conduct this study and write the manuscript.

Authors' contributions
ALV and EC were involved in the study design, data analysis and interpretation, and manuscript writing. KD and BC analysed and interpreted the data. CP reviewed the manuscript. All authors read and approved the final manuscript.

Consent for publication
Not applicable.

Competing interests
CP is an employee of Thea Pharmaceuticals, EC and ALV are employees of Creativ-Ceutical.

Author details
[1]Calderdale and Huddersfield NHS Foundation Trust, Huddersfield, UK. [2]Leeds Teaching Hospitals NHS Trust, Leeds, UK. [3]Thea Pharmaceuticals, Keele, UK. [4]Creativ-Ceutical, Paris, France.

References
1. Minassian DC, Reidy A, Desai P, Farrow S, Vafidis G, Minassian A. The deficit in cataract surgery in England and Wales and the escalating problem of visual impairment: epidemiological modelling of the population dynamics of cataract. Br J Ophthalmol. 2000;84(1):4–8.
2. Reidy A, Minassian DC, Vafidis G, Joseph J, Farrow S, Wu J, Desai P, Connolly A. Prevalence of serious eye disease and visual impairment in a North London population: population based, cross sectional study. BMJ. 1998;316(7145):1643–6.
3. National Health Service Hospital Episode Statistics, Admitted Patient Care - England, 2014–15 [http://digital.nhs.uk/catalogue/PUB19124].
4. Lundstrom M, Barry P, Leite E, Seward H, Stenevi U. 1998 European cataract outcome study: report from the European Cataract Outcome Study Group. J Cataract Refract Surg. 2001;27(8):1176–84.
5. Liou SW, Yang CY. The effect of intracameral adrenaline infusion on pupil size, pulse rate, and blood pressure during phacoemulsification. J Ocul Pharmacol Ther. 1998;14(4):357–61.
6. Meyer SM, Fraunfelder FT. 3. Phenylephrine hydrochloride. Ophthalmology. 1980;87(11):1177–80.
7. Behndig A, Cochener-Lamard B, Guell J, Kodjikian L, Mencucci R, Nuijts R, Pleyer U, Rosen P, Szaflik J, Tassignon MJ. Surgical, antiseptic, and antibiotic practice in cataract surgery: results from the European observatory in 2013. J Cataract Refract Surg. 2015;41(12):2635–43.
8. Lundstrom M, Roos P, Brege KG, Floren I, Stenevi U, Thorburn W. Cataract surgery and effectiveness. 2. An index approach for the measurement of output and efficiency of cataract surgery at different surgery departments. Acta Ophthalmol Scand. 2001;79(2):147–53.

9. Labetoulle M, Findl O, Malecaze F, Alio J, Cochener B, Lobo C, Lazreg S, Hartani D, Colin J, Tassignon MJ, et al. Evaluation of the efficacy and safety of a standardised intracameral combination of mydriatics and anaesthetics for cataract surgery. Br J Ophthalmol. 2015;

10. Henderson BA, Kim JY, Ament CS, Ferrufino-Ponce ZK, Grabowska A, Cremers SL. Clinical pseudophakic cystoid macular edema. Risk factors for development and duration after treatment. *J Cataract Refract Surg.* 2007; 33(9):1550–8.

11. Sivaprasad S, Bunce C, Patel N. Non-steroidal anti-inflammatory agents for treating cystoid macular oedema following cataract surgery. Cochrane Database Syst Rev. 2005;1:CD004239.

12. Slade J: Eye health data summary - A review of published data in England.; 2014.

13. Reindl S, Mönch L, Mönch M, Scheider A. Modeling and simulation of cataract surgery processes. In: Rossetti MD, Hill RR, Johansson B, Dunkin A, Ingalls RG, editors. Proceedings of the 2009 winter simulation conference; 2009. p. 2009.

14. Pharmaceuticals T: Clinical study report of Phase II RCT of Mydrane. 2014.

15. Office for National Statistics [http://www.ons.gov.uk].

16. Unit Costs of Health & Social Care [http://www.pssru.ac.uk/project-pages/unit-costs/].

17. British national formulary [https://www.bnf.org/products/fc/].

Quantitative evaluation of corneal epithelial edema after cataract surgery using corneal densitometry

Sho Ishikawa[1,2]* (ORCID), Naoko Kato[1,2] and Masaru Takeuchi[2]

Abstract

Purpose: The optical density of the cornea can be evaluated quantitatively by "densitometry" using a rotating Scheimpflug camera. Densitometry allows evaluation of corneal opacity in the anterior segment of the eye by quantitative measurement of scattering light. In the present investigation, we evaluate quantitatively minimal subclinical corneal edema after cataract surgery using densitometry.

Methods: Fifty four eyes of 34 patients who underwent cataract surgery were enrolled. Measurement of corneal density was performed using Pentacam® before and on days 1, 3 and 7 after surgery.

Results: Densitometry scores increased from 18.12 ± 1.76 before cataract surgery to 21.03 ± 3.84 on day 1 ($P < 0.001$) and 19.90 ± 2.46 on day 3 ($P = 0.018$), but recovered to 19.44 ± 1.58 on day 7 ($P = 0.131$). Total corneal thickness was 549.1 ± 32.7 μm before surgery and increased to 582.7 ± 46.3 μm on day 1 ($P = 0.001$), but recovered to 566.4 ± 29.7 μm on day 3 ($P = 0.097$). Densitometry reading correlated positively with corneal thickness (correlation coefficient $= 0.13$, $P = 0.003$).

Conclusions: Densitometry is useful to detect corneal edema that is not detectable by slit-lamp examination.

Keywords: Densitometry, Corneal edema, Cataract surgery

Introduction

The Pentacam® (Oculus, Wetzlar, Germany), a corneal tomography using a rotating Scheimpflug camera is a diagnostic tool for the anterior segment of the eye, allows quantitative evaluation of the optical media as "densitometry". The densitometry program that measures scattering light allows quantitative and objective measurement of opacities within the anterior segment of the eyes. Since Smith et al. [1] first reported on the evaluation of healthy cornea by Scheimpflug imaging, densitometry has been used for objective assessment of cataract-associated media opacification.

Several clinical studies have reported the usefulness of densitometry for quantitative evaluation of corneal opacification in various conditions such as corneal dystrophy [2], mucopolysaccharidosis [3], corneal haze after

corneal cross linking for keratoconus [4, 5] or keratectasia [4], laser in situ keratomileusis [6, 7], photorefractive keratectomy [8, 9], and lamellar keratoplasty [10, 11], corneal infection [12], after Descemet's stripping automated endothelial keratoplasty [13] or penetrating keratoplasty [14], increase in corneal light scattering has been detected by densitometry even in cases clinically assessed to be clear by slit-lamp microscopy, indicating the potential use of densitometry for objective measurements as an adjuvant to slit-lamp examination. However, there is no report that densitometry can be used as an indicator of minimal corneal edema.

Phacoemulsification is a standard procedure for cataract surgery, and is the most common procedure performed in recent decades. Even in uneventful cataract surgeries, various intraoperative factors such as ultrasound energy emitted by phacoemulsification, greater infusion volume, mechanical contact of nuclear fragments with the corneal endothelium, and high intraocular pressure may cause

* Correspondence: sho_ijp@yahoo.co.jp
[1]Department of Ophthalmology, Saitama Medical University, 38 Morohongo, Moroyama, Saitama 350-0495, Japan
[2]Department of Ophthalmology, National Defense Medical College, 3-2 Namiki, Tokorozawa, Saitama 359-8216, Japan

subclinical corneal edema, although no significant findings are detected by slit-lamp examination.

The purpose of the present study was to detect quantitatively serial changes of backward light scattering after cataract surgery using the densitometry.

Materials and methods

Fifty four eyes of 34 patients (aged 71 ± 8.4 years, 18 males and 16 females) who underwent cataract surgery at the Department of Ophthalmology, National Defense Medical College between July 2012 and October 2013 were enrolled; a prospective study. All eyes had nuclear cataract of grade 2 or above were included. Eyes with ocular surface diseases before surgery, such as dry eye and superficial punctate keratopathy, were excluded.

In addition to routine ophthalmic examinations, we assessed corneal densitometry readings and corneal thickness by Pentacam® before cataract surgery and on days 1, 3 and 7 after surgery. Examination with Pentacam® was conducted as recommended in the instruction manual. After the patient had placed his/her head on the instrument's head and chin rests, the Pentacam® was aligned so that a dim, blue light illuminated the cornea. The instrument was aligned so that the patient's eye and the live Scheimpflug image came into view. The apex of the cornea was marked by positioning a yellow circle, and the patient was asked to open the eye widely. Twenty-five Scheimpflug images were taken automatically in three-dimensional scan mode. The instrument allows full-thickness corneal haze evaluation, and shows the measured maximum density values on a densitogram on a scale from 0 to 100; 0 indicating no clouding and 100 indicating completely opaque.

We measured corneal density with the cornea density mode of Pentacam®. The cornea is divided into 12 portions according to the zone and the depth; namely, four zones in concentric circles from the corneal apex (central 2 mm zone, surrounding 2–6 mm annulus, 6–10 mm annulus, and 10–12 mm annulus) and three depths (anterior layer: from the corneal surface to a depth of 120 μm, center layer: between the anterior and posterior layers, and posterior layer: the deepest 60 μm). The densitometry value is expressed as the average score in each portion. We used the corneal densitometry score in the central 2 mm zone and the anterior layer (0–120 μm depth) for analysis (Fig. 1). Before the surgery, the lid skin was scrubbed with 10% povidone-iodine (Meiji Seika, Tokyo, Japan) and the conjunctiva and cornea within the operative field were disinfected with 1% povidone-iodine. For topical anesthesia, 4% lidocaine eye drops were instilled onto the operated eye. All cataract surgeries were performed by the same surgeon (S.I) using phacoemulsification and aspiration technique via a small incision (2.4 mm). The Infiniti® (Alcon, Fort Worth, Texas) was used as the phacoemulsification instrument. The setting of the instrument was as follows: irrigation pressure 80–90 cmH2O, aspiration rate 20–25 mm/min, aspiration pressure 40–350 mmHg, and phacopower 40–60%.

The study protocol was approved by the ethical committee of the National Defense Medical College and the research was conducted according to the tenets of the Declaration of Helsinki.

Statistical analysis

JMP software version 10 was used for the statistical analysis. Friedman's test with Bonferroni correction as multiple comparison procedure was used as a nonparametric test to compare corneal densitometry score and corneal thickness. The Spearman's correlation coefficient was used to analyze correlation between corneal densitometry score and corneal thickness. P values less than 0.05 were considered statistically significant.

Results

Fifty four eyes of 34 patients (aged 71 ± 8.4 years, 18 males and 16 females) were enrolled. All eyes had nuclear cataract of grade 2 or above. Sixteen eyes had posterior subcapsular opacity, 34 eyes had cortical opacity, and 4 eyes had mature cataract. All cataract surgeries were completed uneventfully, and no perioperative complications were observed. Best corrected visual acuity (BCVA) was improved in all eyes. The average BCVA (Log MAR) was 0.33 ± 0.38 before surgery and 0.05 ± 0.19 on day 1 after surgery. Intraocular pressure was within normal range in all eyes before (10–19 mmHg) and after (7–17 mmHg) surgery (Table 1). Slit-lamp examination detected minimum fold of the Descemet's membrane after surgery in 6 of 54 eyes.

Densitometry readings in the central 2 mm zone within the anterior layer was 18.12 ± 1.76 before surgery, and increased significantly to 21.03 ± 3.84 on day 1 ($P < 0.001$) and 19.90 ± 2.46 on day 3 ($P = 0.017$) but recovered to 19.44 ± 1.58 on day 7 ($P = 0.131$) after surgery (Fig. 1a). Densitometry readings in the 2–6 mm annulus within the anterior layer was 19.11 ± 4.66 before surgery and increased significantly to 22.18 ± 7.40 on day 1 ($P = 0.046$) but declined to 20.73 ± 4.60 on day 3 ($P = 0.296$) and 21.39 ± 4.86 on day 7 ($P = 0.183$) after surgery (Fig. 1e). In the center layer, the densitometry readings showed no significant changes both in the central 2 mm zone and the 2–6 mm annulus throughout the study period (Fig. 1b and f). In the posterior layer, densitometry readings in the central 2 mm zone increased significantly only on day 1 after surgery (10.8 ± 1.3 to 12.4 ± 2.9, $P = 0.003$), but returned to preoperative value on day 3 after surgery (Fig. 1c and g, Fig. 2, Additional file 1).

Total corneal thickness (mean $\pm$ standard deviation) at the corneal apex was 549.1 ± 32.7 μm before surgery

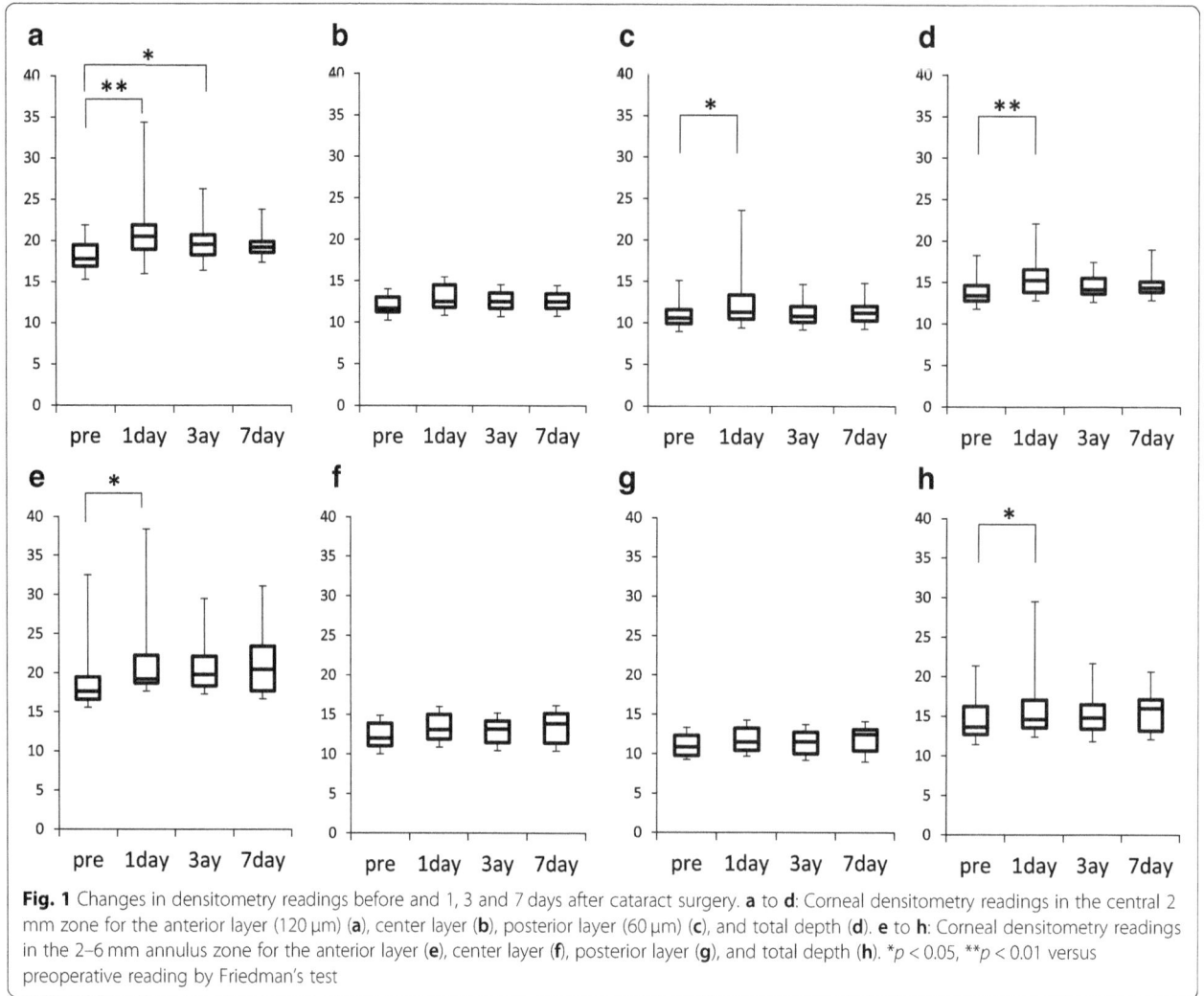

Fig. 1 Changes in densitometry readings before and 1, 3 and 7 days after cataract surgery. **a** to **d**: Corneal densitometry readings in the central 2 mm zone for the anterior layer (120 μm) (**a**), center layer (**b**), posterior layer (60 μm) (**c**), and total depth (**d**). **e** to **h**: Corneal densitometry readings in the 2–6 mm annulus zone for the anterior layer (**e**), center layer (**f**), posterior layer (**g**), and total depth (**h**). *$p < 0.05$, **$p < 0.01$ versus preoperative reading by Friedman's test

and increased to 582.7 ± 46.3 μm on day 1 after surgery ($P = 0.001$), but recovered to 566.4 ± 29.7 μm on day 3 ($P = 0.097$) and 559.4 ± 32.4 μm on day 7 ($P = 0.400$) after surgery (Fig. 3).

Densitometry readings in the central 2 mm zone for the anterior layer correlated positively with the corneal thickness (correlation coefficient $= 0.36$, $P = 0.003$), but the densitometry readings for the center and posterior layers and total depth did not correlate significantly with the corneal thickness (Fig. 4).

Discussion

In the present investigation, we used a rotating Scheimpflug camera to assess the serial changes of corneal densitometry from before cataract surgery to 7 days after surgery. Our results showed transient increases in densitometry reading after uneventful cataract surgeries and a significant correlation between densitometry readings and corneal thickness. These findings may indicate that subclinical corneal epithelial or stromal edema occurs and causes light scattering shortly after cataract surgery.

Table 1 Changes in BVCA, corneal thickness, and intraocular pressure

	Preoperative	Postoperative		
		Day1	Day3	Day7
BVCA (LogMAR)	0.332 ± 0.382	0.050 ± 0.186*		0.008 ± 0.151*
Central corneal thickness (μm)	550.1 ± 32.4	588.3 ± 53.9**	567.8 ± 29.9	561.1 ± 31.9
Intraocular pressure(mmHg)	14.2 ± 2.6	13.2 ± 3.1	11.5 ± 3.1*	12.0 ± 2.5*

BCVA best corrected visual acuity
*$p < 0.05$, **$p < 0.01$ versus preoperative, by Friedman's test

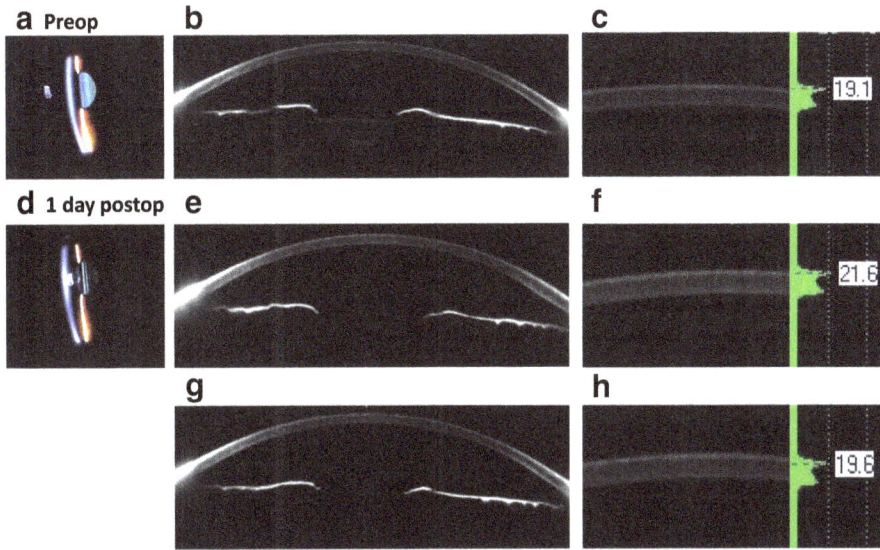

Fig. 2 Representative slit-lamp photographs (left), Scheimpflug images (center), and densitometry readings (right) of central cornea before cataract surgery (**a**) and on day 1 (**b**) and day 3 after surgery (**c**). Slit-lap examination reveals no abnormal finding before (**a**) and 1 day after surgery (**b**). Scheimpflug images show minimal opacity on day 1 and day 3 after surgery. Densitometry score is 19.1 before cataract surgery (**a**), increases to 21.6 on day 1 (**b**) and recovers to 19.6 on day 3 after surgery (**c**)

In this study, densitometry readings in the anterior layer were higher than that in the posterior layer. A similar tendency was also reported in previous investigations using confocal microscopy [15] or scatterometer [16]. According to previous evaluations using atomic force microscopy [17] and second harmonic generation microscopy [18, 19], collagen fibers are interwoven in three dimensions and adhere densely to Bowman's layer and fiber density is less dense in the anterior stroma than in the posterior stroma in healthy cornea [18]. The

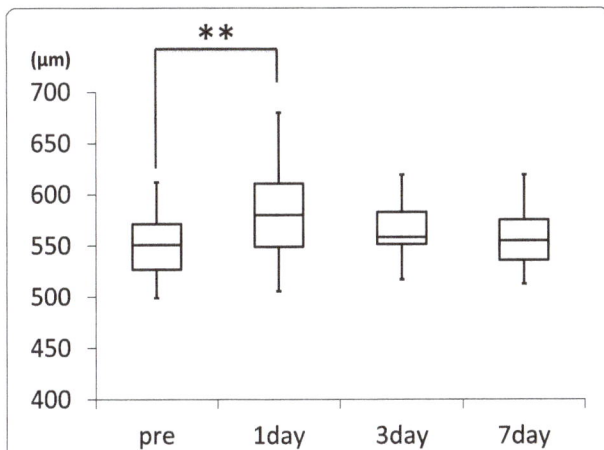

Fig. 3 Changes in central corneal thickness. Total corneal thickness at the corneal apex is 549.1 ± 32.7 μm before surgery and increases to 582.7 ± 46.3 μm on day 1 after surgery ($P = 0.001$ vs. preoperative). Corneal thickness recovers to 566.4 ± 29.7 μm on day 3 ($P = 0.097$ vs. preoperative) and 559.4 ± 32.4 μm on day 7 ($P = 0.400$ vs. preoperative) after surgery

difference in densitometry readings between anterior and posterior corneal layer may reflect the difference in stromal collagen structure between different layers.

Ní Dhubhghaill et al. [20] evaluated corneal densitometry in normal Caucasian eyes using Scheimpflug camera. According to their study, densitometry reading in the central 2 mm zone in the anterior layer (up to 120 μm in depth) was 22.87 ± 2.91, and densitometry reading in the central 2 mm zone for total depth was 16.76 ± 1.87. In the present study, however, the densitometry reading in the central 2 mm zone was 18.1 ± 1.8 in the anterior layer, and was 14.0 ± 1.7 for total corneal depth. We speculate that the difference in scores may reflect racial difference, because all patients enrolled in our study were Asian. Corneal thickness was reported to differ between races, and the central corneal thickness is thicker in Caucasian eyes compared to Asian eyes [21–24]. Age also changes the value of densitometry. The densitometry readings of central and posterior layer increased with age but not anterior layer [25]. According to their study, densitometry reading of 60–69 years old in the central 2 mm zone in the anterior layer was 18.31, center was 15.21, posterior was 12.23 and total depth was 15.37 in Caucasian eyes. In this study, light scattering may increase when the number of corneal collagen fibers is larger, possibly resulting in increase in densitometry reading. It is reported that the ability to detect changes in backscatter was superior with Scheimpflug camera to confocal microscopy [26].

Another possibility is that we excluded eyes with corneal surface diseases including dry eye and superficial

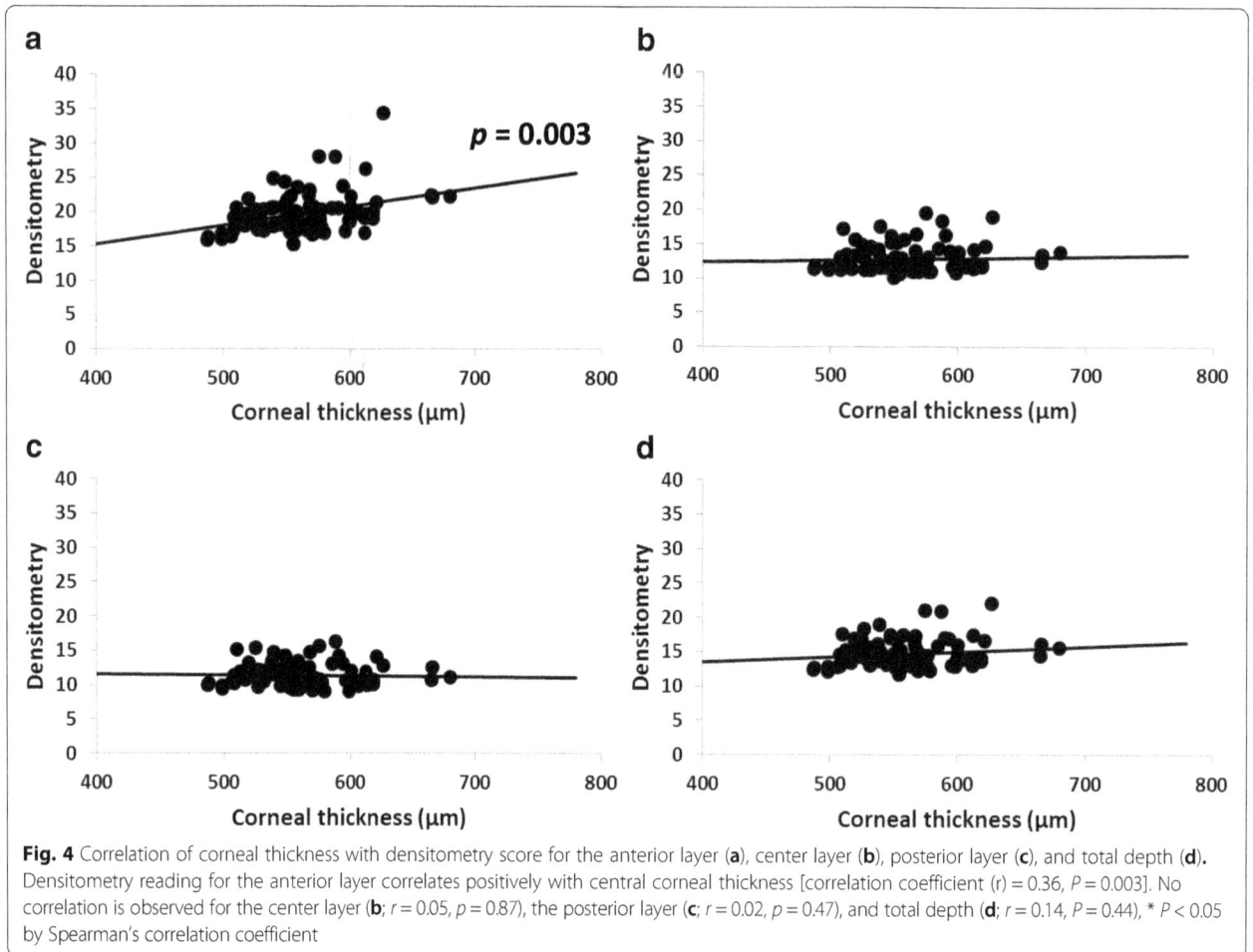

Fig. 4 Correlation of corneal thickness with densitometry score for the anterior layer (**a**), center layer (**b**), posterior layer (**c**), and total depth (**d**). Densitometry reading for the anterior layer correlates positively with central corneal thickness [correlation coefficient (r) = 0.36, $P = 0.003$]. No correlation is observed for the center layer (**b**; $r = 0.05$, $p = 0.87$), the posterior layer (**c**; $r = 0.02$, $p = 0.47$), and total depth (**d**; $r = 0.14$, $P = 0.44$), * $P < 0.05$ by Spearman's correlation coefficient

punctate keratopathy both before and after the surgery in the present investigation. Such ocular surface distintegrity could cause light scattering and possibly influence the densitometry readings. The densitometry readings might increase due to corneal epithelial damage, while increase of densitometry readings in the anterior layer cannot distinguish the light scattering of the epithelial or superficial stromal layer. There are some reports that some drugs using during surgery caused corneal epithelial damage. 5% povidone iodine may cause corneal epithelial damage [27] and 10% povidone iodine with presurgical skin antiseptics are toxic for cornea [28]. We used 1% povidone iodine the conjunctiva and cornea within the operative field, but 10% povidone iodine was used with skin. We cannot deny possibility that 10% povidone iodine has exposed to the cornea and affected densitometry readings. Topical anesthesia may also corneal epithelial damage. When the cornea becomes edematous, intra- and inter-cellular fluid accumulation occurs in the epithelial layer, and is followed by subsequent accumulation of fluid within and between the stromal lamellae within the underneath stroma. These edematous changes of epithelial

and underneath stromal structure may cause light scattering, which is partially reflected by the increase in densitometry reading.

The correlation between corneal thickness and light scattering of the cornea was first reported in 1982 by Olsen [29], who applied slit-lamp fluorophotometry to measure light scattering of the whole cornea in eyes that underwent cataract surgery within 1 week prior to study. He speculated that light scattering increases sharply as the tissue swells; the space between collagen fibrils becomes less regular, thereby increasing the amount of light scattered. These findings may support our theory that the elevation of densitometry reading is due to increase in light scattering caused by corneal epithelial and stromal edema, although the surgical procedure used in Olsen's study was supposed to be extracapsular extraction, which is more invasive than the small incision phacoemulsification used in the present study.

Interestingly, corneal edema occurred shortly after surgery not only around the incision but also in central cornea. However, the edema was transient and improved quickly in subsequent several days. The densitometry readings in the central 2 mm zone improved faster than in the surrounding 2–6 mm zone, probably reflecting centripetal processes of wound healing [30, 31] and endothelial cell migration [32]. Further investigations on the topographical changes of densitometry reading and corneal edema may contribute to elucidate the mechanisms of water distribution and its relation with wound healing in the cornea.

This study had some limitations. First, we did not use confocal microscopy in this study, so we cannot confirm more detailed corneal change. Second, we did not assessed quality of vision such as glare, halos and blurring. None of the patients complained symptoms after the surgery, but there is a possibility that patient did not feel symptoms the several days after surgery. Third, corneal densitometry readings of posterior segment are influenced from the anterior corneal haze. As the anterior densitometry readings increases, the values of central and posterior densitometry readings may be inaccurate. In this study, there was no patient who had very high densitometry readings compared to previous reports such as corneal surgery [8–11], densitometry readings of anterior segment may influence the readings of central and posterior segment.

Conclusions

In summary, densitometry using the Scheimpflug device for measuring corneal scattering may be a useful tool to detect minimal subclinical corneal edema usually undetectable by slit-lamp examination. There is a possibility that densitometry helps to detect subtle edema of the cornea particularly in experimental studies.

Additional file

Additional file 1: Corneal densitometry readings pre and postoperative surgery. Densitometry readings in the central 2 mm zone within the anterior layer before and postoperative on day 1, day 3 and day 7 were 18.1 ± 1.8, 21.3 ± 3.8, 19.9 ± 2.5, 19.4 ± 1.6. Densitometry readings in the 2–6 mm annulus within the anterior layer before and postoperative on day 1, day 3 and day 7 were 19.1 ± 4.7, 22.1 ± 7.4, 20.7 ± 4.6, 21.3 ± 4.9. Densitometry readings in the central 2 mm zone within the center layer before and postoperative on day 1, day 3 and day 7 were 12.2 ± 1.5, 13.7 ± 2.6, 12.8 ± 1.5, 13.0 ± 1.8. Densitometry readings in the 2–6 mm annulus within the center layer before and postoperative on day 1, day 3 and day 7 were 12.6 ± 2.0, 14.2 ± 3.8, 13.1 ± 1.8, 13.5 ± 2.1. Densitometry readings in the central 2 mm zone within the posterior layer before and postoperative on day 1, day 3 and day 7 were 10.8 ± 1.3, 12.4 ± 2.9, 11.2 ± 1.4, 11.4 ± 1.5. Densitometry readings in the 2–6 mm annulus within the posterior layer before and postoperative on day 1, day 3 and day 7 were 11.3 ± 1.6, 12.3 ± 2.4, 11.5 ± 1.5, 11.9 ± 1.7. Densitometry readings in the central 2 mm zone before and postoperative on day 1, day 3 and day 7 were 14.0 ± 1.7, 15.7 ± 2.8, 14.6 ± 1.6, 14.8 ± 1.6. Densitometry readings in the 2–6 mm annulus before and postoperative on day 1, day 3 and day 7 were 14.6 ± 2.8, 16.4 ± 4.3, 15.1 ± 2.3, 15.6 ± 2.6. (DOCX 82 kb)

Abbreviation
BCVA: Best corrected visual acuity

Acknowledgements
The authors thank to Kanako Tonegawa for her assistance for helping medical examination.

Funding
No funding was received by any of the authors for the writing of this manuscript.

Authors' contributions
All authors made significant contribution for the design of the study. SI drafted the manuscript and performed the literature review and participated in information gathering and editing. NK and MT made contributions to analysis and interpretation of data. NK and MT conceived the idea and supervised writing of the case report. NK revised this manuscript critically for important intellectual content. MT made substantial contributions to conception and design. All authors read and approved the final manuscript.

Consent for publication
Not applicable.

Competing interests
The authors declare that they have no competing interests.

References
1. Smith GT, Brown NA, Shun-Shin GA. Light scatter from the central human cornea. Eye (Lond). 1990;4(4):584–8.
2. Ha BJ, Kim TI, Choi SI, Stulting RD, Lee DH, Kim EK, et al. Mitomycin C does not inhibit exacerbation of granular Corneal dystrophy type ii induced by refractive surface ablation. Cornea. 2010;29:490–6.
3. Elflein HM, Hofherr T, Berisha-Ramadani F, Weyer V, Lampe C, Pitz S, et al. Measuring Corneal clouding in patients suffering from Mucopolysaccharidosis with the Pentacam densitometry Programme. Br J Ophthalmol. 2013;97:829–33.
4. Greenstein SA, Fry KL, Bhatt J, Hersh PS. Natural history of Corneal haze after collagen crosslinking for keratoconus and Corneal ectasia: Scheimpflug and biomicroscopic analysis. J Cataract Refract Surg. 2010;36:2105–14.
5. Gutierrez R, Lopez I, Villa-Collar C, Gonzalez-Meijome JM. Corneal transparency after cross-linking for keratoconus: 1-year follow-up. J Refract Surg. 2012;28:781–6.
6. Rozema JJ, Trau R, Verbruggen KH, Tassignon MJ. Backscattered light from the cornea before and after laser-assisted subepithelial keratectomy for myopia. J Cataract Refract Surg. 2011;37:1648–54.
7. Fares U, Otri AM, Al-Aqaba MA, Faraj L, Dua HS. Wavefront-optimized excimer laser in situ Keratomileusis for myopia and myopic astigmatism: refractive outcomes and Corneal densitometry. J Cataract Refract Surg. 2012;38:2131–8.
8. Takacs AI, Mihaltz K, Nagy ZZ. Corneal density with the Pentacam after photorefractive keratectomy. J Refract Surg. 2011;27:269–77.
9. Cennamo G, Forte R, Aufiero B, La Rana A. Computerized Scheimpflug densitometry as a measure of Corneal optical density after excimer laser refractive surgery in myopic eyes. J Cataract Refract Surg. 2011;37:1502–6.
10. Koh S, Maeda N, Nakagawa T, Nishida K. Quality of vision in eyes after selective lamellar Keratoplasty. Cornea. 2012;31(Suppl 1):S45–9.

11. Bhatt UK, Fares U, Rahman I, Said DG, Maharajan SV, Dua HS. Outcomes of deep anterior lamellar Keratoplasty following successful and failed 'Big bubble. Br J Ophthalmol. 2012;96:564–9.

12. Otti AM, Fares U, Al-Aqaba MA, Dua HS. Corneal densitometry as an Indicator of Corneal health. Ophthalmology. 2012;119:501–8.

13. Patel SV, Baratz KH, Hodge DO, Maquire LJ, Mclaren JW. The effect of Corneal light scatter on vision after Descemet stripping with endothelial Keratoplasty. Arch Ophthalmol. 2009;127:153–60.

14. Patel SV, McLaren JW, Hodge DO, Bourne WM. The effect of Corneal light scatter on vision after penetrating Keratoplasty. Am J Ophthalmol. 2008;146:913–9.

15. Hillenaar T, Cals RH, Eilers PH, Wubbels RJ, van Cleynenbreugel H, Remeijer L. Normative database for Corneal backscatter analysis by in vivo confocal microscopy. Invest Ophthalmol Vis Sci. 2011;52:7274–81.

16. Patel SV, Winter EJ, McLaren JW, Bourne WM. Objective measurement of backscattered light from the anterior and posterior cornea in vivo. Invest Ophthalmol Vis Sci. 2007;48:166–72.

17. Meek KM, Corneal FNJ. Scleral collagens--a Microscopist's perspective. Micron. 2001;32:261–72.

18. Morishige N, Takagi Y, Chikama T, Takahara A, Nishida T. Three-dimensional analysis of collagen lamellae in the anterior stroma of the human cornea visualized by second harmonic generation imaging microscopy. Invest Ophthalmol Vis Sci. 2011;52:911–5.

19. Ruberti JW, Roy AS, Roberts CJ. Corneal Biomechanics and Biomaterials. Annu Rev Biomed Eng. 2011;13:269–95.

20. Ni Dhubhghaill S, Rozema JJ, Jongenelen S, Ruiz Hidalgo I, Zakaria N, Tassignon MJ. Normative values for Corneal densitometry analysis by Scheimpflug optical assessment. Invest Ophthalmol Vis Sci. 2014;55:162–8.

21. Semes L, Shaikh A, McGwin G, Bartlett JD. The relationship among race, Iris color, central Corneal Thickness, and Intraocular Pressure. Optom Vis Sci. 2006;83:512–5.

22. Muir KW, Duncan L, Enyedi LB, Freedman SF. Central Corneal Thickness in children: racial differences (black vs. white) and correlation with measured intraocular pressure. J Glaucoma. 2006;15:520–3.

23. Tomidokoro A, Araie M, Iwase A. Corneal Thickness and Relating factors in a population-based study in Japan: the Tajimi study. Am J Ophthalmol. 2007; 144:152–4.

24. Suzuki S, Suzuki Y, Iwase A, Araie M. Corneal Thickness in an Ophthalmologically Normal Japanese population. Ophthalmology. 2005;112:1327–36.

25. Alzahrani K, Carley F, Brahma A, Morley D, Hillarby MC. Corneal clarity measurements in healthy volunteers across different age groups: observational study. Medicine (Baltimore). 2017;96:e8563.

26. Mclaren JW, Wacker K, Kane KM, Patel SV. Measuring Corneal haze by using Scheimpflug photography and confocal microscopy. Cornea. 2016; 57:227–35.

27. Ridder WH 3rd, Oquindo C, Dhamdhere K, Burke J. Effect of povidone iodine 5% on the cornea, vision, and subjective comfort. Optom Vis Sci. 2017;94:732–41.

28. Mac Rae SM, Brown B, Edelhauser HF. The corneal toxicity of presurgical skin antiseptics. Am J Ophthalmol. 1984;97:221–32.

29. Olsen T. Light scattering from the human cornea. Invest Ophthalmol Vis Sci. 1982;23:81–6.

30. Mort RL, Ramaesh T, Kleinjan DA, Morley SD, West JD. Mosaic analysis of stem cell function and wound healing in the mouse Corneal epithelium. BMC Dev Biol. 2009;9:4.

31. Chang CY, Green CR, McGhee CN, Sherwin T. Acute wound healing in the human central Corneal epithelium appears to be independent of Limbal stem cell influence. Invest Ophthalmol Vis Sci. 2008;49:5279–86.

32. He Z, Campolmi N, Gain P, Ha Thi BM, Dumollard JM, Thuret G, et al. Revisited microanatomy of the Corneal endothelial periphery: new evidence for continuous centripetal migration of endothelial cells in humans. Stem Cells. 2012;30:2523–34.

24

Femtosecond laser-assisted cataract surgery with implantation of a diffractive trifocal intraocular lens after laser in situ keratomileusis

Wei Wang, Shuang Ni, Xi Li, Xiang Chen, Yanan Zhu and Wen Xu[*]

Abstract

Background: We report for the first time, a case of femtosecond laser-assisted cataract surgery (FLACS) with implantation of a diffractive trifocal intraocular lens (IOL) after laser in situ keratomileusis (LASIK).

Case presentation: A 60-year-old man underwent FLACS uneventfully 15 years after myopic LASIK. An AT Lisa tri 839MP IOL was implanted with the expectation of spectacle independence. The Haigis-L formula was chosen for calculation of the IOL power and it provided reliable results. Three months postoperatively, the uncorrected visual acuities were 0.00 logMAR for distance, 0.10 logMAR for intermediate, and 0.10 logMAR for near.

Conclusions: This case suggested that FLACS presents a feasible surgical technique for post-LASIK eyes and that implantation of trifocal IOL can achieve good visual performance in strictly selected cases after myopic LASIK.

Keywords: Femtosecond laser, Cataract surgery, Trifocal intraocular lens, Laser in situ keratomileusis

Background

There are a growing number of patients who wish to be spectacle independent after cataract surgery, and this includes some of the millions of people worldwide who have undergone laser in situ keratomileusis (LASIK). Ophthalmologists will encounter many cataract cases that have had previous LASIK surgery and they should have the knowledge to deal with these cases efficiently to achieve the best possible visual and refractive outcomes [1]. Femtosecond laser–assisted cataract surgery (FLACS) has become increasingly more common for its many advantages offered [2]. At the same time, various kinds of multifunctional intraocular lens (IOL) were designed [3] to provide functional visual restoration after cataract surgery. Nowadays, the combination of FLACS with multifocal IOLs has come to the cutting edge of cataract surgery. However, few studies had shed light on whether post-LASIK patients would benefit from this technique combo. Here we report a case of FLACS with the implantation of a diffractive trifocal IOL after LASIK.

Case presentation

A 60-year-old man was diagnosed with nuclear cataract in his right eye about 15 years after myopic LASIK surgery. His corrected distance visual acuity (CDVA) of the right eye was 0.52 logMAR with the refraction of −4.50/− 0.75*29. He asked for a FLACS and desired spectacle independence after the IOL implantation. Corneal topography (Pentacam, Oculus Optikgerate GmbH, Wetzlar, Germany) showed a uniform, well-centered corneal flap (Fig. 1a, b), with a total corneal astigmatism of 0.9D, and a corneal irregular astigmatism of 0.115 μm. Besides, the 6 mm zone corneal spherical aberration (SA) was 0.392 μm while the angle kappa was 0.15. After a series of thorough assessments, we decided to implant a multifocal IOL with negative SA. For IOL power calculations, the standard IOLMaster (Carl Zeiss Meditec,Jena, Germany) biometry was performed and the Haigis-L formula was chosen to determine an IOL power of +23D for emmetropia. A steep

---

* Correspondence: xuwen2003@zju.edu.cn
Eye Center of the 2nd Affiliated Hospital, School of Medicine, Zhejiang University, No.88 Jiefang Road, Hangzhou, China

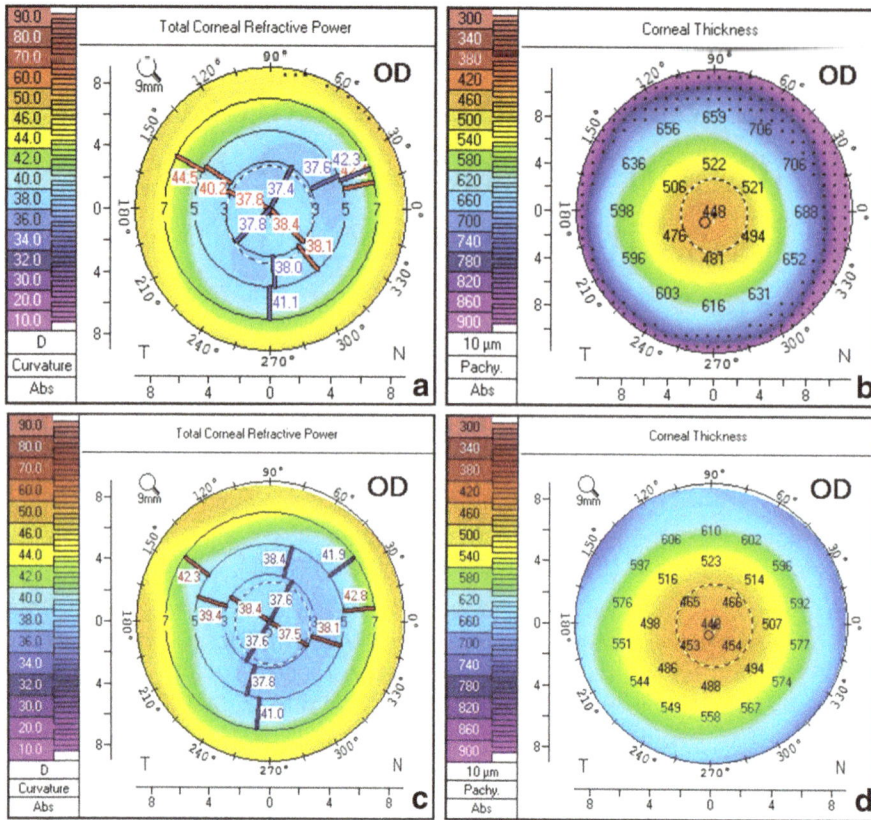

Fig. 1 Corneal topography preoperatively (**a**, **b**) and at 3 months postoperatively (**c**, **d**)

merdian corneal incision was designed at 140 degree according to the Pentacam results.

The LenSx laser system (LenSx Laser; Alcon Laboratories, Inc., Fort Worth,TX, USA) was used to perform the surgery. After the patient's eye was properly docked to the system, the arc cuts of the primary and side port incision were adjusted towards the limbus, anterior to the conjunctival vascular arcades, under the guided of the LenSx real-time imaging system. A 2.0 mm primary corneal incision (Fig. 2a),

a 1.0 mm side port incision and a 5.0 mm capsulotomy were created by the laser. Nuclear prefragmention was performed to obtain 6 pieces in a cross pattern (Fig. 2b). Then phacoemulsification was proceeded in a standard stop-and-chop manner with the Stellaris system (Bausch + Lomb Laboratories, Rochester, NY, USA), and an AT Lisa tri 839MP IOL (Carl Zeiss Meditec AG) was implanted right afterwards. All surgical procedures were uneventful. The patient was instructed to apply topical

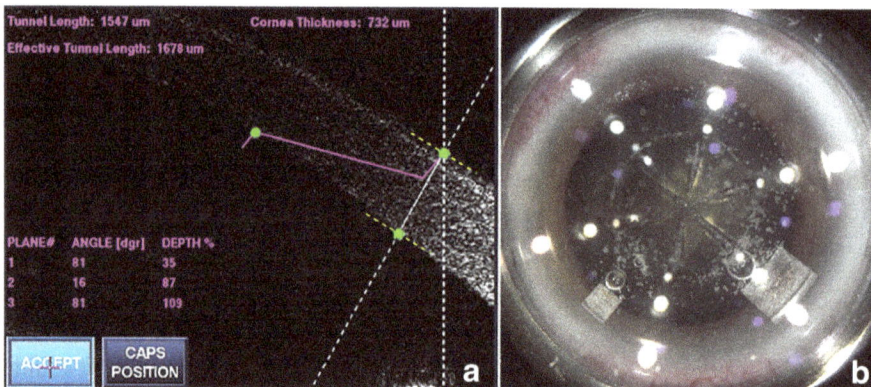

Fig. 2 a AS-OCT image depicts the architecture of clear corneal incision. **b** Screenshot taken after femtosecond laser treatment completed. The primary corneal incision was made at 140 degree, consistent with the steep merdian axis

dexamethasone tobramycin for 2 weeks and pranoprofen for 1 month postoperatively.

Anterior segment optical coherence tomography (AS-OCT, Carl Zeiss Meditec) showed a smooth corneal flap 1 week after FLACS (Fig. 3a). The distance from the external wound opening to the corneal flap edge was 0.15 mm. At 3 months postoperatively, the IOL was well centered in the capsule (Fig. 3b). Pentacam showed a uniform corneal flap (Fig. 1c, d) with slightly decreased total corneal astigmatism and corneal SA (Table 1). Uncorrected visual acuitis were 0.00 LogMAR for distance, 0.10 LogMAR for intermediate at 80 cm, 0.10 LogMAR for near at 40 cm. The defocus curve (Fig. 3c) showed an optimal visual acuity at -3D apart from 0D, but maintained a functional range of visual acuity across from 0D to – 3.5D with visual acuity no less than 0.22 logMAR. Results of ocular aberrations (OPD Scan, Nidek Co., Ltd.) for 5 mm diameter pupils showed 0.831um of high order aberration (HOA), 0.648um of coma, 0.327um of trefoil, 0.119um of tetrafoil, and 0.311um of SA. Contrast sensitivity (CS, CSV-1000, Vector Vision, Greenville, OH) at 4 spatial frequencies (A: 3 cpd, B: 6 cpd, C:12 cpd and D:18 cpd) under both mesopic (3 cd/m^2) and photopic (85 cd/m^2) conditions were at a relatively low level within the normal range (Fig. 4). Despite a mild halo, the patient was very satisfied with his vision.

Discussion

The application of femtosecond laser (FSL) in cataract surgery improves the precision of corneal incision location and extent. FSL also provides a precise and well-centered capsulotomy which contributes to the proper position of the IOL that may be related to refractive outcome improvements [4]. In this patient, the computer-controlled accurate steep merdian incision successfully decreased the total corneal astigmatism and ensured visual outcomes of this patient. Well-centered trifocal IOL with a 360° overlapping capsular edge could reduce the incidence of myopization and HOAs changes. In post-LASIK eyes, postoperative corneal edema after cataract surgery may accumulate in the flap interface and the flap itself, causing early transient central corneal steepening and consequent myopic shift that could disappear after the corneal edema resolves [1]. However, the incidence of this complication could be reduced by FSL assisted lens fragmentation, which helps reduce phacoemulsification energy requirements, protect corneal endothelial cells, and thus shorten the recovery period and improve visual outcomes [5].

As for safety, although vacuum suction during FLACS can lead to an increase of the intraocular pressure, it was proved to be feasible for those with previous corneal surgeries, such as radial keratotomy [6] or even penetrating keratoplasty [7]. In this patient, the docking and suction procession did not have any negative effect on the corneal flap, and no intraoperative complications were observed throughout the surgery either. However, the AS-OCT showed a very short distance between the external wound opening and the corneal flap edge postoperatively. Zhu et al. found that laser corneal incisions

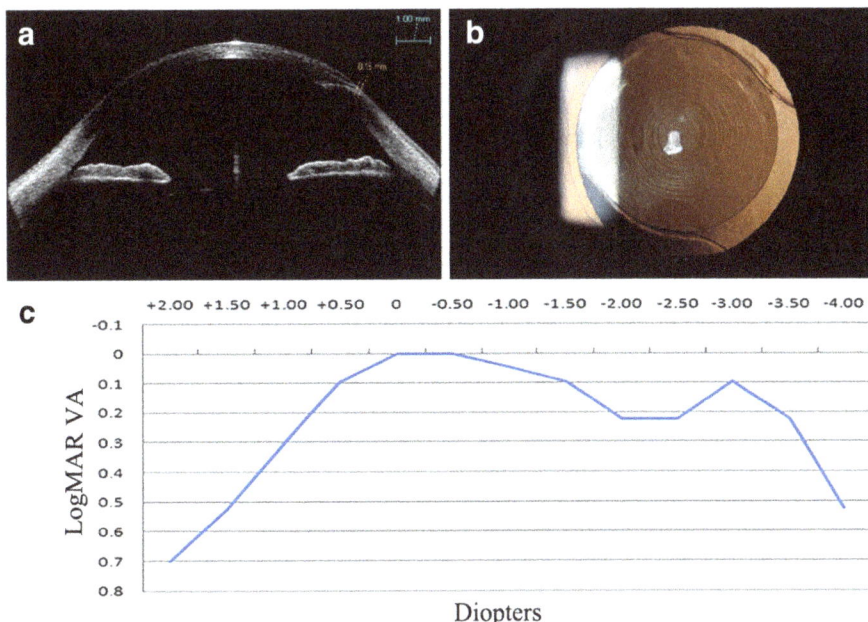

Fig. 3 a AS-OCT taken at 1 week postoperatively. The distance from the external wound opening to the corneal flap edge was 0.15 mm. Bar,1 mm. **b** Slitlamp examination showed well centered IOL with a 360° overlapping capsular edge at 3 months postoperatively. **c** Defocus curve at 3 months postoperatively

Table 1 Preoperative and postoperative pentacam measurements

	Preoperative	Postoperative	
		1 week	3 months
K1	37.5@49.6	37.2@56.2	37.7@69.2
K2	38.4@139.6	37.6@146.2	38.2@159.2
Total Astig(D)	0.9	0.4	0.5
SA at 6 mm zone(um)	0.392	0.305	0.375
Irregular astig(um)	0.115	0.238	0.161

Pentacam showed slightly decreased postoperative total corneal astigmatism and corneal SA. Besides, there was only a slight change in astigmatism and axial direction at 3 months compared to that of 1 week postoperative

were closer to the center of the cornea than manual corneal incisions, and they thought this may be related to the possible inaccuracy or uncertainty in corneal incision positioning of the LenSx machine [8]. So here we have to point out that a laser-assisted corneal incision may increase the risk of intersection between the incision and the corneal flap. Future studies should be conducted to confirm this hypothesis.

Post-LASIK patients are often focusing on better visual quality and they are keen to take off spectacles, even after developing cataract. A few studies have reported that the implantation of multifocal IOLs in patients who underwent previous myopic LASIK provided good visual acuities for distance and near range [9]. The AT LISA tri839MP, a diffractive trifocal preloaded IOL with an asphericity of – 0.18, provides a near addition (add) of + 3.33 D and an intermediate add of + 1.66D. It was developed to overcome the photic phenomena and the poor level of intermediate vision of traditional multifocal IOLs [10]. It is well known that laser refractive surgery would modify the corneal shape and induce positive spherical aberration (SA) while correcting myopia [11]. The negative SA of AT LISA tri839MP could partially compensate SA and help retain good mesopic distance vision.

Furthermore, thorough preoperative evaluation was fundamental for the success of this operation. The inclusion criteria for multifocal IOL implantation in our eye center are corneal astigmatism of no more than 1.25D, root mean square (RMS) of corneal HOAs within 6.0 mm zone no more than 0.50 mm, and kappa angle no more than 0.29. The criteria are consistent with those in the studies of Monaco [12] and Mojzis [9]. In this case, the patient met all the above requirements despite of his myopic LASIK history. In this case, we propose that post-LASIK eye necessitates a uniform, well-centered and closely-attached corneal flap for multifocal IOL implantation. Another noticeable situation is the possible aggravation of dry eye after FLACS [13], since that LASIK procedure had already potentiate the instability of tear film. Therefore, careful evaluation of dry eye and timely treatment before surgery is recommended.

IOL power calculation remains one of the most difficult parts for cataract operation after refractive surgery. In Wong's study, the Asian eyes with previous myopic LASIK or photorefractive keratectomy (PRK) had cataract surgeries with IOL power calculated by 4 formulas. Haigis-L formula turned out to have the highest percentage of cases that achieved the refraction of targeted SE ±0.50 D and SE ±1.00 D [14]. A meta-analysis by Chen et al. also concluded that the clinical inquiry was inaccurate in predicting postoperative refraction as compared to the Haigis-L formula [15]. In this case, the Haigis-L formula again proved to be reliable to attain emmetropia.

Conclusion

In conclusion, our report shows that, for cataract patients with previous LASIK, FLACS with implantation of the AT LISA tri839MP can be an effective option to obtain spectacle independence.

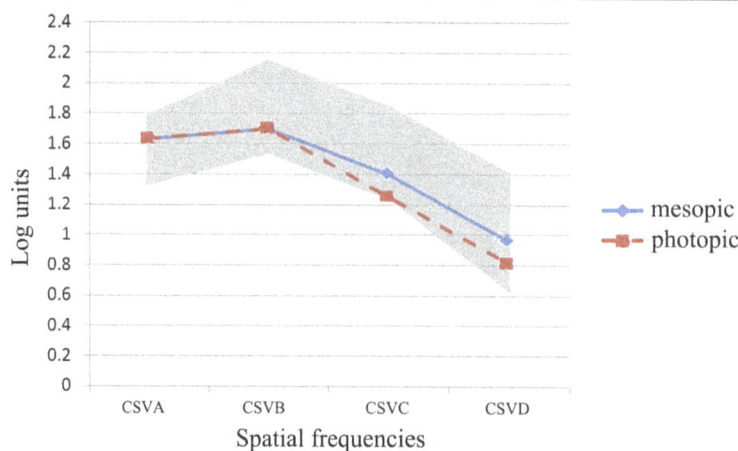

Fig. 4 Contrast sensitivity under mesopic and photopic conditions at 3 months postoperatively. Grey area shows the normal range of contrast sensitivity among 56–75 year-old people

Abbreviations
AS-OCT: Anterior segment optical coherence tomography; CDVA: Corrected distance visual acuity; CS: Contrast sensitivity; FLACS: Femtosecond laser-assisted cataract surgery; FSL: Femtosecond laser; HOAs: Higher-order aberrations; IOL: Intraocular lens; LASIK: Laser in situ keratomileusis; PRK: Photorefractive keratectomy; SA: Spherical aberration; VA: Visual acuity

Funding
This work was supported by the National Natural Science Foundation of China (81600716), the Key Research and Development Plan of Zhejiang Province Science and Technology Hall (2017C03046), General Scientific Research Project of Zhejiang Province Education Department (Y201738741).

Authors' contributions
All authors conceived of and designed the study. All authors were involved in the data analysis. WW and NS did the patient follow-up, collected data and drafted the article. LX and CX reviewed the literature. ZYN revised the manuscript. XW did the surgery and drafted the article. All authors reviewed the manuscript. All authors read and approved the final manuscript.

Consent for publication
Written informed consent was obtained from the patient for publication of this case report and any accompanying images. A copy of the written consent is available for review by the Editor of this journal.

Competing interests
The authors declare that they have no competing interests.

References
1. Alio JL, Abdelghany AA, Abdou AA, Maldonado MJ. Cataract surgery on the previous corneal refractive surgery patient. Surv Ophthalmol. 2016;61(6): 769–77.
2. Grewal DS, Schultz T, Basti S, Dick HB. Femtosecond laser-assisted cataract surgery–current status and future directions. Surv Ophthalmol. 2016;61(2): 103–31.
3. de Vries NE, Nuijts RM. Multifocal intraocular lenses in cataract surgery: literature review of benefits and side effects. J Cataract Refract Surg. 2013;39(2):268–78.
4. Nagy ZZ, McAlinden C. Femtosecond laser cataract surgery. Eye Vis. 2015;2:11.
5. Chen X, Yu Y, Song X, Zhu Y, Wang W, Yao K. Clinical outcomes of femtosecond laser-assisted cataract surgery versus conventional phacoemulsification surgery for hard nuclear cataracts. J Cataract Refract Surg. 2017;43(4):486–91.
6. Noristani R, Schultz T, Dick HB. Femtosecond laser-assisted cataract surgery after radial keratotomy. J Refract Surg. 2016;32(6):426–8.
7. Cao D, Wang S, Wang Y. Femtosecond laser-assisted cataract surgery after penetrating keratoplasty: a case report. BMC Ophthalmol. 2017;17(1)
8. Zhu S, Qu N, Wang W, Zhu Y, Shentu X, Chen P, Xu W, Yao K. Morphologic features and surgically induced astigmatism of femtosecond laser versus manual clear corneal incisions. J Cataract Refract Surg. 2017;43(11):1430–5.
9. Chang JS, Ng JC, Chan VK, Law AK. Visual outcomes, quality of vision, and quality of life of diffractive multifocal intraocular Lens implantation after myopic laser in situ Keratomileusis: a prospective, observational case series. J Ophthalmol. 2017;2017:6459504.
10. Mojzis P, Majerova K, Hrckova L, Pinero DP. Implantation of a diffractive trifocal intraocular lens: one-year follow-up. J Cataract Refract Surg. 2015;41(8):1623–30.
11. Iijima K, Kamiya K, Shimizu K, Igarashi A, Komatsu M. Demographics of patients having cataract surgery after laser in situ keratomileusis. J Cataract Refract Surg. 2015;41(2):334–8.
12. Monaco G, Gari M, Di Censo F, Poscia A, Ruggi G, Scialdone A. Visual performance after bilateral implantation of 2 new presbyopia-correcting intraocular lenses: trifocal versus extended range of vision. J Cataract Refract Surg. 2017;43(6):737–47.
13. Yu YH, Hua HX, Wu MH, Yu YB, Yu WS, Lai KR, Yao K. Evaluation of dry eye after femtosecond laser-assisted cataract surgery. J Cataract Refract Surg. 2015;41(12):2614–23.
14. Wong CW, Yuen L, Tseng P, Han DC. Outcomes of the Haigis-L formula for calculating intraocular lens power in Asian eyes after refractive surgery. J Cataract Refract Surg. 2015;41(3):607–12.
15. Chen X, Yuan F, Wu L. Metaanalysis of intraocular lens power calculation after laser refractive surgery in myopic eyes. J Cataract Refract Surg. 2016;42(1):163–70.

25

Antidepressants use and risk of cataract development

Yana Fu[1], Qi Dai[1]* ⓘ, Liwei Zhu[2] and Shuangqing Wu[2]

Abstract

Background: Epidemiological studies suggest that antidepressants use may increase the risk of cataract, but the results are inconclusive. We aimed to examine this association by performing a systematic review and meta-analysis.

Methods: Relevant studies were identified by searching PubMed and Web of Science databases through June 2017. We included studies that reported risk estimates for the association between antidepressants use and cataract risk. A random-effects model was used to calculate the summary odds ratio (OR) with its 95% confidence interval (CI).

Results: We identified seven studies of antidepressants use and risk of cataract involving 447,672 cases and 1,510,391 controls. Overall, the combined ORs (95% CIs) of cataract for selective serotonin reuptake inhibitors (SSRIs), serotonin noradrenalin reuptake inhibitors (SNRIs), and tricyclic antidepressants (TCAs) were 1.12 (1.06–1.19), 1.13 (1.04–1.24), and 1.19 (1.11–1.28), respectively. A certain degree of heterogeneity was observed across studies ($P < 0.001$, $I^2 = 92.2\%$ for SSRIs, $P = 0.026$, $I^2 = 67.5\%$ for SNRIs, and $P = 0.092$, $I^2 = 58.0\%$ for TCAs).

Conclusion: This meta-analysis provides evidence of a significant positive association between antidepressants use and risk of cataract. Because of the heterogeneity and limited eligible studies, further prospective studies are warranted to confirm the preliminary findings of our study.

Keywords: Antidepressants, Cataract, Meta-analysis, Risk

Background

Cataract is defined as partial or complete loss of transparency of the crystalline lens and is considered the primary cause of vision loss worldwide [1]. The high prevalence and incidence of cataract have resulted in a large public health burden. Although the actual mechanism of cataract development remains unclear, several risk factors have been established, including age [2], corticosteroid use [3], hypertension [4], smoking [5], and so on.

Recently, emerging epidemiological studies have focused on the risk of cataract formation of antidepressants. Two population-based studies from Canada [6] and the United States [7] suggested a significant positive association between the use of selective serotonin reuptake inhibitors (SSRIs) and the incidence of cataract.

Beaver Dam Eye study showed a tendency toward an increased risk of cataract in users of amitriptyline, a tricyclic antidepressant (TCA) [8]. On the other hand, Becker et al. [9] failed to find a positive relationship between SSRIs and cataract risk using the UK-based Clinical Practice Research Datalink (CPRD).

Given the inconsistency and conflict of the existing literature and the insufficient statistical power of individual studies, we performed the present meta-analysis based on all eligible epidemiological studies that provided data on the association of antidepressants use with cataract risk.

Methods
Literature search

We performed this meta-analysis in accordance with the Meta-Analysis of Observational Studies in Epidemiology guidelines [10]. A systematic literature search was carried out in PubMed and Web of Science databases through June 2017 by using the following search

* Correspondence: dq@mail.eye.ac.cn
[1]The Eye Hospital of Wenzhou Medical University, 270 Xueyuan West Road, Wenzhou City 325027, Zhejiang Province, People's Republic of China
Full list of author information is available at the end of the article

strategy: ("antidepressant" or "depression" or "selective serotonin reuptake inhibitor" or "SSRI" or "monoaminoxidase inhibitor" or "MAOI" or "tricyclic antidepressant" or "TCA" or "serotonin noradrenalin reuptake inhibitor" or "SNRI" or "serotonin antagonist and reuptake inhibitor" or "SARI" or "norepinephrine dopamine reuptake inhibitor" or "NDRI" or "norepinephrine reuptake inhibitor" or "NRI" or "noradrenergic and specific serotonergic antidepressant" or "NaSSA") and "Cataract", with no restrictions. Cited references of the retrieved articles and reviews were also checked.

Study selection

Studies included in this meta-analysis met the following criteria: 1) had cohort, nested case-control or case-control study design; 2) the exposure of interest was antidepressants use, including SSRIs, TCAs, serotonin noradrenalin reuptake inhibitors (SNRIs), and so on; 3) the endpoint of interest was cataract incidence; and 4) the risk estimate and the corresponding 95% confidence interval (CI) were reported. If multiple studies used the same population, we included the study with the largest sample size.

Data extraction and quality assessment

We extracted the following data using a standardized data-collection form: last name of the first author, publication year, study region, number of cases and controls, method of exposure and endpoint assessment, types of antidepressants, risk estimates from the most fully adjusted model and the corresponding 95% CIs, matched or adjusted potential confounders.

We assessed the quality of individual studies using Newcastle-Ottawa Scale (NOS), a 9-star system which consists of three dimensions: selection (four items), comparability (one item), and exposure/outcome (three items) (http://www.ohri.ca/programs/clinical_epidemiology/oxford.asp). Two authors (QD and YF) independently performed the literature search, study selection, data extraction, and quality assessment. Any disagreements were resolved by consensus.

Statistical analysis

A DerSimonian and Laird random-effects model [11], which considered both within- and between-study variation, was used to calculate the combined estimate of effect size. For studies that separately provided estimated risk estimates for a number of categories of exposure compared with a single reference category, we combined these risk estimates within each study using the method reported by Hamling et al.'s study [12]. Homogeneity across included studies was tested by Q statistics at the $P < 0.10$ level of significance [13]. The I^2 score, a quantitative measure of inconsistency across studies, was also calculated [13]. Potential publication bias was assessed by a visual funnel plot [14]. All analyses were performed by using STATA version 10.0 (StataCorp, College Station, TX). A P value < 0.05 was considered statistically significant, except where otherwise specified.

Results

Literature search and study characteristics

A flow chart showing the study selection process in detail is presented in Fig. 1. Seven studies [6–9, 15–17] were finally included in this meta-analysis. Of these, five studies were performed in North America, one in Europe, and one in Asia. All individual studies were case-control studies, of which four were nested case-

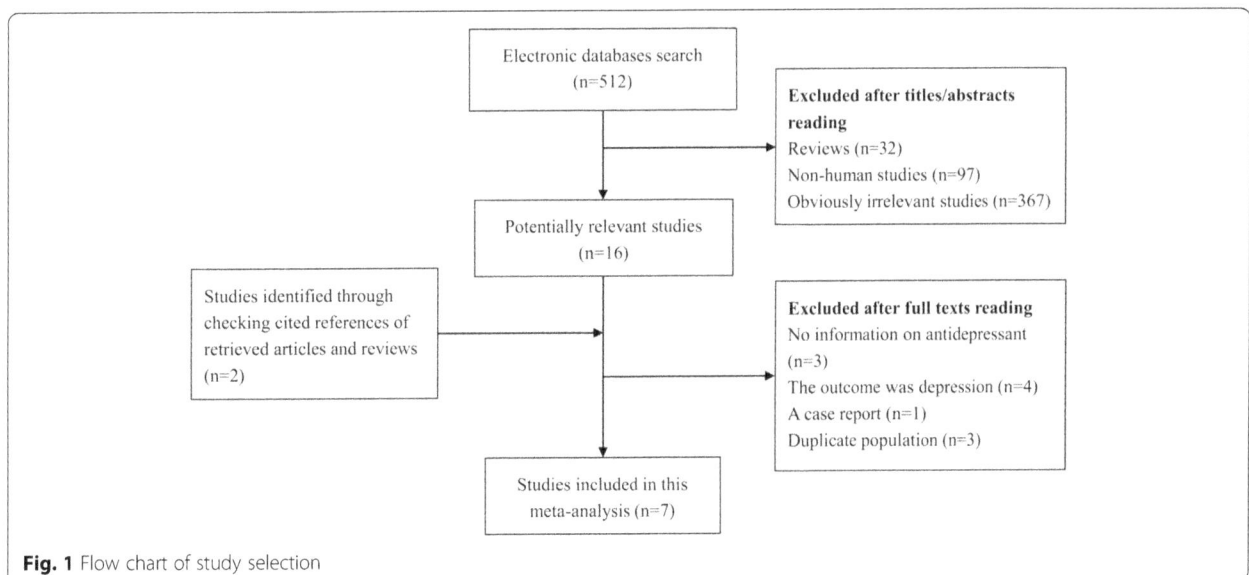

Fig. 1 Flow chart of study selection

Table 1 Main characteristics of the studies included in this meta-analysis

Author	Year	Region	Design	Drug type	No. of cases	No. of controls	Exposure measurement	Outcome ascertainment	NOS	Matched or adjusted variables
Becker et al.	2017	United Kingdom	Case-control	SSRI, TCA, SNRI, and MAOI	206,931	206,931	Computer records (CPRD)	Computer records (CPRD)	8	Calendar time (same index date), age, sex, general practice, and number of years of active history in the CPRD before the index date, BMI, smoking, diabetes hypertension, and systemic steroids
Chou et al.	2017	Taiwan	Nested case-control	SSRI, TCA, and SNRI	7651	6637	Computer records (NHIRD)	Computer records (NHIRD)	8	Age, sex, index date, patient's demographics, mental illness characteristics, propensity score derived from comorbid conditions, and concomitant medications
Erie et al.	2014	United States	Case-control	SSRI	6024	6024	Medical records	Medical records	7	Age, sex, and date of surgery
Wise et al.	2014	United States	Nested case-control	SSRI	45,065	450,650	Medical records (IMS LifeLink database)	Medical records (IMS LifeLink database)	6	Age, time of cohort entry, and follow-up time
Pakzad-Vaezi et al.	2013	Canada	Nested case-control	SSRI	162,501	650,004	Medical records (British Columbia Ministry of Health)	Medical records (British Columbia Ministry of Health)	6	Age, time of cohort entry, and follow-up time
Etminan et al.	2010	Canada	Nested case-control	SSRI and SNRI	18,784	187,840	Medical records	Medical records	6	Age, cohort entry, gender, hypertension, antihypertensive, antidiabetics, statins, and all forms of corticosteroids
Klein et al.	2001	United States	Case-control	TCA	716	2305	Medical history questionnaire	Diagnosed by an ophthalmologist	6	Age and gender

No. number, *NOS* Newcastle-Ottawa Scale, *y* year, *SSRI* selective serotonin reuptake inhibitor, *TCA* tricyclic antidepressant, *SNRI* serotonin noradrenalin reuptake inhibitor, *MAOI* monoaminoxidase inhibitor, *NHIRD* National Health Insurance Research Database, *BMI* body mass index, *CPRD* Clinical Practice Research Datalink

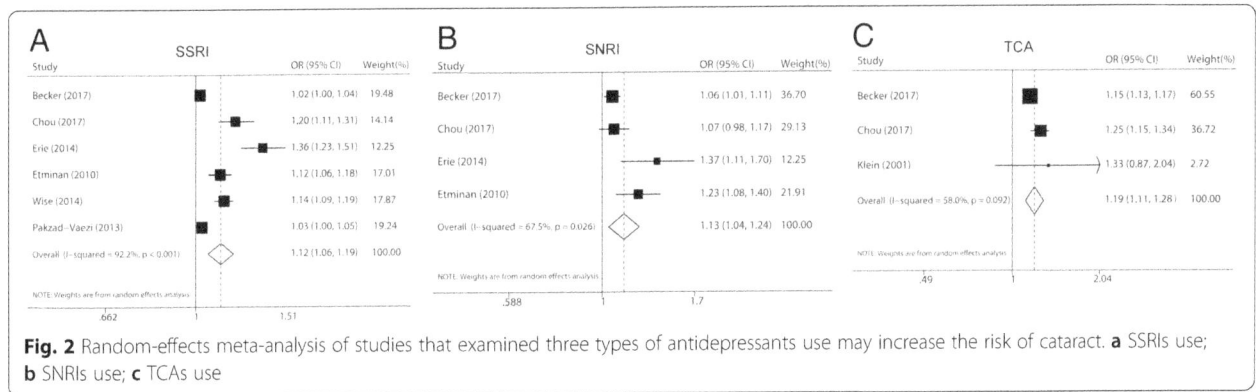

Fig. 2 Random-effects meta-analysis of studies that examined three types of antidepressants use may increase the risk of cataract. **a** SSRIs use; **b** SNRIs use; **c** TCAs use

control studies. Results for SSRIs were presented in six of these studies, four for SNRIs, and three for TCAs. These studies were published between 2001 and 2017. Information on exposure and endpoint were mainly collected from medical records. The NOS scores ranged from six to eight, with a mean value of 6.7. The main characteristics of all included studies have been summarized in Table 1.

Main analysis by antidepressant classifications

The multivariable-adjusted odds ratios (ORs) for each study and the pooled ORs for the any exposure versus none of antidepressants are presented in Fig. 2. Overall, the combined ORs (95% CIs) of cataract for SSRIs, SNRIs, and TCAs were 1.12 (1.06–1.19), 1.13 (1.04–1.24), and 1.19 (1.11–1.28), respectively. Obvious heterogeneity was found across studies ($P < 0.001$, $I^2 = 92.2\%$ for SSRIs, $P = 0.026$, $I^2 = 67.5\%$ for SNRIs, and $P = 0.092$, $I^2 = 58.0\%$ for TCAs).

Subgroup analyses by individual antidepressant drugs

The results of subgroup analysis according to individual antidepressant drugs are presented in Fig. 3. For SSRIs antidepressant drugs, a significantly direct association with cataract incidence was observed for fluoxetine (RR 1.08, 95% CI 1.03–1.12) and fluvoxamine (RR 1.22, 95% CI 1.06–1.40). No evidence of association was found for the rest of SSRIs drugs. For SNRIs antidepressant drugs, the combined ORs (95% CIs) of cataract for any exposure versus none were 1.35 (0.77–2.36), 2.33 (0.94–5.74), and 1.30 (1.18–1.43) for duloxetine, milnacipran, and venlafaxine, respectively.

Publication bias

As only seven studies were included in the present meta-analysis, Begg's test [18] and Egger's test [14] were not eligible for publication bias analysis. Hence we adopted a visual funnel plot to qualitatively assess the publication bias. As shown in Fig. 4, a certain degree of

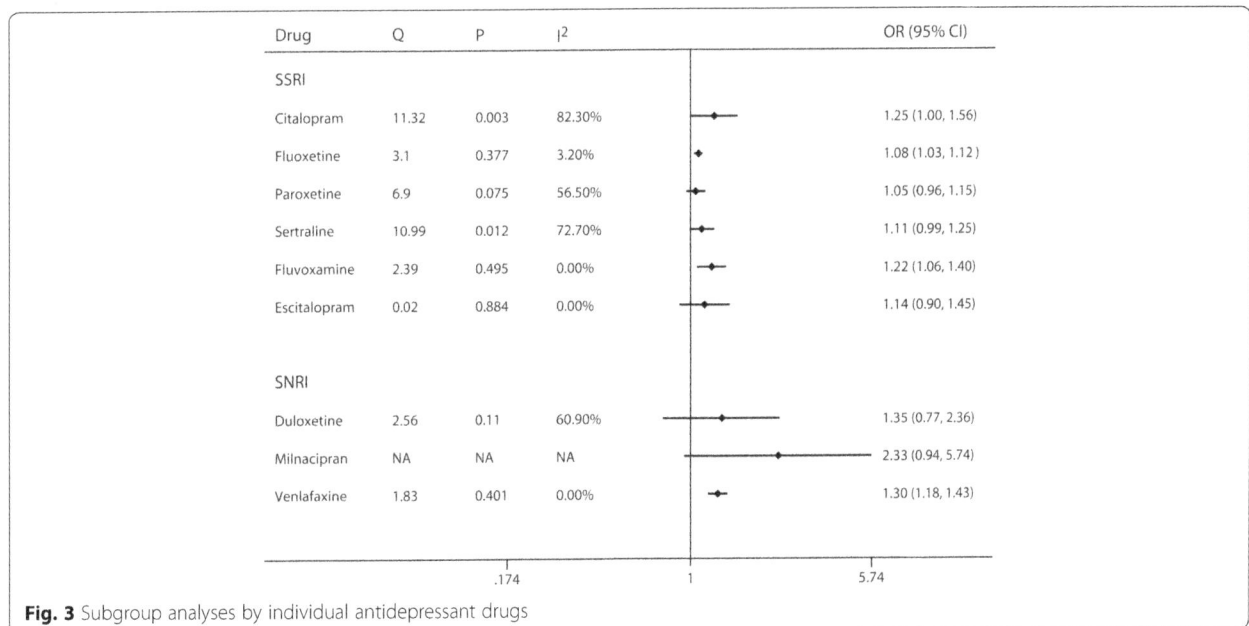

Fig. 3 Subgroup analyses by individual antidepressant drugs

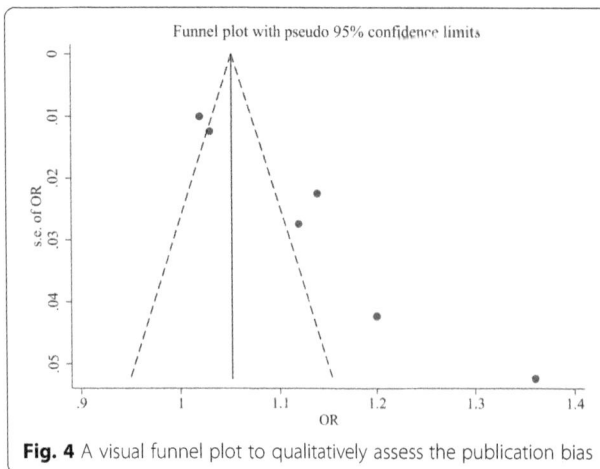

Fig. 4 A visual funnel plot to qualitatively assess the publication bias

asymmetry was observed, which indicated slight publication bias.

Discussion

This meta-analysis of seven eligible studies involving 447,672 cases and 1,510,391 controls supports a significant positive association of SSRIs, SNRIs and TCAs use with risk of cataract. To the best of our knowledge, this is the first systematic review and meta-analysis aimed to evaluate the relationship between antidepressants use and risk of cataract development.

Heterogeneity is often a concern in a meta-analysis. In the present study, obvious heterogeneity was observed among most analyses, which was partially explained by the following factors: study design was different. Although most included studies were performed in Western countries, population characteristics still varied in genetic and environmental background, antidepressants use, and matched or adjusted confounders.

Several mechanisms may be involved in the positive association of antidepressants use with cataract risk. In animal models, serotonin has been reported to play a crucial role in lens transparency [19]. Elevated serotonin levels have been shown to lead to lens opacity in rats [20]. Similarly, cataract and glaucoma patients also had increased levels of serotonin in the aqueous humor [21]. In addition, serotonin 5-HT1A, 5-HT2A/2C, and 5-HT7 receptors have been identified in the crystalline lens, which participate in regulation of intraocular pressure (IOP) homeostasis [22]. Increased IOP is able to contribute to glaucoma, which is a risk factor for cataract formation [23]. TCAs use is reported to be related with photosensitivity to ultraviolet or sunlight. This latter exposure has been suggested to be associated with cortical cataract in Beaver Dam Eye Study [24]. On the other hand, TCAs is able to inhibit norepinephrine uptake, which may also have cataractogenic properties [25].

Our study had some important strengths. Considering individual studies had limited statistical power, this meta-analysis of seven studies involving a large number of cases and controls improved the power to detect a potential association and provided more robust estimates. Most of the original studies matched or adjusted a series of variables, which greatly reduced the likelihood of confounding bias.

Potential limitations of our study should be considered. First, the number of eligible studies was limited, especially in some subgroup analyses, which might influence the reliability of the results. Second, significant heterogeneity was observed among included studies, which might distort the conclusion of our study. Third, a certain degree of publication bias was observed. Gray literature (e.g., conference abstract) was difficult to find and studies with null results were less likely to be published. Finally, random misclassification of antidepressants might influence the results.

Conclusion

Use of antidepressants, including SSRIs, SNRIs and TCAs, is associated with an increased risk of cataract development. Considering the huge heterogeneity and limited included studies, further large well-designed prospective studies are warranted to confirm the preliminary findings of our study.

Abbreviations
95% CI: 95% Confidence Interval; NOS: Newcastle-Ottawa Scale; OR: Odds Ratio; SNRIs: Serotonin noradrenalin reuptake inhibitors; SSRIs: Selective serotonin reuptake inhibitors; TCAs: Tricyclic antidepressants

Acknowledgements
Not Applicable.

Funding
This study was supported by grants from the Natural Science Foundation of Zhejiang Province (LY17H120009, LY17H120008).

Authors' contributions
QD, YF, SW and LZ gave work in the process of designing the study, revising and deciding the final edition of the manuscript. YF and LZ were in charge of data collection, analysis and drafting the manuscript. SW and LZ provided assistance in the data collection. QD and YF provided aids for literature screening. The content of the final version was read and approved by all the authors.

Consent for publication
Not applicable.

Competing interests
The authors declare that they have no competing interests.

Author details

[1]The Eye Hospital of Wenzhou Medical University, 270 Xueyuan West Road, Wenzhou City 325027, Zhejiang Province, People's Republic of China.
[2]Department of Ophthalmology, Hangzhou Red Cross Hospital, Hangzhou City 310003, Zhejiang Province, People's Republic of China.

References

1. Bourne RR, Stevens GA, White RA, Smith JL, Flaxman SR, Price H, et al. Causes of vision loss worldwide, 1990-2010: a systematic analysis. Lancet Glob Health. 2013;1(6):e339–49.
2. Mitchell P, Cumming RG, Attebo K, Panchapakesan J. Prevalence of cataract in Australia: the Blue Mountains eye study. Ophthalmology. 1997;104(4):581–8.
3. Weatherall M, Clay J, James K, Perrin K, Shirtcliffe P, Beasley R. Dose-response relationship of inhaled corticosteroids and cataracts: a systematic review and meta-analysis. Respirology. 2009;14(7):983–90.
4. Yu X, Lyu D, Dong X, He J, Yao K. Hypertension and risk of cataract: a meta-analysis. PLoS One. 2014;9(12):e114012.
5. Ye J, He J, Wang C, Wu H, Shi X, Zhang H, et al. Smoking and risk of age-related cataract: a meta-analysis. Invest Ophthalmol Vis Sci. 2012;53(7):3885–95.
6. Etminan M, Mikelberg FS, Brophy JM. Selective serotonin reuptake inhibitors and the risk of cataracts: a nested case-control study. Ophthalmology. 2010;117(6):1251–5.
7. Erie JC, Brue SM, Chamberlain AM, Hodge DO. Selective serotonin reuptake inhibitor use and increased risk of cataract surgery: a population-based, case-control study. Am J Ophthalmol. 2014;158(1):192–7. e1
8. Klein BE, Klein R, Lee KE, Danforth LG. Drug use and five-year incidence of age-related cataracts: the beaver dam eye study. Ophthalmology. 2001;108(9):1670–4.
9. Becker C, Jick SS, Meier CR. Selective Serotonin Reuptake Inhibitors and Cataract Risk: A Case-Control Analysis. Ophthalmology. 2017;124(11):1635–9.
10. Moher D, Liberati A, Tetzlaff J, Altman DG. Preferred reporting items for systematic reviews and meta-analyses: the PRISMA statement. Ann Intern Med. 2009;151(4):264–9. W64
11. DerSimonian R, Laird N. Meta-analysis in clinical trials. Control Clin Trials. 1986;7(3):177–88.
12. Hamling J, Lee P, Weitkunat R, Ambuhl M. Facilitating meta-analyses by deriving relative effect and precision estimates for alternative comparisons from a set of estimates presented by exposure level or disease category. Stat Med. 2008;27(7):954–70.
13. Higgins JP, Thompson SG. Quantifying heterogeneity in a meta-analysis. Stat Med. 2002;21(11):1539–58.
14. Egger M, Davey Smith G, Schneider M, Minder C. Bias in meta-analysis detected by a simple, graphical test. BMJ. 1997;315(7109):629–34.
15. Pakzad-Vaezi KL, Etminan M, Mikelberg FS. The association between cataract surgery and atypical antipsychotic use: a nested case-control study. Am J Ophthalmol. 2013;156(6):1141–6. e1
16. Wise SJ, Nathoo NA, Etminan M, Mikelberg FS, Mancini GB. Statin use and risk for cataract: a nested case-control study of 2 populations in Canada and the United States. Can J Cardiol. 2014;30(12):1613–9.
17. Chou PH, Chu CS, Chen YH, Hsu MY, Huang MW, Lan TH, et al. Antidepressants and risk of cataract development: a population-based, nested case-control study. J Affect Disord. 2017;215:237–44.
18. Begg CB, Mazumdar M. Operating characteristics of a rank correlation test for publication bias. Biometrics. 1994;50(4):1088–101.
19. Vivekanandan S, Lou MF. Evidence for the presence of phosphoinositide cycle and its involvement in cellular signal transduction in the rabbit lens. Curr Eye Res. 1989;8(1):101–11.
20. Boerrigter RM, Siertsema JV, Kema IP. Serotonin (5-HT) and the rat's eye. Some pilot studies. Doc Ophthalmol. 1992;82(1–2):141–50.
21. Zanon-Moreno V, Melo P, Mendes-Pinto MM, Alves CJ, Garcia-Medina JJ, Vinuesa-Silva I, et al. Serotonin levels in aqueous humor of patients with primary open-angle glaucoma. Mol Vis. 2008;14:2143–7.
22. Costagliola C, Parmeggiani F, Sebastiani A. SSRIs and intraocular pressure modifications. CNS Drugs. 2004;18(8):475–84.
23. Hodge WG, Whitcher JP, Satariano W. Risk factors for age-related cataracts. Epidemiol Rev. 1995;17(2):336–46.
24. Cruickshanks KJ, Klein BE, Klein R. Ultraviolet light exposure and lens opacities: the beaver dam eye study. Am J Public Health. 1992;82(12):1658–62.
25. Trope GE, Sole M, Aedy L, Madapallimattam A. Levels of norepinephrine, epinephrine, dopamine, serotonin and N-acetylserotonin in aqueous humour. Can J Ophthalmol. 1987;22(3):152–4.

26

Ascorbic acid concentrations in aqueous humor after systemic vitamin C supplementation in patients with cataract

Young-Sool Hah[1†], Hye Jin Chung[2†], Sneha B. Sontakke[2], In-Young Chung[3,4], Sunmi Ju[5], Seong-Wook Seo[3,4], Ji-Myong Yoo[3,4] and Seong-Jae Kim[3,4*] (iD)

Abstract

Background: To measure ascorbic acid concentration in aqueous humor of patients with cataract after oral or intravenous vitamin C supplementation.

Methods: Forty-two eyes of 42 patients with senile cataract who underwent uncomplicated cataract surgery were enrolled. Patients ($n = 14$ each) were administered oral vitamin C (2 g), intravenous vitamin C (20 g) or no treatment (control group) on the day before surgery. Samples of aqueous humor (0.1 cm^3) were obtained by anterior chamber aspiration at the beginning of surgery and stored at −80 °C. Ascorbic acid concentration in aqueous humor was measured by high-pressure liquid chromatography.

Results: The mean age at surgery was 62.5 years, with no difference among the three groups. The mean ± standard deviation concentrations of ascorbic acid in aqueous humor in the control and oral and intravenous vitamin C groups were 1347 ± 331 μmol/L, 1859 ± 408 μmol/L and 2387 ± 445 μmol/L, respectively. Ascorbic acid concentration was significantly lower in the control than in the oral ($P < 0.01$) and intravenous ($P < 0.001$) vitamin C groups and was significantly higher in the intravenous than in the oral vitamin C group ($P < 0.05$).

Conclusions: Ascorbic acid concentration in aqueous humor is increased by systemic vitamin C supplementation, with intravenous administration being more effective than oral administration.

Keywords: Antioxidant, Ascorbic acid, Aqueous humor, Cataract, Vitamin C

Background

Vitamins are essential nutrients required for various biological processes in the body. Because they cannot be synthesized in the body, vitamins must be ingested in foods. Vitamin C (ascorbic acid) facilitates the conversion of cholesterol into bile acids and increases the absorption of iron in the gut. Vitamin C is also an antioxidant, protecting the body from the deleterious effects of free radicals, pollutants and toxins [1]. Deficiencies in vitamin C have been associated with anaemia, infections, bleeding tendency and delayed wound healing [2].

The concentration of ascorbate is about 15 times greater in the aqueous humor of the eye than in plasma, suggesting that vitamin C may protect against harmful factors within the eye [3]. However, the concentration of vitamin C in aqueous humor of patients with age-related cataract decreases with age of the patient (from 50 to 70 years old), suggesting that this decrease may play a role in susceptibility to cataract formation in older people [4, 5]. Vitamin C concentrations in aqueous humor are also lower in patients with various ophthalmic diseases. For example, the concentration of vitamin C in the anterior chamber has been reported lower in

* Correspondence: maya12kim@naver.com

†Equal contributors

[3]Department of Ophthalmology, Gyeongsang National University Hospital, Gyeongsang National University School of Medicine, Jinju, South Korea

[4]Gyeongsang Institute of Health Science, Gyeongsang National University, Jinju, South Korea

Full list of author information is available at the end of the article

patients with Lowe's syndrome and exfoliation syndrome than in age-matched controls [6–8]. Moreover, reduced levels of vitamin C in aqueous humor may be associated with glaucoma [8, 9]. Thus, measuring vitamin C concentrations in aqueous humor may be useful for studying the pathogenesis of several ocular diseases.

Systemic oral administration of 2.0 g of vitamin C resulted in saturation of aqueous humor, with additional vitamin C, up to 5 g, not further increasing its concentration [10]. That study, however, did not assess whether intravenously administered vitamin C resulted in higher concentrations in the anterior chamber. This study therefore investigated ascorbic acid concentration in aqueous humor, as measured by high-pressure liquid chromatography (HPLC), after systemic (oral and intravenous) vitamin C supplementation in patients with cataract.

Methods

This study was approved by the Institutional Review Board of the Gyeongsang National University Hospital (no. 2016–04–012-002) and complied with the guidelines of the Declaration of Helsinki. All subjects provided written informed consent.

Patients and sampling of aqueous humour

This study prospectively enrolled cataract patients with no previous ocular morbidities who had not undergone previous intraocular surgery or procedures. Patients with chronic systemic diseases (e.g., of the liver or kidneys), uncontrolled diabetes mellitus or hypertension, history of renal calculi or gout, hypersensitivity to vitamin C or history of vitamin C supplements were excluded, as were pregnant or lactating women. Participants were classified into control, oral vitamin C and intravenous vitamin C groups. The latter two groups were administered oral vitamin C (2 g/day) or intravenous vitamin C (20 g/day) on the day before cataract surgery. To minimize the effect of time on ascorbic acid concentration, 1 g (oral group) or 10 g (intravenous group) of vitamin C was administered twice at 8 h interval to complete the total dose of 2 g or 20 g to the patients on the day before surgery. And, on the day of surgery, the collection of aqueous humor was completed within at least 2 h from 8 am. Samples of aqueous humor (0.1 cm^3) were obtained by anterior chamber aspiration into a syringe using a 26-gaugeze needle at the beginning of the surgery, prior to the injection of viscoelastic. All samples were stored at –80 °C in amber tubes.

Materials

L-Ascorbic acid and metaphosphoric acid (MPA) were purchased from Sigma-Aldrich Co. (St Louis, MO, USA) and Kanto Chemicals Co. Inc. (Tokyo, Japan), respectively. HPLC-grade acetonitrile and water were purchased

from Fisher Scientific (Pittsburgh, PA, USA). All other chemicals were of analytical grade.

Measurement of ascorbic acid in aqueous humour

Ascorbic acid concentrations in aqueous humour were measured by HPLC, as previously described with slight modifications [11]. Briefly, 100 µL of cold 10% MPA solution was added to a 100 µL aliquot of sample, vortexed and kept at 4 °C for 10 min for protein precipitation and ascorbic acid stabilization. The samples were centrifuged at 4 °C for 5 min at 10,000 g, and 20 µL of supernatant was transferred to a clean tube and diluted with 180 µL of 0.9% MPA. A 10 µL aliquot of each sample was injected into the HPLC. All solutions were carefully protected from light during sample preparation and analysis. Ascorbic acid was determined using an Agilent 1260 HPLC system (Agilent, Singapore) and a Synergi Hydro-RP column (4 µm, 4.6 × 150 mm; Phenomenex, CA, USA) maintained at 20 °C. The mobile phase consisted of 0.9% MPA (A) and acetonitrile (B), with gradient elution at a flow rate of 0.7 mL/min. The initial composition of 100% A was kept for 5 min, increased from 0% to 90% B for 3 min and maintained at 90% B for 2 min. The gradient was then changed back to the initial condition over 1 min and kept at the initial condition for 6 min. The total run time was 17 min. Effluent was monitored using a UV detector set at 265 nm. Representative HPLC chromatograms after stabilization of vitamin C are presented in Fig. 1. The calibration curves of ascorbic acid were linear over the ranges studied, with $r^2 > 0.995$.

Data were summarized using mean and standard deviation. Statistical analyses comparing three groups were performed using a one-way analysis of variance (ANOVA), and post hoc analysis with Bonferonni correction was used to evaluate the difference between the two groups using SPSS ver 18.0 (SPSS Inc., Chicago, IL, USA). Statistical significance was set at 0.05.

Results

Table 1 shows the baseline characteristics of the 42 study subjects (42 eyes) enrolled from February to July 2015. The mean age of this cohort was 62.5 ± 10.1 years. Mean age, gender and status of cataract (Lens Opacities Classification System III, LOCS III) were similar ($P > 0.05$) in the three groups.

Ascorbic acid concentrations in aqueous humour are presented in Fig. 2. The mean ± standard deviation concentrations of ascorbic acid in the aqueous humor of the control, oral vitamin C and intravenous vitamin C groups were 1347 ± 331 µmol/L, 1859 ± 408 µmol/L and 2387 ± 445 µmol/L, respectively. Ascorbic acid concentration was significantly lower in the control than in the oral ($P < 0.01$) and intravenous ($P < 0.001$) vitamin

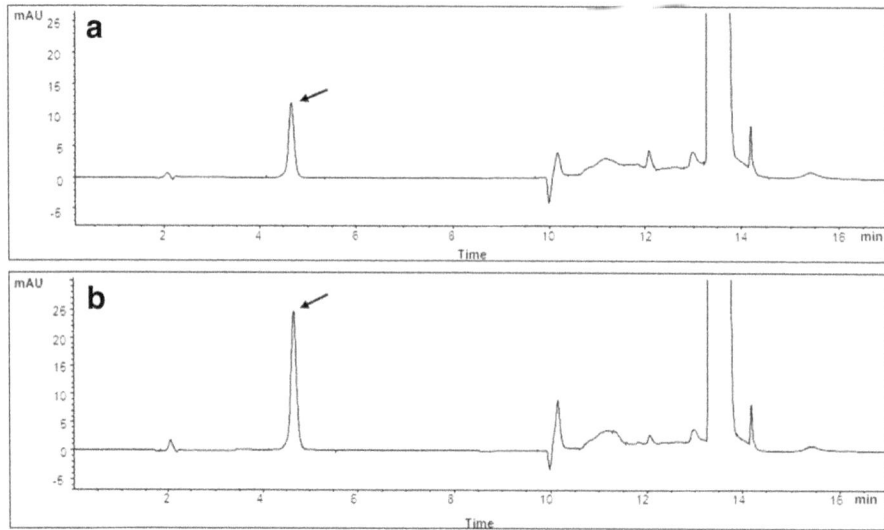

Fig. 1 Representative HPLC chromatograms after stabilization of vitamin C. **a** vitamin C standard solution (1000μM) (**b**) human aqueous sample collected after intravenous administration of vitamin C. The arrows indicate vitamin C. UV absorption at 265nm is shown in milliabsorption units (mAU)

C groups and was significantly higher in the intravenous than in the oral vitamin C group (*P* < 0.05).

Discussion

To our knowledge, no previous study has investigated the effects of oral and intravenous vitamin C supplementation on ascorbic acid concentrations in aqueous humor. Our results indicate that both types of systemic vitamin C supplementation increased ascorbic acid concentrations in aqueous humor, with intravenous administration being more effective than oral administration.

Previous studies show that ascorbic acid concentrations are much higher in aqueous humor than in plasma [12, 13]. This concentration gradient is a result of active transport in the ciliary epithelium [14]. In eyes, ascorbic acid protects against the effects of ultraviolet rays and oxidants, thereby preventing cataract formation [5, 15]. Lower than normal ascorbic acid concentrations in aqueous humor have been reported in various ophthalmic diseases. For example, the concentration of vitamin C was

reported to decrease with age in patients with age-related cataract, suggesting that reductions in ascorbic acid may play an important role in cataract formation [4, 5]. Lower levels of vitamin C in aqueous humor may be associated with glaucoma, including in patients with primary open angle glaucoma and secondary glaucoma [8, 9, 16]. Finally, patients with Lowe's syndrome and exfoliation syndrome have significantly lower levels of ascorbic acid in aqueous humor than age-matched controls [6, 8]. These findings suggest that vitamin C concentrations may provide clues to the pathogenesis and treatment of several ocular diseases.

High ascorbic acid concentrations in aqueous humor may protect the lens against the cataractogenic effects of UV radiation [17, 18]. Moreover, oral, topical or intravenous application of vitamin C lowers intraocular pressure in glaucoma patients [8, 9, 19]. The Age-Related Eye Disease Study (AREDS) found that long-term supplementation with vitamin C (500 mg/day) and other vitamins was effective in retarding the progression of

Table 1 Clinical characteristics of the study population

		Intravenous vitamin C	Oral vitamin C	Control	*P* value	Total
Number of patients		14	14	14		42
Age, yr (mean±SD)		64 ± 10.9	62.6 ± 10.3	60.5 ± 6.7	0.541	62.5 ± 10.1
Sex (M/F)		7/7	6/8	8/6	0.741	21/21
Grade of Cararact (LOCS III)	NO2NC2	0	1	1		2
	NO3NC3	8	8	9		25
	NO4NC4	5	4	4		13
	NO5NC5	1	1	0		2

LOCS Lens Opacities Classification System, *NO* Nuclear Opalescence, *NC* Nuclear Color

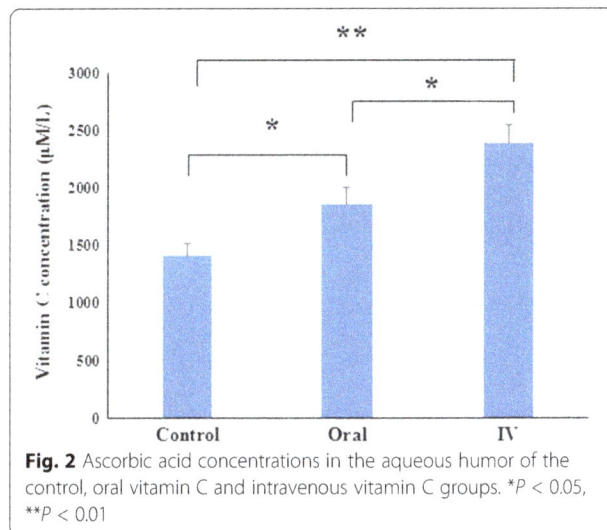

Fig. 2 Ascorbic acid concentrations in the aqueous humor of the control, oral vitamin C and intravenous vitamin C groups. *$P < 0.05$, **$P < 0.01$

ascorbic acid level in the aqueous humor. Future studies assessing the impact of vitamin C on various ocular diseases should include direct administration of various concentrations of vitamin C and measurements of vitamin C in aqueous humor. Large, long-term clinical studies are warranted to establish the optimal dose, route of administration, duration of treatment and frequency of administration of vitamin C for various ophthalmic diseases.

Conclusion

In conclusion, the results of this study suggest that systemic administration of vitamin C increased ascorbic acid concentration in aqueous humor, with intravenous administration being more effective than oral administration.

Abbreviations
AREDS: Age-Related Eye Disease Study; HPLC: High-pressure liquid chromatography; LOCS: Lens opacities classification system

Acknowledgements
Not applicable.

Funding
This research was supported by Basic Science Research Program through the National Research Foundation of Korea (NRF) funded by the Ministry of Science, ICT & Future Planning (NRF-2015R1C1A1A02037702).

Authors' contributions
SJK: Patients interaction, diagnosis, data analysis, manuscript drafting and supervision. YSH, HJC, and SBS: Perfomed the HPLC and analyzed the patient data. IYC, SJ, SWS and JMY: Patient interaction, diagnosis and data analysis. All authors read and approved the final manuscript.

Consent for publication
Not applicable.

Competing interests
The authors declare that they have no competing interests.

age-related macular degeneration (AMD) [20] and in delaying the progression of lens opacities [4, 18]. Supplementation with low- and high-dose vitamin C was found to be associated with decreased risk of glaucoma [21]. However, the optimal concentrations and routes of administration remain unclear.

Our findings are largely consistent with those of earlier studies. A 10% increase in plasma ascorbate concentration was found to increase ascorbate concentrations in aqueous humor by 48% [13] and 66% [22]. Oral administration of 2.0 g of vitamin C was found to saturate the aqueous humor, with further vitamin C supplementation having no effect on its concentration in aqueous humor [10]. By contrast, this study showed that intravenous administration was more effective than oral administration at increasing the ascorbic acid concentration in aqueous humor. Intravenous supplementation with high-dose vitamin C and its increased concentration in aqueous humor may protect normal ocular structures against harmful reactive oxygen radicals and may treat diseases associated with these radicals. Our previous study found that systemic (oral or intravenous) vitamin C supplementation reduced the size of corneal opacities resulting from infectious keratitis, with intravenous vitamin C being more effective than oral vitamin C [23]. Additional studies are needed to determine the effect of vitamin C in patients with severe uveitis, glaucoma, cataract and other inflammatory diseases.

This study had several limitations, including its small sample size. In addition, serum concentrations of vitamin C were not measured. And, the subjects were not randomly divided into three groups, so there could be a selections bias. Finally, there is no standardization of ascorbic intake of the individual patients, so, it can affect

Author details
[1]Biomedical Research Institute, Gyeongsang National University Hospital, Jinju, South Korea. [2]College of Pharmacy and Research institute of Pharmaceutical Sciences, Gyeongsang National University, Jinju, South Korea. [3]Department of Ophthalmology, Gyeongsang National University Hospital, Gyeongsang National University School of Medicine, Jinju, South Korea. [4]Gyeongsang Institute of Health Science, Gyeongsang National University, Jinju, South Korea. [5]Division of Pulmonology and Allergy, Department of Internal Medicine, Gyeongsang National University Hospital, Jinju, South Korea.

References

1. Buettner GR, Schafer FQ. Albert Szent-Gyorgyi. Vitamin C identification Biochemist. 2006;28:31-3.
2. Graumlich JF, Ludden TM, Conry-Cantilena CLR Jr, Wang Y, Levine M. Pharmacokinetic model of ascorbic acid in healthy male volunteers during depletion and repletion. Pharm Res. 1997;14:1133-9.
3. Reiss GR, Werness PG, Zollman PE, Brubaker RF. Ascorbic acid levels in the aqueous humor of nocturnal and diurnal mammals. Arch Ophthalmol. 1986;104:753-5.
4. Wei L, Liang G, Cai C, Ly J. Association of vitamin C with the risk of age-related cataract: a meta-analysis. Acta Ophthalmol. 2016;94:e170-6.
5. Canadananovic V, Latinovic S, Barisic S, Babic N, Jovanovic S. Age-related changes of vitamin C level in aqueous humor. Vojnosanit Pregl. 2015;72:823-6.
6. Hayasaka S, Yamada T, Nitta K, Kaji Y, Hiraki S, Tachinami K, Matsumoto M, Yamammoto S, Yamammoto S. Ascorbic acid and amino acid values in the aqueous humor of a patient with Lowe's syndrome. Graefes Arch Clin Exp Ophthalmol. 1997;235:217-21.
7. Ferreira SM, Lerner SF, Brunzini R, Evelson PA, Llesuy SF. Antioxidant status in the aqueous humor of patients with glaucoma associated with exfoliation syndrome. Eye (Lond). 2009;23:1691-7.
8. Koliakos GG, Kontas AG, Schlotzer-Scherhardt U, Bufidis T, Georgiadis N, Ringvold A. Ascorbic acid concentration is reduced in the aqueous humor of patients with exfoliation syndrome. Am J Ophthalmol. 2002;134:879-83.
9. Leite MT, Prata TS, Kera CZ, Miranda DV, de Moraes Barros SB, Melo LA Jr. Ascorbic acid concentration is reduced in the secondary aqueous humor of glaucomatous patients. Clin Experiment Ophthalmol. 2009;37:402-26.
10. Iqbal Z, Midgley JM, Watson DG, Karditsas SD, Dutton GN, Wilson WS. Effect of oral administration of vitamin C on human aqueous humor ascorbate concentration. Zhongguo Yao Li Xue Bao. 1999;20:879-93.
11. Ross MA. Determination of ascorbic acid and uric acid in plasma by high-performance liquid chromatography. J Chromatogr B Biomed Appl. 1994;657:197-200.
12. Badhu B, Baral N, Lamsal M, Das H, Dhital BA. Plasma and aqueous humor ascorbic acid levels in people with cataract from diverse geographical regions of Nepal. Southeast Asian J Trop Med Public Health. 2007;36:277-83.
13. Taylor A, Jacques PF, Nowell T, Perrone G, Blumberg J, Handelman G, Jozwiak B, Nadler D. Vitamin C in human and guinea pig aqueous, lens and plasma in relation to intake. Curr Eye Res. 1997;16:857-64.
14. To CH, Kong CW, Chan CY, Shahidullah M, Do CW. The mechanism of aqueous humor formation. Clin Exp Optom. 2002;85:335-49.
15. Babizhayev MA. Mitochondria induce oxidative stress, generation of reactive oxygen species and redox state unbalance of the eye lens leading to human cataract formation: disruption of redox lens organization by phospholipid hydroperoxides as a common basis for cataract disease. Cell Biochem Funct. 2011;29:183-206.
16. Xu P, Lin Y, Porter K, Liton PB. Ascorbic acid modulation of iron homeostasis and lysosomal function in trabecular meshwork cells. J Ocul Pharmacol Ther. 2014;30:246-53.
17. Reddy VN, Giblin FJ, Lin LR, Chakrapani B. The effect of aqueous humor ascorbate on ultraviolet-B-induced DNA damage in lens epithelium. Invest Ophthalmol Vis Sci. 1998;39:344-50.
18. Age-Related Eye Disease Study Research Group. A randomized, placebo-controlled, clinical trial of high-dose supplementation with vitamins C and E and beta carotene for age-related cataract and vision loss: AREDS report no. 9. Arch Ophthalmol. 2001;11:1439-52.
19. Lee PF, Fox R, Henrick I, Lam WK. Correlation of aqueous humor ascorbate with intraocular pressure and outflow facility in hereditary buphthalmic rabbits. Invest Ophthalmol Vis Sci. 1978;17:799-802.
20. Chew EY, Clemons TE, Agron E, Sperduto RD, Sangiovanni JP, Davis MD, Ferris FL. 3rd; age-related eye disease study research group. Ten-year follow-up of age-related macular degeneration in the age-related eye disease study AREDS report no.36. JAMA Ophthalmol. 2014;132:272-7.
21. Wang SY, Singh K, Lin SC. Glaucoma and vitamins a, C, and E supplement intake and serum levels in a population-based sample of the United States. Eye (Lond). 2013;27:487-94.
22. Taylor A, Jacques PF, Nadler D, Morrow F, Sulsky SI, Shepard D. Relationship in humans between ascorbic acid consumption and levels of total and reduced ascorbic acid in lens, aqueous humor, and plasma. Curr Eye Res. 1991;10:751-9.
23. Cho YW, Yoo WS, Kim SJ, Chung IY, Seo SW, Yoo JM. Efficacy of systemic vitamin C supplementation in reducing corneal opacity resulting from infectious keratitis. Medicine. 2014;93:e125.

27

Differences in serum oxidative status between glaucomatous and nonglaucomatous cataract patients

Wojciech Rokicki[1][*] (iD), Jolanta Zalejska-Fiolka[2], Dorota Pojda-Wilczek[1], Alicja Hampel[2], Wojciech Majewski[3], Serap Ogultekin[1] and Ewa Mrukwa-Kominek[1]

Abstract

Background: Oxidative stress contributes to both intraocular pressure regulation and glaucomatous neuropathy. The systemic redox status (solitary determination) was examined in primary open-angle glaucoma (POAG) patients with cataract and nonglaucomatous cataract patients. Cataract-matched group comparisons appear more precise in the context of oxidative stress evaluation. The aim of this study was to establish if systemic oxidative status in POAG patients was elevated compared with the cataract only subjects.

Methods: The study included patients with primary open angle glaucoma (POAG group, $n = 30$) and controls (non POAG group, $n = 25$). Serum concentration of lipofuscine (LPS), malondialdehyde (MDA) and activity of total superoxide dismutase (SOD), and its mitochondrial (Mn-SOD) and cystolic (Cu,Zn-SOD) isoform were measured. Total oxidant state (TOS) and total antioxidant capacity (TAC) in blood were also evaluated.

Results: Significant increase of LPS ($p = 0.0002$) and MDA ($p = 0.005$) concentration was observed in glaucomatous patients as compared with controls. Total SOD activity was significantly lowered in the glaucoma group ($p = 0.003$); serum level of Mn-SOD was significantly lower in glaucoma patients ($p = 0.048$) however, Cu,Zn-SOD was not. Glaucoma patients presented elevated mean TOS ($p = 0.016$). Both groups presented with comparable TAC.

Conclusion: Systemic redox balance of cataract patients was significantly altered in the course of glaucoma.

Keywords: Glaucoma, Oxidative stress, Serum, Neurodegenerative disease

Background

Glaucoma refers to several disorders having the same clinical features. Characterized by progressive retinal ganglion cell (RGC) and axon loss; glaucoma causes damage to the optic nerve and results in gradual visual field loss. Subsequently, this leads to irreversible blindness. Despite well-developed diagnostic tools and relatively efficient treatment, glaucoma still remains the world's leading cause of irreversible blindness. Glaucomatous neuropathy may progress with elevated or normal (arbitrarily estimated) intraocular pressure (IOP). Therefore, elevated IOP, the main known risk factor for glaucoma, is neither enough nor necessary to trigger

glaucomatous neuropathy. Research suggests a multifactorial etiology of glaucoma pathogenesis; nevertheless, the trigger(s) initiating glaucomatous pathology still remains unidentified. Primary glaucoma should not be considered solely as an ocular pathology [1]. Data suggests oxidative stress in glaucomatous disturbances do not conflict with other observations but complements mechanical, vascular, genetic and immunologic theories in the pathogenesis of glaucoma. Oxidative stress presumably plays an important role in increasing IOP, producing trabecular meshwork alterations and promoting neuronal cell death affecting retinal ganglion cells in glaucoma [2, 3]. Furthermore, an increase in IOP is understood to generate oxidative stress in retina [4]. POAG in the context of oxidative stress presents two main front lines of oxidation and defense against oxidative stress. The first front line in the anterior segment

* Correspondence: wojtek.rokicki@gmail.com
[1]Department and Clinic of Ophthalmology, School of Medicine in Katowice, Medical University of Silesia, Ceglana 35, 40-514 Katowice, Poland
Full list of author information is available at the end of the article

functions when UV and visible light are the main resources of exogenous ROS, produced mostly in aqueous humor. The second front line is in the well vascularized posterior segment and functions when endogenous and systematic ROS are delivered with blood [5]. Additionally, there is an age-dependent increase in production of endogenous free radicals and ROS. Therefore, both POAG occurrence and age dependent systemic redox balance deterioration presumably have common pathways.

In this research serum oxidative state represented by oxidative degradation products (malonyl dialdehyde - MDA, lipofuscine - LPS) and selected antioxidant enzymatic defense (total superoxide dismutase - SOD, and its isoenzymes: Mn-SOD and Cu,Zn-SOD) were studied. We also evaluated the oxidant and antioxidant status by measurement of total oxidant status (TOS) and total antioxidant capacity (TAC) respectively.

MDA, widely regarded as a marker of a peroxidative damage to cell membranes, is induced by physical and/ or chemical oxidative stress. Nucci et al. demonstrated that glaucoma patients had significantly higher levels of serum and humor aqueous MDA as compared with non-glaucomatous controls [6].

LPS - Lipofuscin (called age pigment) is a marker of normal aging. Lipofuscin tends to accumulate throughout life in post-mitotic cells, such as neurons and glia. Dolman et al. in 1980 reported the presence of lipofuscin in the optic nerve [7]. The subsequent investigations linked LPS accumulation with age-related disorders, especially with POAG [8].

As previously reported, human and animal ocular fluids and tissues contain one of the major antioxidant enzymes - superoxide dismutase (SOD, EC1.15.1.1) which plays a key role in protecting against oxidative damage [9]. SOD activity alteration was previously reported in aqueous humor of glaucoma patients [10].

The aim of this present research was to assess serum oxidative stress in glaucoma/cataract patients compared with cataract only controls.

Methods
The study protocol was approved by the Ethics Committee of School of Medicine in Katowice, Poland (permission number: KNW/0022/KB1/123/10) and adhered to the tenets of the Declaration of Helsinki for experiments involving human tissue and samples.

Participants
The POAG group was comprised only of Caucasians. Only patients whose eye was scheduled for antiglaucomatous drainage surgery due to progressive visual field loss and whose target IOP was not reached pharmacologically, was taken under analysis.

Patients with previous history of IOP over 23 mmHg within the last 6 months before examination and on sampling day were excluded. We set the threshold of 23 mmHg, arbitrary (21 mmHg + 10%). We presuppose, IOP ≤ 23 mmHg is not yet in the acute phase of intraocular hypertension, and a limitation of 21 mmHg would reduce our examined group. All patients presented bilateral visual field defect.

The Controls group included Caucasians who were scheduled for cataract surgery.

Sequential inclusion criteria both for POAG and for the Controls group were as follows:

(1) no previous intrabulbar surgery, (2) between 65 and 75 years old, (3) best corrected visual acuity of 0.5 or better (Snellen's charts) (4) no myopia or hyperopia >3D (dioptres) (5) non-smokers, (6) no documented, diagnosed, treated ophthalmic and organic diseases (only treated arterial hypertension was accepted), (7) no abnormalities in the routine preoperative laboratory tests especially in C-reactive protein (CRP), complete blood count (CBC) and differential, (8) body mass index (BMI) < 30.

Patients for examined groups were chosen, according to above mentioned criteria, and from patients consecutively admitted to The Cataract/Glaucoma Station of The Department of Ophthalmology, Medical University of Silesia for planned surgery.

Ophthalmic examination
Clinical evaluation of POAG included gonioscopy, detailed ophthalmoscopy, central corneal thickness measurement, tonometry (Goldmann's, Haag-Streit, Bern, Switzerland; 0.5% Alcaine) visual field examination (Octopus 301 HS, Interzeag) and policlinic history analysis. The average IOP for each patient was determined by three measurements (the day before admission, day of admission and the day of surgery). All IOP measurements were taken during morning hours (between 8 AM and 11 AM). The IOP policlinic history (within the last 6 months) together with our measurements guided us to exclude POAG patients in the acute IOP phase.

The patients were examined on the day of blood sample collection.

Blood sample collection
Blood samples were collected into chemically clean tubes to obtain serum. After coagulation samples were centrifuged at room temperature for 10 min at 3000 rpm, serum was retracted and transferred into clean tubes for biochemical analysis. Pending analysis, serum samples were frozen at −80 ° C for further studies.

Electrophysiological Examination
The transient pattern electroretinogram (PERG) was examined using Reti-Port equipment (Roland Consult,

Germany). The study conditions were performed as per the recommendations and standards of the ISCEV (International Society for Clinical Electrophysiology of Vision) [11]. Square checks with check size 30', contrast 97%, reversal rate four reversals per second were used. Two trials for each stimulus condition were obtained to confirm reproducibility, 200 sweeps were collected and averaged. Fiber electrodes as recording electrodes, gold-cup as a reference, and ground electrodes were used. The patients wore best optical correction for the distance of examination (1 m). Implicit time (the time to peak) and amplitude of the negative wave N95 (from the peak of P50 to the trough of N95) were measured.

Biochemistry

Determination of superoxide dismutase activity (SOD, Mn-SOD, Cu,Zn-SOD)

Oyanagui's method [12] was used to measure the activity of SOD in blood serum. In this method, xanthine oxidase produces superoxide anions, which react with hydroxylamine forming nitric ions. These ions react with naphthalene diamine and sulfanilic acid generating a colored product. Concentration of this product is proportional to the amount of superoxide anions produced and is negatively proportional to the activity of SOD. Absorbance was measured using an automated Perkin Elmer analyzer at a wavelength of 550 nm. The enzymatic activity of SOD was expressed in nitric units. The isoenzymes of SOD, Mn-SOD and CuZn-SOD, were also indicated using KCN as the inhibitor of the CuZn-SOD activity. The activity of SOD is equal to one nitric unit (NU) when it inhibits nitric ion production by 50%. Activities of SOD in blood serum were expressed in NU/ml.

Determination of malondialdehyde (MDA) concentration

The product of lipid peroxidation - MDA was measured fluorometrically as 2-thiobarbituric acid-reactive substance (TBARS) in blood serum according to Ohkawa [13] with modifications. Samples were mixed with 8,1% sodium dodecyl sulfate, 20% acetic acid and 0,8% 2-thiobarbituric acid. After vortexing, samples were incubated for 1 h at 950 C and butanol-pyridine 15:1 (v/v) was added. The mixture was shaken for 10 min. and then centrifuged. The butanol- pyridine layer was measured fluorometrically at 552 nm and 515 nm excitation (Perkin Elmer, USA). TBARS values are expressed as malondialdehyde (MDA) equivalents. Tetraethoxypropane was used as the standard. Concentrations are given in µmol/l plasma.

Determination of Total Oxidation Status (TOS)

Total oxidant status was measured according to Erel [14] in blood serum. The assay is based on the oxidation of ferrous ion to ferric ion in the presence of various oxidant species in acidic medium. The change in color of the ferric ion by xylenol orange was measured as a change in absorbance at 560 nm. This process was applied to an automated Perkin Elmer analyzer and calibrated with hydrogen peroxide. Data is shown in µmol/l.

Determination of Total Antioxidant Capacity (TAC)

Total antioxidant capacity was measured according to Erel [15] in blood serum. In this colorimetric method, radicals are generated and the antioxidant activity of blood serum reduces radical formation. The change in color of ABTS+ ions (2,2'-azinobis(3-ethylbenzothiazoline-6-sulfonate) was measured as the change in absorbance at 660 nm. This method was conducted in an automated Perkin Elmer analyzer calibrated with Trolox. Data is shown in mmol/l.

Determination of lipofuscin concentration

In blood serum, the LPS concentration was determined according to Jain [16]. Fluorescence was measured using an LS45 spectrofluorimeter Perkin Elmer at wavelengths of 360 nm (absorbance) and 440 nm (emission). Values are presented as relative units (relative fluorescence lipid extract, RF), where X corresponds to a fluorescence solution of 0.1 mg/mL quinidine sulfate in 0.1 N sulfuric acid.

Statistical

The statistical analysis was performed with a Statistica package. The comparison between groups was performed either with parametrical t-test or with non-parametrical Mann-Whitney test if assumptions of a parametrical test were not met.

Results

Baseline patient characteristics are summarized in Table 1.

Only one eye per patient was included in the study. Number of patients with IOP $< =21$ was 17 and with IOP > 21 was 13.

No significant differences between groups in BMI was recorded.

Serum concentration of malondialdehyde (MDA), the indicator of lipid peroxidation was significantly raised in the glaucoma group (1.16 µmol/l; SD: 0.54; 95% CI: 0.96–1.36) as compared with controls (0.757 µmol/l; SD: 0.13 95% CI: 0.70–0.81) $p = 0.005$ (Table 2).

The serum lipofuscin varied between compared patients (Table 2). In glaucomatous subjects the mean concentration of "age pigment" was elevated to 1636.27 RF; SD: 325.03 95% CI: 1514.90–1757.64 while nonglaucomatous participants were about 1298.84 RF; SD: 241.59 95% CI: 1201.26–1396.42 ($p = 0.0002$).

Table 1 Patients characteristics

	Glaucoma + Cataract	Vs	Cataract
Sex (men/female)	♂ = 14 n = 30 ♀ = 16	N/S	♂ = 10 n = 25 ♀ = 15
Age (years)	68 ± 5,42	p = 0.21	69 ± 3,72
Median duration of known glaucoma (years)	5–12 8,6 ± 3,3	∅	∅
Intraocular pressure (IOP)	21,0 mmHg SD: 2,35 95% CI: 20,12–21,88	p = 0.000	16,3 mmHg SD: 1,43 95% CI: 15,69–16,85
BCVA (best corrected visual acuity)	0,72 SD: 0,18	NS	0,66 SD: 0,16
N95 amplitude (pattern electroretinography PERG)	2,05 SD: 1,09 95% CI:1,64–2,45	p = 0.000	3,3 SD: 1,48 95% CI: 2,70–3,89
N95 implicit time (pattern electroretinography PERG)	97,93 SD: 9,41 95% CI: 94,42–101,45	NS	97,15 SD: 7,63 95% CI: 94,01–100,24

As recorded, the first line of antioxidant defense represented by total SOD activity in POAG patients (17.48 NU/ml; SD: 3,12 95% CI: 16,3–18,6) was decreased as compared with healthy controls (20,43 NU/ml; SD: 4,03 95% CI: 18,80–22,06) - Table 2. The differences reached statistical significance ($p = 0.003$). When SOD isoform activities were assessed separately significant diversification of examined groups were noted only in mitochondrial SOD2 (Mn-SOD) (glaucoma: 8.61 NU/ml; SD: 2.04 vs controls: 10.59 NU/ml; SD: 3.49. $p = 0.048$) – Table 2. The differences between compared groups in the mean

Table 2 Differences in oxidative stress markers between groups

	Glaucoma + Cataract	Cataract	p
Malondialdehyde	1.16 μmol/l SD: 0.54; 95% CI: 0.96–1.36	0.757 μmol/l SD: 0.13 95% CI: 0.70–0.81	p = 0.005
Lipofuscine	1636.27 RF SD: 325.03 95% CI: 1514.90–1757.64	1298.84 RF SD: 241.59 95% CI: 1201.26–1396.42	p = 0.000
Total SOD[a]	17.48 NU/ml SD: 3,12 95% CI: 16,3–18,6	20,43 NU/ml SD: 4,03 95% CI: 18,80–22,06	p = 0.003
Cytosolic SOD[a]	8.87 NU/ml SD: 2.44	9.84 NU/ml SD: 2.20	NS
Mitochondrial SOD[a]	8.61 NU/ml SD: 2.04	10.59 NU/ml SD: 3.49	p = 0.048
Total Oxidative State	22.81 μmol/l SD: 26,44; 95% CI: 12,94–32,68	8.08 μmol/l SD: 5,82; 95% CI: 4,71–9,35	p = 0.016
Total Antioxidant Capacity	1.03 mmol/l SD: 0,19; 95% CI: 0,96–1,10	1.02 mmol/l SD: 0,09; 95% CI: 0,98–1,06	NS

[a]*SOD* Superoxide dismutase

cytosolic SOD1 (Cu,Zn-SOD) activity failed to reach significance (glaucoma: 8.87 NU/ml; SD: 2.44 vs controls: 9.84 NU/ml; SD: 2.20. $p = 0.13$).

No correlation between concentration of MDA ($p = 0.29$), LPS ($p = 0.14$), activity of total SOD ($p = 0.4$), Mn-SOD ($p = 0.2$), Cu,Zn-SOD ($p = 0.99$), TOS ($p = 0.45$), TAC ($p = 0.23$) and N95 amplitude was found.

Total oxidative state (TOS) showed intensification in the glaucoma group as compared with controls (22.81 μmol/l; SD: 26,44; 95% CI: 12,94–32,68 vs 8.08 μmol/l; SD: 5,82; 95% CI: 4,71–9,35; $p = 0.016$). Total antioxidant capacity (TAC) was comparable in examined patients (1.02 mmol/l; SD: 0,09; 95% CI: 0,98–1,06 in controls and 1.03 mmol/l; SD: 0,19; 95% CI: 0,96–1,10 in glaucoma, $p = 0.31$).

Discussion

In this study, we found increased oxidative stress in patients with primary glaucoma. Changes in redox state were observed by enzymatic defense (SOD), accumulation of oxidative stress products (LPS and MDA) and total oxidant state.

Slightly different from previous experimental protocols, we designed this study model to select from participants scheduled for surgical procedures. Medical pre-operative evaluation was conducted in the hospital, which provided well-documented medical history of those involved in the study as compared with e.g., policlinic research model(s). Primary glaucoma is rather generalized than just an ocular disorder. Therefore, we believe, to examine primary glaucoma precisely, the general clinical condition of patients should be carefully studied.

We have included patients with documented visual field (VF) damage progression in the POAG group. Although performed, visual field analysis of participants was intentionally precluded. To evaluate glaucomatous damage in the course of oxidative stress precisely, in our study, we chose the transient pattern electroretinogram (PERG). The PERG is less depended on lens opacification than visual field examination. In glaucoma, both PERG amplitude reduction and implicit time increase have been reported in various studies, however the implicit time increase is relatively small and amplitude reduction have drawn the most interest. Results from experimental studies (primate model) indicate that PERG amplitude reduction precede the development of significant changes in the optic nerve head, and are related to the degree of cupping and nerve fiber loss, and are not diminished when IOP is reduced pharmacologically [17].

Therefore, for patient comparisons and RGC vitality assessment PERG is more precise, and less dependent on physician interpretation. Optic nerve diseases preferentially affect N95 and its amplitude is decreased or absent in optic atrophy [18]. In this current study, no significant differences in the N95 implicit time between the study groups were found. The N95 amplitude was notably significantly lower in the POAG group than in the control group, which reflects advanced glaucomatous atrophic changes of the optic nerve. No correlation between the N95 amplitude and serum level of analyzed substances indicates that PERG does not reflect rapid local changes in ganglion cells' activity in the presence of oxidative stress (Fig. 1).

Mittag et al. demonstrated the developing changes in optic nerve atrophy experimentally in a rat glaucoma model. Their research suggests ERG responses begin to decline after 3 to 4 months of about 100% increase in IOP [19].

As described, glaucomatous pathological processes fluctuate over stable and progressive states [20]. Our glaucoma group patients were scheduled for surgery due to glaucomatous neuropathy exacerbation. Therefore, our examined patients were presenting in the active phase of neuropathy. The examined group of patients presented with oscillating IOP around is upper limit and comparable among themselves.

We decided to include patients presenting with cataract in both the examined group and the control. Oxidative stress has long been involved in the pathogenesis of cataract [21]. As suggested by Nucci et al. [6], comparing the age-matched and cataract-matched groups is more precise in the context of oxidative stress.

Noteworthy to mention, we sampled one tube of blood serum for the measurement of redox status, incidentally selecting an instant of the glaucomatous process. Thus, we should include this determination as a screening test. On the other hand, we included this eye in the research

that revealed progressive neuropathy; this was assessed with visual field and electrophysiology over the last 6 months.

We examined eyes with IOP less or equal to 23 mmHg over the last 6 months. Thus, we assume that primary oxidative stress delivered with blood has a remarkable impact on the glaucomatous process than topical oxidative stress: that could be produced by intraocular pressure ≤23 mmHg.

We intentionally analyzed only one eye per patient because the second eye in many cases was after intrabulbar surgery (drainage or/and cataract) which could have additional impacts on the glaucomatous process in this eye.

The serum concentration of lipofuscin in POAG was significantly higher as compared with controls. Considered together with the research of Fernandez de Castro et al. [8], when lipofuscin concentration was recorded proportionally higher in the optic nerve of glaucomatous subjects, this suggests the age-related lipopigment involvement in the exacerbation of a glaucomatous neuropathy in the course of age-related POAG.

Significant increase in MDA serum concentration (almost two fold) corresponds with results as a marker of oxidation degradation products evaluated in serum [22], aqueous humor [23] and both, serum and humor [6], erythrocytes [5] and even in the optic nerve head [24]. This supports that systemic pathological processes are reflected in the glaucomatous eye, both by increasing IOP and exacerbation of RGC death. It should be mentioned that lipid metabolism has an impact on the amount of MDA formation, thus we have included patients with comparable body mass index into our study.

Activity of the total superoxide dismutase in our research model was significantly decreased in glaucomatous patients and corresponds with observations of Engin et al. [22]. Presumably, this decrease results from the depletion of the antioxidant defense system due to long exposure of oxidative stress. Glaucomatous patients in our research presented with exacerbated oxidative stress as indicated by TOS differences between groups. When focused on isoenzymes separately, only SOD2 presented significant deficiency. Emerging evidence suggests that SOD2 (mitochondrial), not SOD1 has a protective role against neuronal cell death induced by glutamate excitotoxicity and oxidative stress [24].

Finally, we collated our results with other previous observation regarding accumulation of MD, LPS and tSOD activity in serum, aqueous humor, lamina cribrosa and optic nerve of patients with POAG (Table 3).

In our study, the antioxidative reserves (TAC) were comparable with controls and oxidative stress. TOS was higher in glaucomatous participants. It should be recognized that only some antioxidative enzymes could play a key role in a glaucomatous pathology.

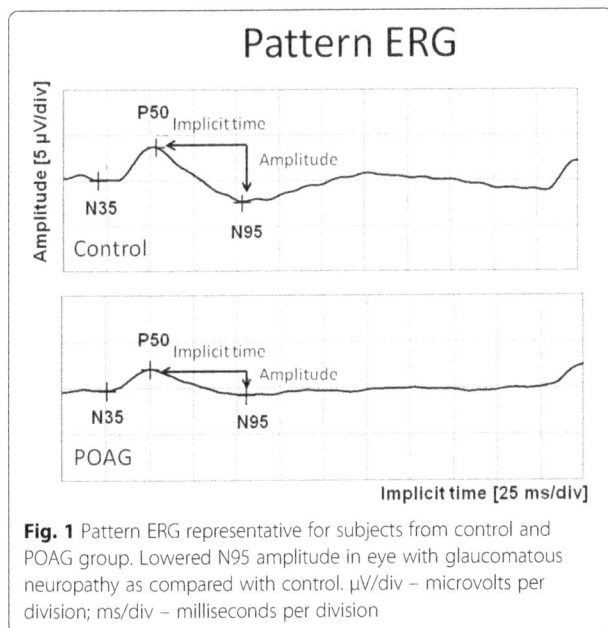

Fig. 1 Pattern ERG representative for subjects from control and POAG group. Lowered N95 amplitude in eye with glaucomatous neuropathy as compared with control. µV/div – microvolts per division; ms/div – milliseconds per division

Table 3 Previously reported LPS, MDA accumulation and tSOD activity in POAG group as compared with non-glaucoma patients

	Increased	Decreased	Not affected
LPS accumulation	SERUM[present study] LAMINA CRIBROSA [25] OPTIC NERVE [8]	Not reported	Not reported
MDA accumulation	SERUM [present study] + [22, 26] AH[b] [23, 27] SERUM + AH [6] LAMINA CRIBROSA [28][a]	Not reported	Not reported
tSOD activity	SERUM [26] AH [10, 27, 29]	SERUM[present study +] [22]AH [30]	Not reported

[a]unclear type of glaucoma
[b]AH aqueous humour

Finally, the biggest limitations of present study should be mentioned. This study model made it impossible to compare progressing with nonprogressing glaucomatous subjects in the context of oxidative stress. For such a comparison, a long-term prospective study with detailed monitoring of systemic and topic conditions is most suitable. Examined groups are small. However, the results are encouraging enough for designing a larger study. Groups were not genetically investigated.

Conclusion
Systemic redox balance of cataract patients was significantly altered in the course of glaucoma.

Abbreviations
AM: Ante meridiem; BMI: Body mass index; CBC: Complete blood count; CI: Confidence interval; CRP: C-reactive protein; Cu,Zn-SOD (SOD1): Cystolic superoxide dismutase; ERG: Electroretinogram; IOP: Intraocular pressure; KCN: Potassium Cyanide; LPS: Lipofuscine; MDA: Malondialdehyde; Mn-SOD (SOD2): Mitochondrial superoxide dismutase; NU: Nitric unit; PERG: Pattern electroretinogram; POAG: Primary open-angle glaucoma; RF: Relative fluorescence lipid extract; RGC: Retinal ganglion cell; ROS: Reactive oxygen species; RPM: Revolutions per minute; SD: Standard deviation; SOD: Superoxide dismutase; TAC: Total antioxidant capacity; TBARS: 2-thiobarbituric acid-reactive substance; TOS: Total oxidant state; VF: Visual field

Acknowledgement
Not applicable.

Funding
Medical University of Silesia, Katowice, Poland covered publishing costs.

Authors' contributions
WR – conception and design, the clinical examinations, acquisition of data, drafting manuscript. JZ-F - conception and design, biochemical determinations, drafting biochemical section. DP-W – patients classification for study, electrophysiology examinations, data analysis, drafting electrophysiological section. HA – coordination of the study, policlinic data collection, primary selection patients for study. WM – analysis and interpretation of data, figures creation, drafting sections with statistical comments. SO – study the history of patients, drafting and editing manuscript, collection and analysis of publications. EM-K – carried out the clinical examinations, final edition of manuscript. All authors have read and approved the final version of the manuscript.

Competing interests
The authors declare that they have no competing interests.

Consent for publication
Not applicable.

Author details
[1]Department and Clinic of Ophthalmology, School of Medicine in Katowice, Medical University of Silesia, Ceglana 35, 40-514 Katowice, Poland. [2]Department of Biochemistry, School of Medicine with the Division of Dentistry in Zabrze, Medical University of Silesia, Katowice, Poland. [3]Radiotherapy Department, Maria Sklodowska-Curie Memorial Cancer Center and Institute of Oncology, Gliwice Branch, Poland.

References
1. Gupta N, Ang LC, De Tilly NL, Bidaisee L, Yücel YH. Human glaucoma and neural degeneration in intracranial optic nerve, lateral geniculate nucleus, and visual cortex. Br J Ophthalmol. 2006;90:674–8.
2. Awai-Kasaoka N, Inoue T, Kameda T, Fujimoto T, Inoue-Mochita M, Tanihara H. Oxidative stress response signaling pathways in trabecular meshwork cells and their effects on cell viability. Mol Vis. 2013;19:1332–40.
3. Izzotti A, Bagnis A, Saccà SC. The role of oxidative stress in glaucoma. Mutat Res. 2006;612:105–14.
4. Moreno MC, Campanelli J, Sande P, Sánez DA, Keller Sarmiento MI, Rosenstein RE. Retinal oxidative stress induced by high intraocular pressure. Free Radic Biol Med. 2004;37:803–12.
5. Rokicki W, Zalejska-Fiolka J, Pojda-Wilczek D, Kabiesz A, Majewski W. Oxidative stress in the red blood cells of patients with primary open-angle glaucoma. Clin Hemorheol Microcirc. 2016;62:369–78.
6. Nucci C, Di Pierro D, Varesi C, Ciuffoletti E, Russo R, Gentile R, Cedrone C, Pinazo Duran MD, Coletta M, Mancino R. Increased malondialdehyde concentration and reduced total antioxidant capacity in aqueous humor and blood samples from patients with glaucoma. Mol Vis. 2013;19:1841–6.
7. Dolman CL, McCormick AQ, Drance SM. Aging of the optic nerve. Arch Ophthalmol. 1980;98:2053–8.
8. Fernandez de Castro JP, Mullins RF, Manea AM, Hernandez J, Wallen T, Kuehn MH. Lipofuscin in human glaucomatous optic nerves. Exp Eye Res. 2013;111:61–6.
9. Behndig A, Svensson B, Marklund SL, Karlsson K. Superoxide dismutase isoenzymes in the human eye. Invest Ophthalmol Vis Sci. 1998;39:471–5.
10. Ferreira SM, Lerner SF, Brunzini R, Evelson PA, Llesuy SF. Oxidative stress markers in aqueous humor of glaucoma patients. Am J Ophthalmol. 2004; 137:62–9.
11. Bach M, Brigell MG, Hawlina M, Holder GE, Johnson MA, McCulloch DL, Meigen T, Viswanathan S. ISCEV standard for clinical pattern electroretinography (PERG): 2012 update. Doc Ophthalmol. 2013;126:1–7.
12. Oyanagui Y. Reevaluation of assay methods and establishment of kit for superoxide dismutase activity. Anal Biochem. 1984;142:290–6.
13. Ohkawa H, Ohishi N, Yagi K. Assay for lipid peroxides in animal tissues by thiobarbituric acid reaction. Anal Biochem. 1979;95:351–8.
14. Erel O. A new automated colorimetric method for measuring total oxidant status. Clin Biochem. 2005;38:1103–11.
15. Erel O. A novel automated direct measurement method for total antioxidant capacity using a new generation, more stable ABTS radical cation. Clin Biochem. 2004;37:277–85.

16. Jain SK. In vivo externalization of phosphatidylserine and phosphatidylethanolamine in the membrane bilayer and hypercoagulability by the lipid peroxidation of erythrocytes in rats. J Clin Invest. 1985;76:281–6.

17. Marx MS, Podos SM, Bodis-Wollner I, Howard-Williams JR, Siegel MJ, Teitelbaum CS. Flash and pattern electroretinograms in normal and laser-induced glaucomatous primate eyes. Invest Ophthalmol Vis Sci. 1986;27:378–86.

18. Holder GE. Pattern electroretinography (PERG) and an integrated approach to visual pathway diagnosis. Prog Retin Eye Res. 2001;20:531–61.

19. Mittag TW, Danias J, Pohorenec G, Yuan HM, Burakgazi E, Chalmers-Redman R, Podos SM, Tatton WG. Retinal damage after 3 to 4 months of elevated intraocular pressure in a rat glaucoma model. Invest Ophthalmol Vis Sci. 2000;41:3451–9.

20. Singh K. Is the patient getting worse? Open Ophthalmol J. 2009;3:65–6.

21. Borchman D, Yappert MC. Age-related lipid oxidation in human lenses. Invest Ophthalmol Vis Sci. 1998;39:1053–8.

22. Engin KN, Yemişci B, Yiğit U, Ağaçhan A, Coşkun C. Variability of serum oxidative stress biomarkers relative to biochemical data and clinical parameters of glaucoma patients. Mol Vis. 2010;16:1260–71.

23. Zanon-Moreno V, Marco-Ventura P, Lleo-Perez A, Pons-Vazquez S, Garcia-Medina JJ, Vinuesa-Silva I, Moreno-Nadal MA, Pinazo-Duran MD. Oxidative stress in primary open-angle glaucoma. J Glaucoma. 2008;17:263–8.

24. Fukui M, Zhu BT. Mitochondrial superoxide dismutase SOD2, but not cytosolic SOD1, plays a critical role in protection against glutamate-induced oxidative stress and cell death in HT22 neuronal cells. Free Radic Biol Med. 2010;48:821–30.

25. McElnea EM, Hughes E, McGoldrick A, McCann A, Quill B, Docherty N, Irnaten M, Farrell M, Clark AF, O'Brien CJ, Wallace DM. Lipofuscin accumulation and autophagy in glaucomatous human lamina cribrosa cells. BMC Ophthalmol. 2014;14:153.

26. Erdurmuş M, Yağcı R, Atış Ö, Karadağ R, Akbaş A, Hepşen IF. Antioxidant status and oxidative stress in primary open angle glaucoma and pseudoexfoliativeglaucoma. Curr Eye Res. 2011;36:713–8.

27. Ghanem AA, Arafa LF, El-Baz A. Oxidative stress markers in patients with primary open-angle glaucoma. Curr Eye Res. 2010;35:295–301.

28. McElnea EM, Quill B, Docherty NG, Irnaten M, Siah WF, Clark AF, O'Brien CJ, Wallace DM. Oxidative stress, mitochondrial dysfunction and calcium overload in human lamina cribrosa cells from glaucomadonors. Mol Vis. 2011;17:1182–91.

29. Goyal A, Srivastava A, Sihota R, Kaur J. Evaluation of oxidative stress markers in aqueous humor of primary open angle glaucoma and primary angle closure glaucoma patients. Curr Eye Res. 2014;39:823–9.

30. Bagnis A, Izzotti A, Centofanti M, Saccà SC. Aqueous humor oxidative stress proteomic levels in primary open angle glaucoma. Exp Eye Res. 2012;103:55–62.

28

A case report of Werner's syndrome with bilateral juvenile cataracts

Chun-li Chen[1,4†], Jia-song Yang[3†], Xiang Zhang[2], Tian Tian[2], Rui Zeng[3], Guan-hong Zhang[1*] and Xin-guo Jia[1*] ⓘ

Abstract

Background: To report a case of Werner's syndrome with bilateral juvenile cataracts.

Case presentation: Review of the clinical, laboratory, photographic, genetic testing of the patient.
A 26-year-old Chinese man presented with impaired vision in both eyes for more than a year. Anterior segment examination of both eyes revealed cataract. According to the ocular symptoms and systemic signs, including low body weight, a short stature, a bird-like face, atrophic and scleroderma-like skin, in addition to the juvenile cataracts, the clinical diagnosis of Werner's syndrome was made. Next-generation sequencing identified a homozygous *WRN* mutation in this patient.

Conclusions: The ocular and systemic findings in this patient in combination with the homozygous WRN mutation indicated the definitive Werner's syndrome diagnosis.

Keywords: Werner's syndrome, *WRN* mutation, Premature aging

Background

Werner's syndrome was first described by Werner in 1904; it is also known as adult premature aging syndrome, or progeria of adult. Werner's syndrome is an autosomal recessive and rarely inherited disease characterized by onset of a prematurely aged-appearance (grey hair, scleroderma-like skin) typically starts in the 20–30s followed by age-related disorders like cataracts, diabetes mellitus, atherosclerosis, cancers, and osteoporosis [1, 2]. We present a case diagnosed with Werner's syndrome confirmed by genetic testing, to improve doctors' knowledge of this rare genetic disease.

Case presentation

The patient was a 26-year-old Chinese male with a chief complaint of impaired vision in both eyes for more than a year. An ocular examination revealed that the vision in his right eye was FC/20 cm and left eye was 0.02, intraocular pressure was 18 mmHg in both eyes, ptosis of both upper eyelids, lateral eyelashes touched the cornea. Corneas were transparent in both eyes, central corneal thickness was 547 μm in right eye, and left corneal

* Correspondence: 13905461351@139.com; dongyingjxg@163.com
†Chun-li Chen and Jia-song Yang contributed equally to this work.
¹Department of Ophthalmology, Shengli Oilfield Central Hospital, Shandong Province, Dongying 257000, China
Full list of author information is available at the end of the article

thickness was 540 μm. The central anterior chamber depth of the right eye was 3.25 mm, and the central anterior chamber depth of the left eye was 3.03 mm. The pupils were round, about 3 mm in diameter. The lenses were milky and opaque in both eyes (Fig. 1a). The thickness of the right eye lens was 3.30 mm and the lens of left eye was 3.32 mm. The fundus of both eyes was not clear due to the occlusion of cloudy lens. The right eye axial length was 22.38 mm, and the left eye was 22.17 mm. No obvious vitreoretinal abnormalities were found on ultrosonography. Family history showed that his parents were consanguineous (first cousions). The patient's father died in a traffic accident at 40 years old, and his mother, and sister, uncle, cousin, and niece were in good health. The patient denied any family history of genetic diseases. Developmental retardation occurred when he was 8 years old and Achilles tendon elongation was performed due to Achilles tendon contracture. Physical examination on admission revealed the patient had a spare figure, weighed 40 kg and was 150 cm tall (Fig. 2). Vital signs testing demonstrated his temperature was 36.7 °C, pulse was 98 b/min, respiratory rate 19/min, and the blood pressure was 108/65 mmHg. Heart and lung auscultation found no obvious abnormalities. A complete blood cell count, thyroid hormone levels, hepatic function,

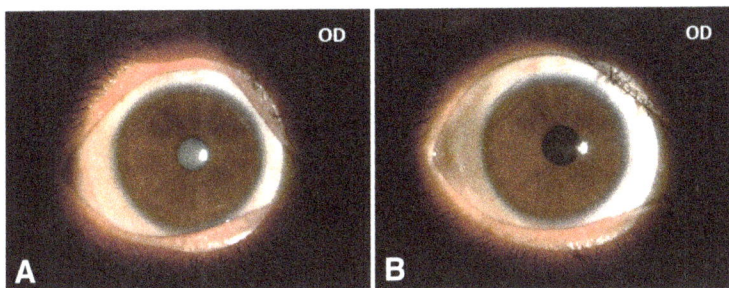

Fig. 1 Photograph of the anterior segment of the right eye (OD). **a**, lens was opaque and cloudy; **b**, post-operative appearance showed the clear IOL in place. OD, right eye

and renal function were evaluated, and no abnormalities were found. Figure 2 depicts the patient with the symptoms of short stature, slightly built, gray hair, bird-like face appearance, skin depigmentation, skin drying and atrophy, scleroderma-like skin changes, beak-like nose, and teeth abnormalities.

According to the ocular symptoms and systemic signs, including low body weight, a short stature, a bird-like face, atrophic and scleroderma-like skin, and juvenile cataracts, the clinical diagnosis of Werner's syndrome was made. Next-generation sequencing identified a homozygous *WRN* mutation in this patient. Five bases (c.3460_3461 insTTGTG) were inserted between the 3460 and 3461 nucleotides of *WRN* gene in this patient, resulting in a frame shift mutation of amino acids (p. Y 1157 Cfs * 7) (Fig. 3). After searching the literature, this mutation has not been reported, and does not belong to the polymorphic site, incidence is very low in the population and not reported in the Human Gene Mutation Database (HGMD professional). The *WRN* mutation was the likely pathogenic variant. So the definitive Werner's syndrome diagnosis was established. Besides, the same heterozygous *WRN* mutation was identified in his mother, his father's brother, and sister. The pedigree chart has been constructed in Fig. 4.

The patient underwent phacoemulsification combined with intraocular lens implantation in both eyes. The right eye was implanted with a + 23.0 diopter intraocular lens and the left eye was implanted with a + 24.0 diopter intraocular lens. Post-operative appearance showed the clear IOL in place (Fig. 1b). The post-operative best-corrected visual acuity was 0.6 in both eyes. No vitreoretinal abnormalities were observed in both eyes.

Discussion

The age-related pathophysiology resembles the normal aging [1]. Early susceptibility to a number of major age-related diseases is the key feature of this syndrome. The incidence of Werner's syndrome is one in 20,000–40,000 in Japan and one in 200,000 in the USA [2]. However, the incidence of Werner's syndrome has not been reported in China. Our case presented the characteristic of Werner's syndrome resembling premature aging, including a bird-like face, atrophic skin, scleroderma-like skin, and juvenile cataract.

The definitive diagnosis for Werner's syndrome is based on the genetic analysis for mutations in the *WRN* gene. *WRN* is a RecQ family member with both helicase and exonuclease activities and it participates in several cell metabolic pathways, including DNA repair, and telomere maintenance [3, 4]. The genetic pattern of this

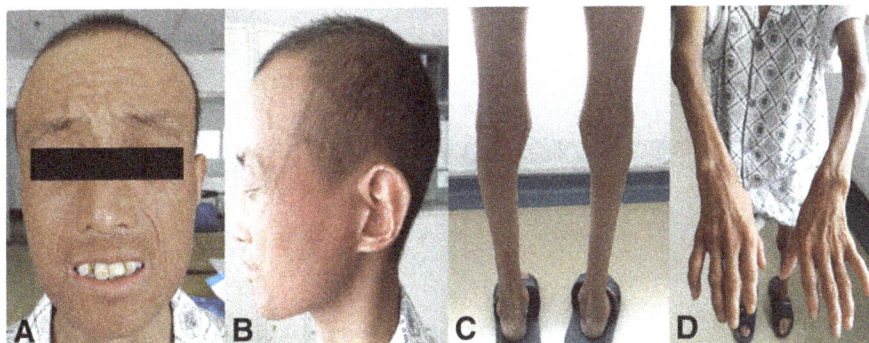

Fig. 2 The appearance of the patient and his form extremely slight. **a**, beak-like nose and teeth abnormalities; **b**, Gray hair, bird-like face appearance; **c&d**, skin depigmentation, skin drying and atrophy, and scleroderma-like skin changes

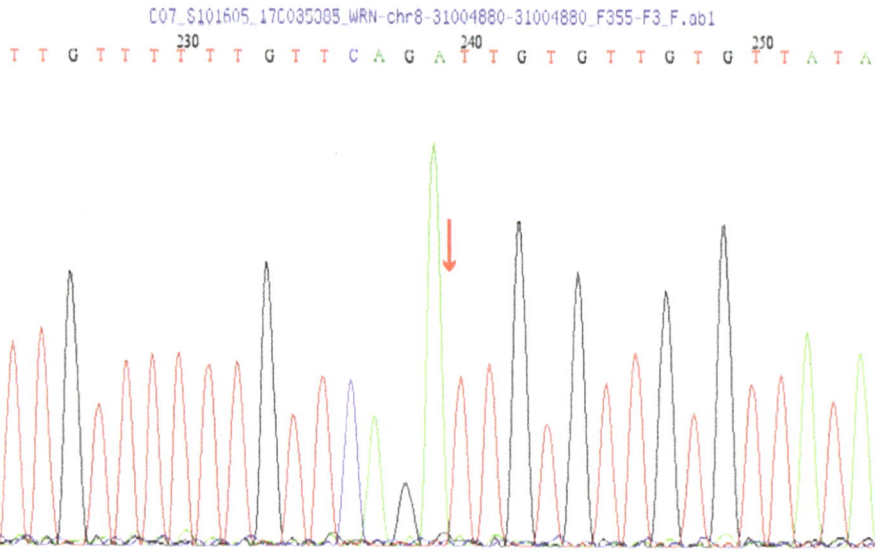

Fig. 3 Next-generation sequencing identified a homozygous WRN mutation in this patient. Five bases (c.3460_3461 insTTGTG) were inserted between the 3460 and 3461 nucleotides of WRN gene in this patient

genetic disease is autosomal recessive. Homozygous mutation of *WRN* was detected, which may be inherited from their parents with consanguineous marriage. Homozygous *WRN* gene mutation (c.3460_3461 insTT GTG) was found in this patient and heterozygous *WRN* gene mutation were found in his close relatives. After physical examination, the relatives of the patient carrying the heterozygous mutations were not found to be associated with Werner's syndrome. Features of early aging which include premature graying or loss of hair, juvenile cataract, type 2 diabetes mellitus, hypogonadism, osteoporosis, and atherosclerosis are very common in patients with Werner's syndrome.

The patients with Werner's syndrome develop a variety of serious diseases, especially atherosclerosis and malignant tumors. Early diagnosis of Werner syndrome is important to enable early serial screening for these associated diseases in the patients. Although there is no definitive therapy that addresses the underlying gene mutation, but many of the signs including cataracts, diabetes, and atherosclerosis are treatable. In our case, the patient was transferred to us due to his poor vision. After performing phacoemulsification and intraocular lens implantation in both eyes, his visual acuity improved significantly.

Conclusions

Both the ocular symptoms and systemic signs combination with the homozygous WRN mutation indicated the definitive Werner's syndrome diagnosis. Our case presented the characteristic of Werner's syndrome resembling premature aging, including bird-like face, atrophic skin, scleroderma-like skin, and juvenile cataract. Genetic testing is important for the accurate diagnosis of inherited diseases and contributes to the early diagnosis and treatment of diseases.

Abbreviation
HGMD: Human Gene Mutation Database

Acknowledgements
We thank Dr. Huan-Jun Shi for her professional editing of the figures. We thank Mr. Cináed Remus Langley, Mrs. Esha Nicole Ramey, and Mr. John Frederick Suckow for their professional manuscript editing.

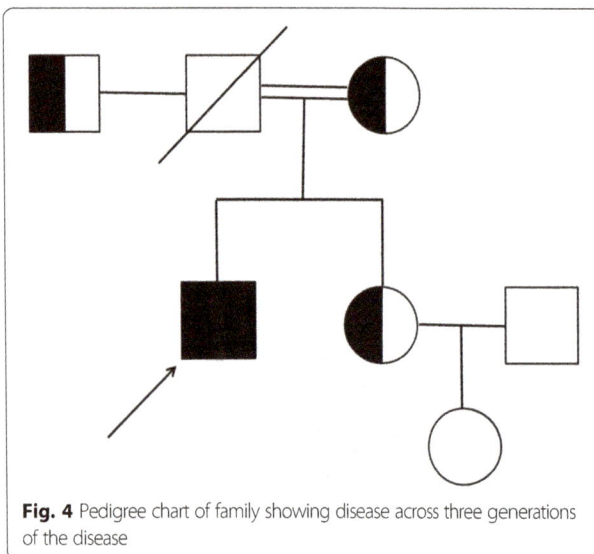

Fig. 4 Pedigree chart of family showing disease across three generations of the disease

Authors' contributions
JSY and CLC contributed equally to this case report and they were both major contributor in writing the manuscript. CLC, TT, XZ and RZ contributed to the literature search and preparation of the manuscript and figures. XGJ and GHZ are responsible for the design of the case report. All authors read and approved the final manuscript.

Consent for publication
Written informed consent was obtained from the patient for publication of this case report and any accompanying images.

Competing interests
The authors declare that they have no competing interests.

Author details
[1]Department of Ophthalmology, Shengli Oilfield Central Hospital, Shandong Province, Dongying 257000, China. [2]Department of Ophthalmology, Xin Hua Hospital Affiliate of Shanghai Jiao Tong University School of Medicine, Shanghai 200092, China. [3]Vitreous & Retinal Department, Apex Eye Hospital, Xincai 463500, Henan Province, China. [4]Department of Ophthalmology, Tianjin Medical University Eye Hospital, Tianjin 30000, China.

References
1. Kyng K, Croteau DL, Bohr VA. Werner syndrome resembles normal aging. Cell Cycle. 2009;8(15):2323.
2. Satoh M, Imai M, Sugimoto M, Goto M, Furuichi Y. Prevalence of Werner's syndrome heterozygotes in Japan. Lancet. 1999;353(9166):1766.
3. Yu CE, Oshima J, Fu YH, Wijsman EM, Hisama F, Alisch R, Matthews S, Nakura J, Miki T, Ouais S, et al. Positional cloning of the Werner's syndrome gene. Science. 1996;272(5259):258–62.
4. Goto M, Imamura O, Kuromitsu J, Matsumoto T, Yamabe Y, Tokutake Y, Suzuki N, Mason B, Drayna D, Sugawara M, et al. Analysis of helicase gene mutations in Japanese Werner's syndrome patients. Hum Genet. 1997;99(2): 191–3.

29

Association of alpha A-crystallin polymorphisms with susceptibility to nuclear age-related cataract in a Han Chinese population

Zhennan Zhao[1†], Qi Fan[1†], Peng Zhou[2†], HongFei Ye[1], Lei Cai[1] and Yi Lu[1*]

Abstract

Background: Alpha A-crystallin (CRYAA) is considered critical for the maintenance of lens transparency and is related to the pathogenesis of age-related cataracts (ARCs), especially the nuclear subtype. As the 5' untranslated region (5' UTR) modulates gene expression, the purpose of current study was to investigate whether single nucleotide polymorphisms (SNPs) in the 5' UTR of *CRYAA* were associated with susceptibility to ARC in a Han Chinese population and to clarify the mechanism of this association.

Methods: SNPs in the 5' UTR (−1 to −1000) of *CRYAA* were identified in 243 nuclear ARC patients and 263 controls using polymerase chain reaction and DNA sequencing. Allele and genotype frequencies were calculated and compared between two groups. Haploview 4.2 was used to calculate the linkage disequilibrium index, and the SHEsis analysis platform was used to infer haplotype construction. A dual-luciferase reporter gene assay was used for transcription of *CRYAA* in the presence of a protective haplotype with individual SNP alteration, Chromatin immunoprecipitation (ChIP) was employed to determine whether SNPs regulated *CRYAA* expression by altering the binding affinity of transcription factors.

Results: Three polymorphisms were identified in the 5' UTR of CRYAA: rs3761381 ($P = 0.000357$, odds ratio [OR] $= 1.837$), rs13053109 ($P = 0.788$, OR $= 1.086$), and rs7278468 ($P = 0.00136$, OR $= 0.652$). The haplotype C-G-T ($P = 0.0014$, OR $= 1.536$) increased the risk of nuclear ARC, whereas the haplotype T-G-G ($P = 0.00029$, OR $= 0.535$) decreased the risk. The haplotype C-G-T decreased CRYAA transcription through rs7278468, which is located in the binding site of specificity protein 1 (Sp1). Furthermore, the G allele of rs7278468 increased CRYAA transcription by enhancing the binding affinity of Sp1.

Conclusions: These data indicate that the CRYAA polymorphism is a genetic marker of inter-individual differences in the risk of nuclear ARC.

Keywords: Alpha A-crystallin, Age-related cataract, 5' untranslated region, Single nucleotide polymorphisms, Transcriptional activity

* Correspondence: luyieent@126.com
†Equal contributors
[1]Department of Ophthalmology, Eye and ENT Hospital of Fudan University, 83 Fenyang Road, Shanghai 200031, People's Republic of China
Full list of author information is available at the end of the article

Background

Age-related cataracts (ARCs), which are a major cause of blindness worldwide, are characterized by lens opacities and visual impairment due to degenerative changes in the lens in the elderly [1]. The causes of ARCs are multifactorial, with both environmental and genetic variations implicated in the disease [2]. A study of twins strongly implicated genetic factors in the pathogenesis of ARCs, demonstrating heritability of 48% for the nuclear subtype [2]. Recent studies also indicated that several genes, such as galactokinase and eph-receptor tyrosine kinase-type A2 [3, 4], were genetic risk factors for cataracts. Although the importance of genetic risk factors for ARC has been highlighted, the pathophysiology is far from clearly understood.

As a major structural protein component expressed in the lens, alpha A-crystallin (CRYAA) is considered critical for the maintenance of lens transparency [5]. Many studies showed that CRYAA was related to the pathogenesis of ARC, including a study conducted by our research group [6–8]. The chaperone-like activity of CRYAA enables it to protect other crystallins against thermally induced inactivation or aggregation [9]. In addition, CRYAA can trap aggregation-prone denatured proteins, an action that is thought to delay the development of ARC [10]. Although previous research demonstrated that the levels of CRYAA decreased in the nuclear capsule of ARC patients compared to those of controls [8], the mechanism underlying the downregulation of CRYAA in the lens was unclear.

Previous research demonstrated that the 5′ untranslated region (5′ UTR) acted as a regulatory element in genes and that it was associated with modulating the expression of gene-coding regions [11]. Single nucleotide polymorphisms (SNPs) in 5′ UTR sequences were shown to play a critical role in regulating gene expression [12]. In addition, previous studies showed that SNPs in the 5′ UTR of the SLC16A12 gene were involved in the pathogenic consequences of ARC [13]. Recently, SNPs that were identified in the CRYAA gene promoter region that were associated with cortical ARC in a Northern Italian population [14]. However, it is unknown whether SNPs in the 5′ UTR of CRYAA contribute to ARC susceptibility in a Han Chinese population, especially the nuclear subtype (the most frequent form).

The present study focuses on polymorphisms within the 5′ UTR of CRYAA (−1 to −1000) and attempts to shed light on the development of nuclear ARC in a Han Chinese population.

Methods

Subjects

Subjects were recruited from the Eye and ENT Hospital of Fudan University. All the subjects underwent a full ophthalmic examination, including visual acuity, slit-lamp microscopic examinations, and ophthalmoscopic examinations. There was no consanguinity between the subjects (at least not among all four grandparents). All the enrolled subjects self-identified as Han Chinese (all four grandparents were ethnic Han Chinese). This research was approved by the Institutional Review Board and followed the tenets of the Declaration of Helsinki. All the subjects signed informed consent forms.

Lens opacity grading

After pupil dilation with 1% tropicamide, a trained ophthalmologist graded the lens opacity of each right eye according to the Lens Opacity Classification System (LOCS) III. Opacity was classified as nuclear opalescence (NO), nuclear color (NC), cortical (C), and posterior subcapsular (P). The grading consisted of six standards for NO and NC (standards 1 to 6) and five standards for C and P (standards 1 to 5). Each standard was assigned using decimals to interpolate between the reference standards, with the assigned scores ranging from 0.1 to 6.9 for NO and NC and 0.1 to 5.9 for C and P. The subtype of the cataract was then classified as nuclear (NO or NC ≥3), cortical (C ≥ 2), posterior subcapsular cataract (PSC) ($P \geq 2$), or mixed type (i.e., the presence of more than one type in one eye).

ARC group and control group

All subjects with nuclear cataract were enrolled. Subjects with cortical and posterior subcapsular cataracts were excluded from this study. For the mixed type, only subjects with NO or NC scores higher than C and P scores were enrolled. Cases and controls were then recruited based on their NO and NC grading scores. The cases included subjects with NO and NC grading scores ≥3.0, and the controls included those with NO and NC grading scores <2.0.

The exclusion criteria for the cases and controls included: (1) subjects younger than 45 years; (2) pseudophakia or aphakia in either eye; (3) the presence of other eye diseases, such as dislocated lens, trauma, uveitis, high myopia, glaucoma, macular diseases, and retinal detachment; (4) previous ocular surgery in either eye; and (5) a history of diabetes, kidney disease, respiratory disease, cancer, or tumors.

Blood sample collection and DNA isolation

Five milliliters of peripheral blood samples were collected in EDTA tubes from all the subjects was and stored at −80 °C until use. DNA was isolated from whole blood cells using a Mammal Blood Genomic DNA Extraction Kit (LifeFeng Biotech Co., Shanghai, China), following the manufacturer's protocol, and was stored at −20 °C until used for genotyping.

Identification and genotyping of SNPs

For analyzing the polymorphism in the 5′ UTR (−1 to −1000) of *CRYAA*, the polymerase chain reaction (PCR) and DNA direct sequencing were performed. A set of primers (forward: GGTGACACAGCAAGACTCCA and reverse: CACGTCCATGTTCAGCTTTG) from Generay Biotechnology Co., Ltd. (Shanghai, China) was used to amplify the target fragment. The PCR reactions were performed in 50 μl reaction mixtures, consisting of 25 μl of PrimeSTAR Max Premix (Takara), 20 μl of RNase-free water, 1 μl of the forward primer, 1 μl of the reverse primer, and 1 μl of extracted genomic DNA. The PCR program included a 94 °C activation step for 3 min, followed by 30 cycles of 94 °C for 20 s, 60 °C for 20 s, 72 °C for 40 s, and 72 °C for 65 s. The PCR products were sequenced using ABI 3730xl (Generay Biotechnology Co., Ltd).

Cell culture and transfection

The human lens epithelium (HLE) B3 cell line obtained from American Type Culture Collection (ATCC; Rockville, MD, USA) was cultured in Dulbecco's Modified Eagle Medium (DMEM) containing 20% fetal bovine serum (FBS). Before transfection, the cells were seeded in six-well plates and grown overnight, so that the cell density reached approximately 70%. A mixture of 2 μg of plasmid DNA and 4 μl of Lipofectamine™ 2000 (Invitrogen) reagent in 2 ml of serum-free medium was then added in a six-well plate. The cells were collected for luciferase activity testing and chromatin immunoprecipitation (ChIP) analysis 72 h and 48 h later, respectively.

Plasmid construction

The human *CRYAA* 5′ UTR (−1 to −1000) was amplified using primers, as described above and then inserted into the PGL3-Basic vector (Invitrogen) using the restriction enzymes Hind III and KpnI (Takara). The *CRYAA* 5′ UTR containing each SNP mutation was constructed using site–directed mutagenesis, with the following primers: rs3761381-mut forward: ATCATGTGGGTGGTGGG TCT, reverse: ATGCCTTGATGTAACATCCCC; rs1305 3109-mut forward: GGTGAGACTCTGAGGACGATG TGT, reverse: ACACATCGTCCTCAGAGTCTCACC; rs7278468-mut forward: GGGTGTGTGCTCTCCCTC CTCT, reverse: AGAGGAGGGAGAGCACACACCC.

Luciferase assay

The HLE cells were cultured in six-well plates with 2 μg of either PGL3-Basic-CRYAA 5′ UTR or PGL3-Basic plasmid and 20 ng of pRL-TK and then transfected into cells, as described above. Then, 72 h after transfection, luciferase activities were checked by a Dual-luciferase Reporter (DLR™) Assay System (Promega), according to the manufacture's protocol.

In silico analysis

The transcription factor binding sites of the identified SNPs of CRYAA 5′UTR were predicted by MEME SUITE as described previously [15].

Chromatin immunoprecipitation (ChIP) analysis

ChIP analysis of HLE cells transfected with a plasmid containing the *CRYAA* 5′ UTR was conducted 48 h after transfection using a Pierce Agarose ChIP Kit (Thermo Scientific), according to the manufacture's protocol. The antibodies used for ChIP included anti-human IgG (Abcam) and anti-specificity protein 1 (Sp1) (Abcam). The captured genomic DNA fragments were then purified with Premix Taq™ (Takara). The primers used for the ChIP PCR were as follows: CRYAA ChIP forward: CTGAG GACGATGTGTCTAACCTC, reverse: AGGCCTGGA CTCAGCTGA. CRYAA ChIP NC: forward: ACCCTGA CAGGAGCAGCCCA, reverse: TCCTCCAGGGGTCA CATGC. The ChIP-quantitative PCR (qPCR) data relative to Sp1 were calculated using the $2^{-\Delta\Delta Ct}$ methods and presented as % input.

Statistical analysis

Differences between the values were evaluated using a two-tailed Student's *t*-test or Fisher's chi-squared test, depending on the variables types. SPSS for Windows, version 17.0 (SPSS, IBM Inc., Chicago, IL, USA) was used in the statistical analysis of the above data and for the calculation of odds ratios (ORs). The Hardy–Weinberg equilibrium (HWE), linkage disequilibrium (LD) and the haplotype analysis was conducted using the SHEsis software platform [16]. The experiments were all repeated at least three times. A value of $P < 0.05$ was considered statistically significant.

Results

Participant characteristics

In total, 243 unrelated ARC patients and 263 control subjects were included in this study. The mean ages of the ARC patients and controls were 70.06 ± 6.22 years and 69.01 ± 4.64 years, respectively ($p = 0.667$).

The SNPs identified in the CRYAA 5′ UTR

Three polymorphisms were identified in the 5′ UTR of CRYAA: rs3761381 (C > T), rs13053109 (G > C), and rs7278468 (T > G) (Fig. 1). The allele and genotype distributions of each identified SNP are shown in Table 1 and Table 2, respectively. All three SNPs were in Hardy Weinberg equilibrium ($P > 0.05$). The frequencies of the rs3761381 T allele ($P = 0.000357$, OR = 1.837,95% confidence interval [95% CI] = 1.312–2.572) and rs7278468 G allele ($P = 0.00136$, OR = 0.652,95% CI = 0.501–0.847) were significantly higher in the control group compared to the ARC group. With regard to rs13053109, there

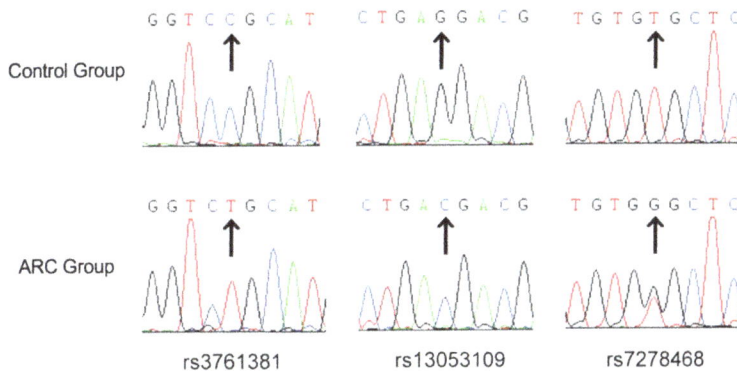

Fig. 1 Sequence analysis of the 5′UTR region of *CRYAA* in the ARC group and the control group. The arrows point to the SNP sites

were no significant differences in the genotype or allele frequency between the ARC patients and the controls.

LD analysis and haplotype construction

The D′ values for the LD of the three SNPs are shown in Fig. 2 (D′ values: all >0.9). As seen, there were very strong levels of LD in all three SNPs. Five possible haplotypes were constructed (Table 3). The haplotype C-G-T appeared to confer a high risk of ARC ($P = 0.0014$, OR = 1.536, 95% CI = 1.180–1.997), whereas the haplotype T-G-G ($P = 0.00029$, OR = 0.535, 95% CI = 0.381–0.753) seemed to confer protection against ARCs.

The transcriptional activity of CRYAA in the presence of the haplotypes

Based on the position of these three SNPs, we constructed luciferase reporter vectors containing the CRYAA 5′ UTR and either T-G-G (protective haplotype) or C-G-T (risk haplotype) and evaluated whether they could influence the transcriptional activity of the gene. Seventy-two hours after transfection of the HLE cells, a dual-luciferase reporter assay showed that the luciferase activity of the cells transfected with the vector containing the CRYAA 5′ UTR (Fig. 3) was more than

11 times higher than that of the cells transfected with the vector alone, demonstrating that the CRYAA 5′ UTR exhibited positive transcriptional activity in the HLE cells. The transcriptional activity of the CRYAA 5′ UTR with the risk-associated haplotype C-G-T was approximately 17% lower than that of the protective T-G-G haplotype (Fig. 3a). This finding indicated that the C-G-T haplotype reduced CRYAA transcriptional activity in HLE cells and that this haplotype might cause nuclear ARC by decreasing the transcriptional efficiency of CRYAA.

The transcriptional activity of *CRYAA* in the presence of the protective haplotype with individual SNP alteration

To distinguish which individual SNPs of the haplotypes in the CRYAA 5′ UTR were predominantly responsible for the regulation of transcriptional activity, site-directed mutagenesis was employed to alter the single base of each individual SNP present in the protective T-G-G haplotype, one by one. Subsequent transcriptional activity was then analyzed. As shown by a dual-luciferase reporter assay, 72 h after transfection, the transcriptional activities of the 5′ UTR containing the individual alleles of rs3761381 and rs13053109 occurring as a single base variation were not significantly different from those of

Table 1 Allele frequencies of SNPs in the CRYAA gene among the ARC group and the control group

SNPs	Allele	ARC group n (%)	Control group n (%)	P value	OR for minor allele (95% CI)
rs3761381				0.000357	1.837 (1.312–2.572)
	C	423 (87.0%)	413 (78.5%)		
	T	63 (13.0%)	113 (21.5%)		
rs13053109				0.788	1.086 (0.594–1.988)
	G	464 (95.5%)	504 (95.8%)		
	C	22 (4.5%)	22 (4.2%)		
rs7278468				0.00136	0.652 (0.501–0.847)
	T	344 (70.8%)	322 (61.2%)		
	G	142 (29.2%)	204 (38.8%)		

SNPs Single Nucleotide Polymorphisms, *ARC* Age-Related Cataract, *OR* Odds Ratio, *CI* Confidence Interval

Table 2 Genotype frequencies of SNPs in the CRYAA gene among the ARC group and the control group

SNPs	Genotype	ARC group n (%)	Control group n (%)	P value
rs3761381				0.0011
	C C	182 (74.9%)	161 (61.2%)	
	C T	59 (24.3%)	91 (34.6%)	
	T T	2 (0.8%)	11 (4.2%)	
rs13053109				0.965
	G G	222 (91.4%)	242 (92.0%)	
	G C	20 (8.2%)	20 (7.6%)	
	C C	1 (0.4%)	1 (0.4%)	
rs7278468				0.0054
	T T	120 (49.4%)	99 (37.6%)	
	T G	104 (42.8%)	124 (47.1%)	
	G G	19 (7.8%)	40 (15.2%)	

SNPs Single Nucleotide Polymorphisms, *ARC* Age-Related Cataract

the protective T-G-G haplotype (Fig. 3b). However, when the G allele of rs7278468 replaced with the T allele, the consequent transcriptional activity of the *CRYAA* 5′ UTR with the T-C-T haplotype decreased approximately 11% ($P < 0.05$) compared with that of the protective T-G-G haplotype. These data indicated that the allelic change in rs7278468 affected CRYAA expression.

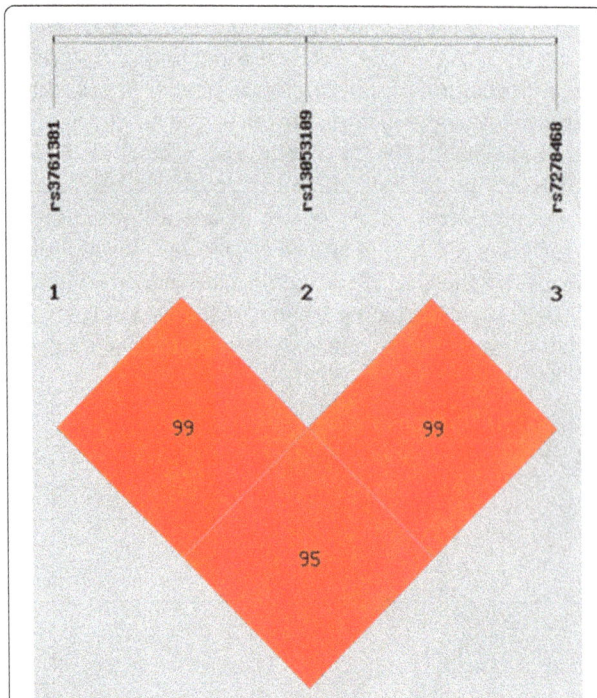

Fig. 2 LD status of the three SNPs in *CRYAA 5′UTR*. Each square represents a pair-wise comparison between the 2 SNPs, and the respective D′ is given within each square. The darker colored squares indicate higher values of D′

The rs7278468 G allele increased *CRYAA* transcription by enhancing the binding affinity of Sp1

Previous data showed that the rs7278468 alleles affected *CRYAA* transcriptional activity, as it lies upstream of the transcription start site. It is feasible that it might influence the binding affinity of one or more transcription factors and affect the transcriptional activity of *CRYAA*. Thus, using the MEME SUITE, transcription factor binding prediction of the sequence around rs7278468 was performed. The rs7278468 T allele is located in the binding motifs of several transcription factors, including specificity protein 1 (Sp1) (Additional file 1: Table S1). Sp1 is a transcriptional factor that applies its activity via binding to a GC-rich element in the promoter region of target genes. The methylation within the CpG sites of the CRYAA promotor might decrease the DNA-binding capacity of Sp1, leading to epigenetic repression in nuclear ARC lenses. The aforementioned factors make Sp1 a good candidate for further studies. To determine whether rs7278468 regulated *CRYAA* by altering the binding affinity of Sp1, ChIP-PCR was used to analyze the binding affinity of Sp1 in HLE cells (Fig. 4). With the ChIP-NC primers, bands were detected only in the input lanes and not in any of the immunoprecipitated samples. As shown by the ChIP-PCR, bands were detected in both the HLE cells alone and in the HLE cells transfected with the CRYAA_T-G-T or *CRYAA*_T-G-G plasmid. However, a higher strength ChIP-PCR band was detected in the *CRYAA*_T-G-G transfected cells (Fig. 4b), and the ChIP-qPCR confirmed this tendency (Fig. 4c). These data showed that Sp1 binds directly to the CRYAA 5′ UTR and that the rs7278468 G allele increased this binding. These findings implied that Sp1 might regulate the transcription of *CRYAA* by direct interaction with the 5′ UTR and that the rs7278468 G allele increased this interaction and enhanced transcriptional activity.

Discussion

This study demonstrated evidence of the involvement of alleles, genotypes, and haplotypes of SNPs in the 5′ UTR of *CRYAA* in the susceptibility to nuclear ARC. Similar results were reported previously in the case of all types of ARC (especially the cortical subtype) in a northern Italian population [14]. However, in the Han Chinese population with nuclear ARC in the current study, the sites of the SNP (rs3761381) and allelic frequency (rs7278468) were significantly different than those reported. In the present study, the frequency of the T allele of rs7278468 was higher (70.8%) than that (49.5%) reported in a previous study of patients with ARC. Numerous studies have demonstrated a population-specific and subtype-specific effect of SNPs, and ARC is no exception [17–19]. The increased frequency of the T allele of

Table 3 Haplotype analysis of the ARC group and the control group

Haplotypes	ARC group (freq)	Control group (freq)	P value	OR (95% CI)
C-C-G	22.00 (0.045)	22.00 (0.042)	0.788	1.087 (0.594–1.989)
C-G-G	59.31 (0.122)	71.32 (0.6136)	0.522	0.886 (0.613–1.282)
C-G-T	341.69 (0.703)	319.68 (0.608)	0.0014	1.536 (1.180–1.997)
T-G-G	60.69 (0.125)	110.68 (0.210)	0.00029	0.535 (0.381–0.753)
T-G-T	2.31 (0.005)	2.32 (0.004)	0.695	1.247 (0.816–1.457)

ARC Age-Related Cataract, *OR* Odds Ratio *CI* Confidence Interval

rs7278468 observed in the present study might indicate an increased risk of the progression of ARC in the Han Chinese population, which was similar to epidemiological findings that the incidence rate of nuclear cataract in the Chinese population is higher than that in the Caucasian population [20, 21]. Furthermore, as rs7278468 has been found to be associated with cataracts in different populations, which points to the importance of the rs7278468 locus in the pathogenesis of cataracts, providing a potential target for future gene therapy. Additionally, the difference of allelic frequency between ours and Ma's study might be caused by selection bias. They included all types of ARC, but our study included only nuclear ARC. Therefore, further studies with all types of ARC should be considered.

As a molecular chaperone, CRYAA protects other crystallins from aggregation or inactivation and to traps aggregation-prone denatured proteins, which are suggested to delay the progression of ARC [10]. Studies with CRYAA-knockout animals and our previous reports demonstrated the importance of CRYAA in lens clarity [7, 22]. In a previous study, we showed that CRYAA expression decreased in the lens capsules of individuals with age-related nuclear cataracts compared to age-matched controls and confirmed lower CRYAA levels in samples with greater lens opacity severity [8]. The decrease in CRYAA expression may be one cause of lens opacity and also contributes to cataract pathology.

SNPs in the 5′ UTR play a critical role in gene expression and are involved in the pathophysiology of disease. Seshadri identified a SNP, rs366316, in the 5′ UTR of CD1a that was strongly associated with CD1a expression [23]. SNPs identified in the 5′ UTR of the *SLC16A12* gene affected the pathogenic consequences of ARC [13]. As shown in the current study, Sp1 appeared to regulate *CRYAA* via binding to the binding motif in the 5′ UTR of CRYAA, with an increase in the binding strength of the Sp1 binding motif in the rs7278468 G allele increasing CRYAA transcription. The resulting increased in CRYAA transcription seemed to enhance the expression of the alpha A-crystallin protein in the lens, making individuals with the rs7278468 G allele invulnerable to the development of nuclear ARC.

Sp1 is a ubiquitously expressed transcription factor, which plays a critical role in regulating plenty of genes required for normal cell function [24, 25]. In human cells, SP1 acts as gene activator [25]. The DNA-binding affinity of Sp1 can be regulated both by altering protein interactions and by post-translational modification [26]. Recently, Liu reported that the methylation of CpG sites of the CRYAA promotor directly decreased the DNA-binding capacity of Sp1, leading to a reduction in the expression of CRYAA in HLE cells [27]. In the current study, Sp1 bound directly to the CRYAA 5′ UTR, and the rs7278468 G allele increased the binding affinity of Sp1, suggesting a mechanism for Sp1 regulation of CRYAA transcription.

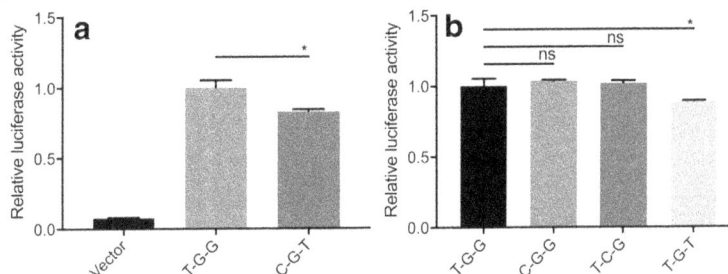

Fig. 3 Allelic variation of the rs7278468 alters the transcription of CRYAA. **a** The luciferase activity of CRYAA 5′UTR within either the T-C-G or C-G-T haplotype after being transfected into HLE cells. **b** Site–directed mutagenesis was applied to discern the impact of rs3761381, rs13053109 and rs7278468. The allele rs7278468 is mainly accounted for the transcriptional activity alteration of the CRYAA 5′UTR. The CRYAA 5′UTR with T-C-G were set to 1, to which other values were normalized. The results are shown as the mean ± SD. (*p < 0.05)

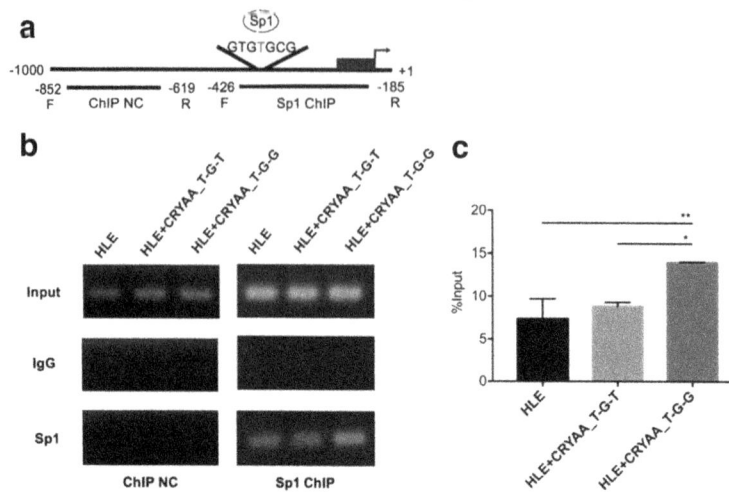

Fig. 4 The rs7278468 G allele increases *CRYAA* transcription through enhancing Sp1 binding capacity. **a** Diagram of the CRYAA 5'UTR shows the Sp1 binding site within rs7278468. **b** ChIP analyses showing the rs7278468 G allele enhanced Sp1 binding. Right panel shows Sp1 binding to its responsive elements; left panel represents the control, which shows the DNA beyond Sp1 binding sites. Additionally, input is the positive control for the total genomic DNA extract before precipitation, and IgG is the negative control for nonspecific binding. A stronger PCR band was detected in the *CRYAA*_T-G-G transfected cells. **c** Levels of HLE cells alone and CRYAA_C-G-T and CRYAA_T-G-G transfected cells immunoprecipitated using Sp1 antibodies were measured following q-PCR. Signals from IgG controls used for each ChIP were subtracted from each of the Sp1 immunoprecipitation signals and the fold enrichment ratios of ChIP enriched vs total input were represented. The results are shown as the mean ± SD. (*$p < 0.05$). Gel photographs presented here are cropped and the originals are available in the Additional file 2: Figures S1 and S2)

To address the limitation of the sample size, larger sample studies are required to validate the association we have observed. Further studies could also be focused on the association of SNPs with cortical and PSC cataracts.

Conclusions

This study identified three SNPs and their haplotypes in the 5′ UTR of CRYAA that appeared to be associated with nuclear ARC. As shown by the analysis of the effects of the individual SNP alleles on *CRYAA* transcription, rs7278468 appeared to be mainly responsible for the alteration in the transcriptional activity of the 5′ UTR of CRYAA. It exerted this effect through its G allele, which strengthened the binding affinity of Sp1. Manipulating these polymorphisms may provide a strategy to prevent or slow the progression of ARC.

Additional files

Additional file 1: The transcription factor binding sites overlapping rs7278468. This is the raw data of the in-silico analysis. (DOCX 52 kb)

Additional file 2: Figures S1 and S2. The whole gels of the NC and Sp1 ChIPs respectively. This is the raw data of the chromatin immunoprecipitation (ChIP) analysis described above. (DOCX 645 kb)

Abbreviations

5′UTR: 5′ untranslated region; ARC: Age-related cataract; C: Cortical; ChIP: Chromatin immunoprecipitation; CI: Confidence interval; CRYAA: Alpha A-crystallin; DMEM: Dulbecco's Modified Eagle Medium; FBS: Fetal bovine serum; HLE: Human lens epithelium; HWE: Hardy–Weinberg equilibrium; LD: Linkage disequilibrium; LOCS: Lens Opacity Classification System; NC: Nuclear color; NO: Nuclear opalescence; OR: Odds ratio; PCR: Polymerase chain reaction; PSC: Posterior subcapsular cataract; SNPs: Single nucleotide polymorphisms; Sp1: Specificity protein 1

Funding

This work was supported by the National Natural Science Foundation of China Grant (No. 81270989 and No. 81200669).

Authors' contributions

ZNZ carried out the Luciferase assay and ChIP analysis and drafted the manuscript. QF collected the blood sample and graded the lens opacity and participated in data collection. PZ and YL designed this study and helped in revising the manuscript. LC and HFY participated in design this study and analyzed the data. All authors read and approved the final manuscript.

Consent for publication

Not applicable. This research did not involve individual participants.

Competing interests

The authors declare that they have no competing interests.

Author details
[1]Department of Ophthalmology, Eye and ENT Hospital of Fudan University, 83 Fenyang Road, Shanghai 200031, People's Republic of China. [2]Department of Ophthalmology, Parkway Health Hong Qiao Medical Center, Shanghai 200336, People's Republic of China.

References

1. Congdon NG, Friedman DS, Lietman T. Important causes of visual impairment in the world today. JAMA. 2003;290(15):2057–60.
2. Hammond CJ, Snieder H, Spector TD, Gilbert CE. Genetic and environmental factors in age-related nuclear cataracts in monozygotic and dizygotic twins. N Engl J Med. 2000;342(24):1786–90.
3. Singh R, Ram J, Kaur G, Prasad R. Galactokinase deficiency induced cataracts in Indian infants: identification of 4 novel mutations in GALK gene. Curr Eye Res. 2012;37(10):949–54.
4. Yang J, Luo J, Zhou P, Fan Q, Luo Y, Lu Y. Association of the ephreceptor tyrosinekinase-type A2 (EPHA2) gene polymorphism rs 3754334 with age-related cataract risk: a meta-analysis. PLoS One. 2013;8(8):e71003.
5. Thampi P, Hassan A, Smith JB, Abraham EC. Enhanced C-terminal truncation of alphaA- and alphaB-crystallins in diabetic lenses. Invest Ophthalmol Vis Sci. 2002;43(10):3265–72.
6. Andley UP. Crystallins in the eye: function and pathology. Prog Retin Eye Res. 2007;26(1):78–98.
7. Chen Y, Yi L, Yan GQ, Jang YX, Fang YW, Wu XH, Zhou XW, Wei LM. Decreased chaperone activity of alpha-crystallins in naphthalene-induced cataract possibly results from C-terminal truncation. J Int Med Res. 2010;38(3):1016–28.
8. Zhou P, Luo Y, Liu X, Fan L, Lu Y. Down-regulation and CpG island hypermethylation of CRYAA in age-related nuclear cataract. FASEB J. 2012;26(12):4897–902.
9. Horwitz J. Alpha-crystallin. Exp Eye Res. 2003;76(2):145–53.
10. Andley UP. Effects of alpha-crystallin on lens cell function and cataract pathology. Curr Mol Med. 2009;9(7):887–92.
11. Reynolds PR. In sickness and in health: the importance of translational regulation. Arch Dis Child. 2002;86(5):322–4.
12. Chavez-Mardones J, Valenzuela-Munoz V, Nunez-Acuna G, Maldonado-Aguayo W, Gallardo-Escarate C. Concholepas concholepas Ferritin H-like subunit (CcFer): molecular characterization and single nucleotide polymorphism associated to innate immune response. Fish Shellfish Immunol. 2013;35(3):910–7.
13. Zuercher J, Neidhardt J, Magyar I, Labs S, Moore AT, Tanner FC, Waseem N, Schorderet DF, Munier FL, Bhattacharya S, et al. Alterations of the 5'untranslated region of SLC16A12 lead to age-related cataract. Invest Ophthalmol Vis Sci. 2010;51(7):3354–61.
14. Ma X, Jiao X, Ma Z, Hejtmancik JF. Polymorphism rs7278468 is associated with age-related cataract through decreasing transcriptional activity of the CRYAA promoter. Sci Rep. 2016;6:23206.
15. Shi YY, He L. SHEsis, a powerful software platform for analyses of linkage disequilibrium, haplotype construction, and genetic association at polymorphism loci. Cell Res. 2005;15(2):97–8.
16. Bailey TL, Boden M, Buske FA, Frith M, Grant CE, Clementi L, Ren J, Li WW, Noble WS. MEME SUITE: tools for motif discovery and searching. Nucleic Acids Res. 2009;37(Web Server issue):W202–8.
17. Guven M, Unal M, Sarici A, Ozaydin A, Batar B, Devranoglu K. Glutathione-S-transferase M1 and T1 genetic polymorphisms and the risk of cataract development: a study in the Turkish population. Curr Eye Res. 2007;32(5):447–54.
18. Juronen E, Tasa G, Veromann S, Parts L, Tiidla A, Pulges R, Panov A, Soovere L, Koka K, Mikelsaar AV. Polymorphic glutathione S-transferases as genetic risk factors for senile cortical cataract in Estonians. Invest Ophthalmol Vis Sci. 2000;41(8):2262–7.
19. Alberti G, Oguni M, Podgor M, Sperduto RD, Tomarev S, Grassi C, Williams S, Kaiser-Kupfer M, Maraini G, Hejtmancik JF. Glutathione S-transferase M1 genotype and age-related cataracts. Lack of association in an Italian population. Invest Ophthalmol Vis Sci. 1996;37(6):1167–73.
20. Klein BE, Klein R, Lee KE, Gangnon RE. Incidence of age-related cataract over a 15-year interval the beaver dam eye study. Ophthalmology. 2008;115(3):477–82.
21. Xu L, Cui T, Zhang S, Sun B, Zheng Y, Hu A, Li J, Ma K, Jonas JB. Prevalence and risk factors of lens opacities in urban and rural Chinese in Beijing. Ophthalmology. 2006;113(5):747–55.
22. Brady JP, Garland D, Duglas-Tabor Y, Robison WG Jr, Groome A, Wawrousek EF. Targeted disruption of the mouse alpha A-crystallin gene induces cataract and cytoplasmic inclusion bodies containing the small heat shock protein alpha B-crystallin. Proc Natl Acad Sci U S A. 1997;94(3):884–9.
23. Seshadri C, Shenoy M, Wells RD, Hensley-McBain T, Andersen-Nissen E, McElrath MJ, Cheng TY, Moody DB, Hawn TR. Human CD1a deficiency is common and genetically regulated. J Immunol. 2013;191(4):1586–93.
24. Suske G. The sp-family of transcription factors. Gene. 1999;238(2):291–300.
25. Li L, He S, Sun JM, Davie JR. Gene regulation by Sp1 and Sp3. Biochem Cell Biol. 2004;82(4):460–71.
26. Li L, Davie JR. The role of Sp1 and Sp3 in normal and cancer cell biology. Ann Anat. 2010;192(5):275–83.
27. Liu X, Zhou P, Fan F, Li D, Wu J, Lu Y, Luo Y. CpG site methylation in CRYAA promoter affect transcription factor Sp1 binding in human lens epithelial cells. BMC Ophthalmol. 2016;16:141.

30

Siderotic cataract with no signs of intraocular foreign body

Ke-Ke Zhang[1,2,3,4†], Wen-Wen He[1,2,3,4†], Yi Lu[1,2,3,4*] and Xiang-Jia Zhu[1,2,3,4*]

Abstract

Background: Ocular siderosis is a clinical condition induced by deposition of an iron-containing intraocular foreign body. We report a unique case of histopathologically proven lens siderosis in a young woman with a preceding history of trauma but no signs of retained intraocular foreign body.

Case presentation: A 32-year-old woman presented with an opacified lens showing brownish deposits on the anterior capsule and underwent cataract surgery. Preoperative ophthalmic examination did not show any retained intraocular foreign body. Histopathologic staining of the anterior capsule confirmed the presence of iron deposits and macrophages. Electroretinography examination performed in the postoperative period showed the changes characteristic of retinal degeneration in ocular siderosis.

Conclusion: This case illustrates the importance of close monitoring of patients with a history of trauma or previous penetrating injury to the eye, even if there is no intraocular foreign body, because they might develop ocular siderosis at a later stage. This case report underscores the importance of electroretinography and histopathologic analysis, in addition to ophthalmic examination, in the diagnosis of ocular siderosis.

Keywords: Ocular siderosis, Cataract, Intraocular foreign body, Histopathology, Electroretinography, Case report

Background

Ocular siderosis is a clinical condition caused by deposition of an iron-containing intraocular foreign body [1] and may occur 18 days to 8 years after ocular injury [2]. Clinical findings include iris heterochromia, pupillary mydriasis, iron deposition on the corneal endothelium and anterior lens capsule, cataract formation, lens subluxation, secondary glaucoma, uveitis, and retinal pigment changes or degeneration [3, 4]. Patients usually present with a history of ocular trauma, although some may remain asymptomatic and present only later when their visual acuity has decreased [2, 5]. We report a rare case of histopathologically proven lens siderosis in a young woman with a history of trauma but no signs of retained intraocular foreign body.

Case presentation

A 32-year-old Chinese woman presented to the outpatient department on May 13, 2016 complaining of a

* Correspondence: luyieent@126.com; zhuxiangjia1982@163.com
†Equal contributors
[1]Eye Institute, Eye and Ear, Nose, and Throat Hospital, Fudan University, Shanghai 200031, China
Full list of author information is available at the end of the article

6-month history of progressive blurring of vision in her right eye. She has no past medical history of note, but gave an uncertain history of a foreign body made of iron hitting her right eye 1 year earlier. After being given eyedrops by a doctor at a local hospital, she did not seek further medical care until she noticed further worsening of her vision.

The patient's visual acuity was 6/20 in the right eye (OD) and 20/20 in the left eye (OS); intraocular pressures were normal (16.9 mmHg OD and 17.2 mmHg OS, by non-contact tonometry). Both pupils were round and there was no relative afferent pupillary defect. Examination of the anterior and posterior segments of the left eye was normal. However, in the right eye, slit-lamp biomicroscopy revealed a corneal macula inferiorly, indicating a possible perforating wound previously. Lens opacification was also observed in the right eye, with clumps of brownish pigment on the anterior lens capsule clinically suggestive of siderotic cataract (Fig. 1). There was no evidence of any breach in the anterior lens capsule. The anterior chamber was clear and of medium depth. As the cataract did not entirely obscured the fundus, it is possible for us to perform the detailed fundus

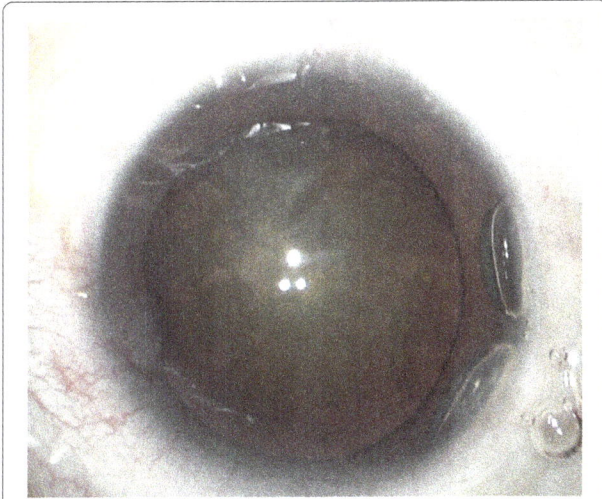

Fig. 1 Anterior segment image of the right eye. This image was taken during cataract surgery and shows an opacified lens with brownish deposits on the anterior lens capsule

examination with a three-mirror lens, which showed no retinal detachment or signs of foreign body. Using slit-lamp examination and gonioscopy, no intraocular foreign body was visualized in the anterior segment of the injured eye before and after mydriasis. Optical coherence tomography vaguely indicated no retinal detachment in the posterior pole region (Additional file 1: Figure S1). An ultrasound B-scan (10 MHz) showed moderately dense, mobile, vitreous opacities with posterior vitreous detachment and no retinal tear or detachment. No intralenticular foreign body was seen on low gain (Figs. 2a and b). An orbital X-ray (Fig. 2c) and a 3.0-mm thin-sliced computed tomography scan (Fig. 2d) did not show any retained intraocular foreign body.

On the basis of the above findings, the patient was diagnosed with siderotic cataract and underwent an uneventful cataract phacoemulsification with implantation of a posterior chamber intraocular lens (IOL) and capsular tension ring under regional anesthesia in her right eye on May 23, 2016. Dilated fundus examination was also performed intraoperatively to determine if there were any siderotic changes on the retina. However, no retained intraocular foreign body, retinal detachment, retinal tear, or vitreous hemorrhage was seen. The anterior lens capsule was obtained during continuous curvilinear capsulorhexis and sent for histopathology. The patient was treated with Cravit Eye Drops (Alcon Laboratories, Inc., Fort Worth, TX, USA) QID OD, Pred Forte Eye Drops (Allergan Pharmaceuticals, Inc., Dublin, Ireland) QID OD, and Diclofenac Sodium Eye Drops (Shenyang Xingqi Pharmaceutical Co. Ltd, Shenyang, China) QID OD. One week after the surgery, her best uncorrected visual acuity improved to 16/20, and her

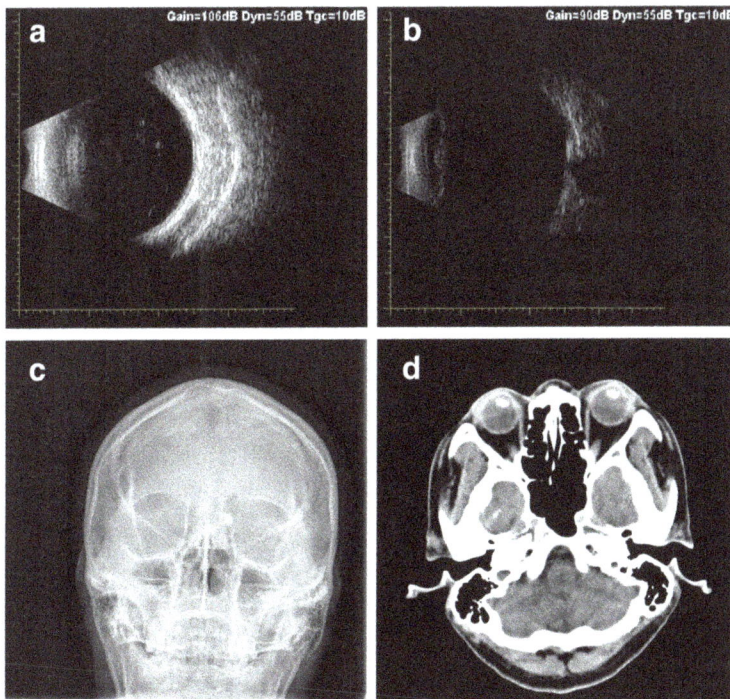

Fig. 2 (**a-b**) Ultrasound B-scan of the posterior segment in low gain settings. The posterior capsule is intact and there is no foreign body seen intraocularly. (**c**) X-ray of orbits showing no radiopaque foreign body in Water's view. (**d**) Computed tomography scan showing normal intact globe with no intraocular foreign body in the right eye

best corrected visual acuity improved to 20/20 with a corneal macula inferiorly, a clear anterior chamber of medium depth, and a well-centered IOL (Fig. 3).

Electroretinography (ERG) examination performed in the postoperative period revealed the changes characteristic of retinal degeneration with reduced A-wave and B-wave amplitudes (Fig. 4). It also showed implicit time delayed and decreased B:A ratio in both rod and cone system. ERG was normal in the left eye for combined, scotopic, and photopic responses, as well as a normal flicker response. However, these responses were decreased in the right eye.

Histopathologic examination using hematoxylin and eosinstain and special stains like Prussian blue and CD18, a classic macrophage marker, were also conducted. Hematoxylin and eosin staining showed scattered hemosiderin deposits in the anterior capsule (Fig. 5a and b). Prussian blue staining confirmed the presence of iron pigments in the anterior capsule (Fig. 5c and d). The cells in the anterior capsule were strongly stained for macrophages, as indicated in Fig. 5e and f.

During the first 3 months of follow-up at our medical center, the patient was satisfied with the surgical outcomes as she obtained a best uncorrected visual acuity of 12/20 and a best corrected visual acuity of 20/20, with an IOL in situ and a stable retina. Six months after the cataract surgery, her best uncorrected visual acuity was still 12/20 and best corrected visual acuity was 20/20. As computed tomography scan cannot detect this tiny foreign body in our case, we conducted serial follow-up examinations 6 months after surgery, including electrophysiology tests, ultrasound biomicroscopy and detailed fundus examination with a three-mirror lens, to check the presence of any intraocular foreign body in this patient. According to the follow-up tests (Figs. 6, 7, and 8), there was no evidence of intraocular foreign body during 6-month postoperative follow-up. At present we recommended the patient to routinely follow up fundus examination and ERG every 3 months.

Discussions

This woman presented with a one-year history of progressive blurring of vision and a preceding uncertain history of being struck in the right eye by foreign body made of iron. Slit-lamp examination showed a corneal macula inferiorly and an opacified lens with brownish deposits on the anterior capsule. Although no solid evidence of ocular foreign body was observed on the ultrasound B-scan, an orbital X-ray, or computed tomography scan before cataract surgery, the possibility of ocular siderosis caused by deposition of an iron-containing intraocular foreign body was not ruled out. With the assistance of ERG and histopathologic analysis after cataract surgery, the patient was finally diagnosed with ocular siderosis, albeit with no intraocular foreign body.

Iron is a frequent component of metallic intraocular foreign bodies and may lead to ocular siderosis, which commonly presents as reduced visual acuity. Intralenticular foreign bodies account for about 8%–10% of all intraocular foreign bodies. Cataract formation may be an indicator of early siderosis and has been associated with intralenticular foreign bodies [2, 5, 6]. Although computed tomography is still considered to be the gold standard for detection of an occult foreign body, a small intraocular foreign body may be missed with this technique. There has been a previous report of lens siderosis due to an intraocular foreign body missed on imaging such as computed tomography and ultrasonography but later detected perioperatively [5].

A complete ophthalmic evaluation including imaging studies is essential. The diagnosis of an intraocular foreign body is often made by direct visualization on slit-lamp examination or ophthalmoscopy. In this case, there was no intraocular or intralenticular foreign body detected clinically or on imaging, but the patient still

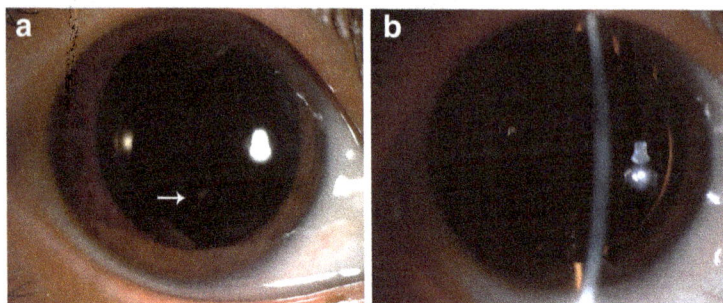

Fig. 3 Postoperative anterior segment images of the right eye after mydriasis through direct diffuse illumination (**a**) and indirect illumination (**b**). Despite a corneal macula inferiorly (*arrow*), the right eye showed no signs of inflammation and had a clear anterior chamber of medium depth with a well-centered intraocular lens

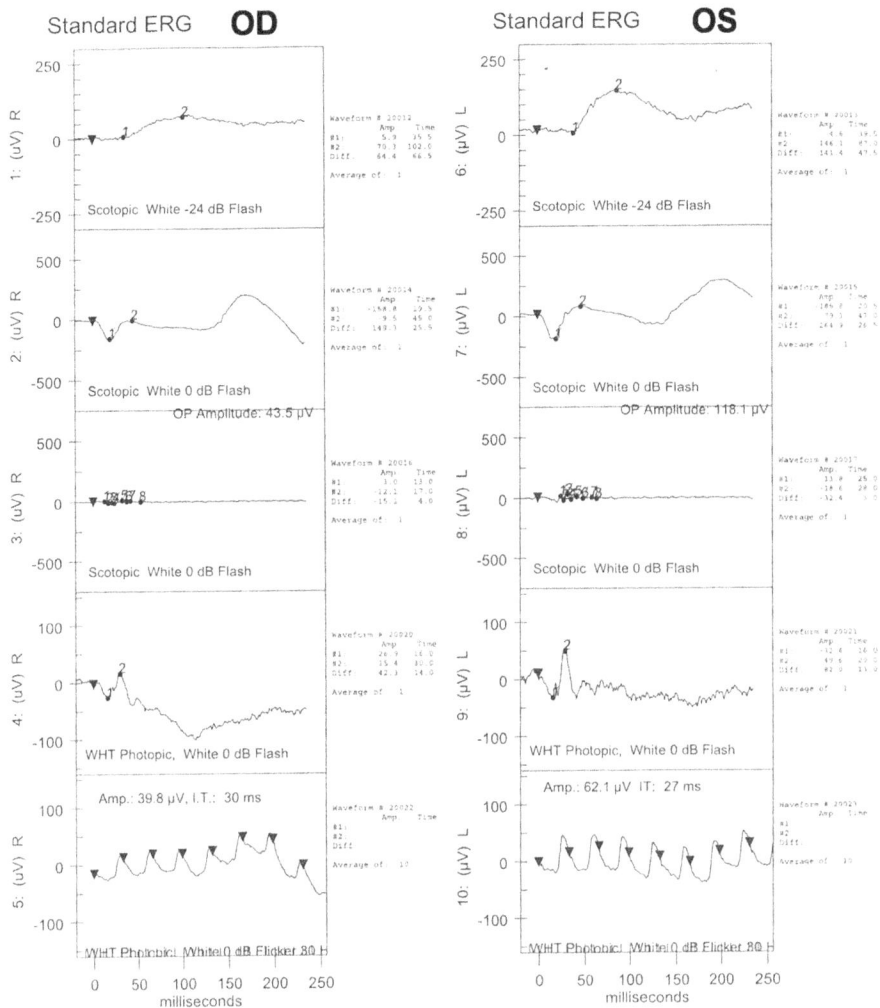

Fig 4 Electroretinography examination of both eyes performed in the postoperative period. Electroretinography was basically normal in the left eye (OS) for combined, scotopic, and photopic responses, as well as a normal flicker response. However, these responses were decreased in the right eye (OD), which demonstrated reduced A-wave and B-wave amplitudes compared with the normal left eye. (From top to bottom: rod, mixed cone-rod, OP, single-flash cone, and 30-Hz flicker ERG responses)

developed lens siderosis. The optic nerve and retina were healthy, so there was no associated afferent papillary defect. However, in the right eye, slit-lamp biomicroscopy revealed a corneal macula inferiorly, which could indicate a possible perforating wound previously. As mentioned in a previous study, the time between ocular trauma and development of ocular siderosis may be related to the severity of the intraocular toxic reaction [7]. This varies depending on the shape and size of the foreign body, its iron content, and the amount of time it remains within the eye [3]. Therefore, we cannot rule out the possibility of a dislodged or resorbed intraocular foreign body. There may have been a lodged intralenticular foreign body immediately after trauma that was resorbed over time.

ERG is the method most commonly used to detect ocular siderosis, and all patients should have this prior

to surgical intervention. Iron retinotoxicity leads to dysfunction of all the layers of the retina, and more severe damage occurs in the inner retina than in the outer retina in the later stages of this condition [8]. Rod-dominated responses are predominantly affected because they are more susceptible to iron toxicity than the cone system. Eventually, responses are progressively reduced in amplitude to become undetectable [7].Our patient underwent cataract surgery prior to ERG due to a delayed ERG appointment at our medical center. ERG recordings remain the reference follow-up examination in patients with ocular siderosis, especially since after the surgery, as previous reports have illustrated, many small particles can be released at the inner retinal surface, potentially inducing further toxicity [4]. Therefore, due to the invisible retinal changes caused by siderosis, it is of great importance to follow up ERG in specific interval in

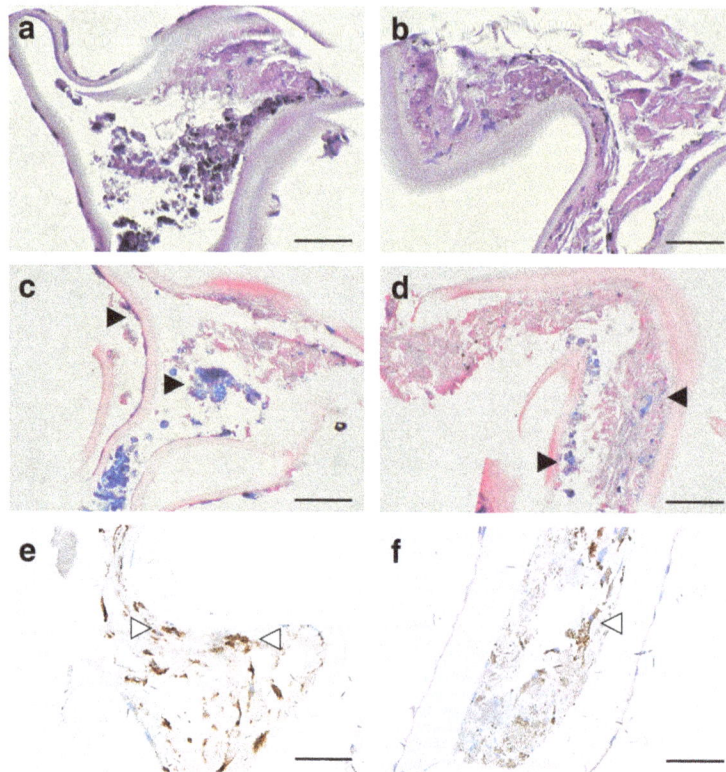

Fig. 5 Histopathologic results for the anterior lens capsule with ocular siderosis. **a, b** Hematoxylin and eosinstaining showed scattered hemosiderin deposits in the anterior capsule. **c, d** Prussian blue staining confirmed the presence of iron pigments in the anterior capsule (black triangle). **e, f** Cells in the anterior capsule stained strongly for CD18, a classic macrophage marker (white triangle)

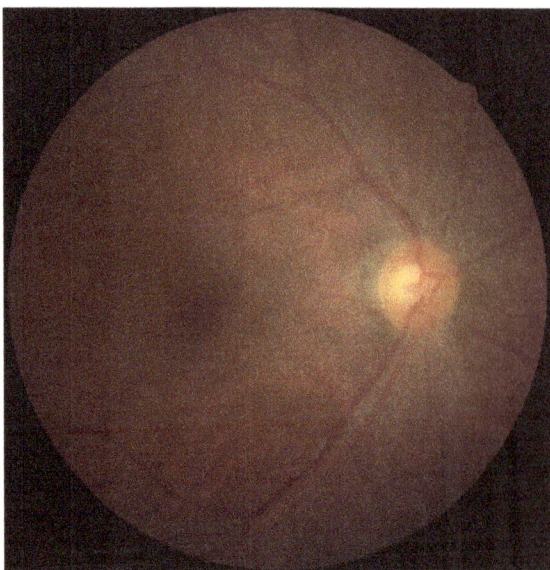

Fig. 6 Posterior segment fundus image after the surgery

a siderosis case that failed to identify intraocular foreign body.

If all means failed to identify the foreign body, the innegligible role of endoscopic ciliary process and ciliary body examination should be addressed. Ophthalmic endoscope has two fundamental surgical advantages, including bypassing anterior segment opacities, and visualizing anteriorly positioned structures such as the ciliary bodies and sub-iris space [9]. It has been reported that endoscope can be applied to observe the ciliary body, periphery retina tear or other pathological changes, the intraocular foreign body at or near ciliary body and the whole retina in the vitrectomy. This makes the extraction of intraocular foreign body at or near the ciliary body and the conduct of cyclophotocoagulation more accurate and simple [10].

Similar to previous studies, histopathologic analysis in our case showed brownish depositions in the epithelial cells of the lens capsule, and iron was identified in the lens capsule by Prussian blue staining. It is noteworthy that we initially used a stain specific for macrophages so that we could see the effect of iron on phagocytosis in the anterior capsule with ocular siderosis. Macrophage activity is closely related to the mechanism and

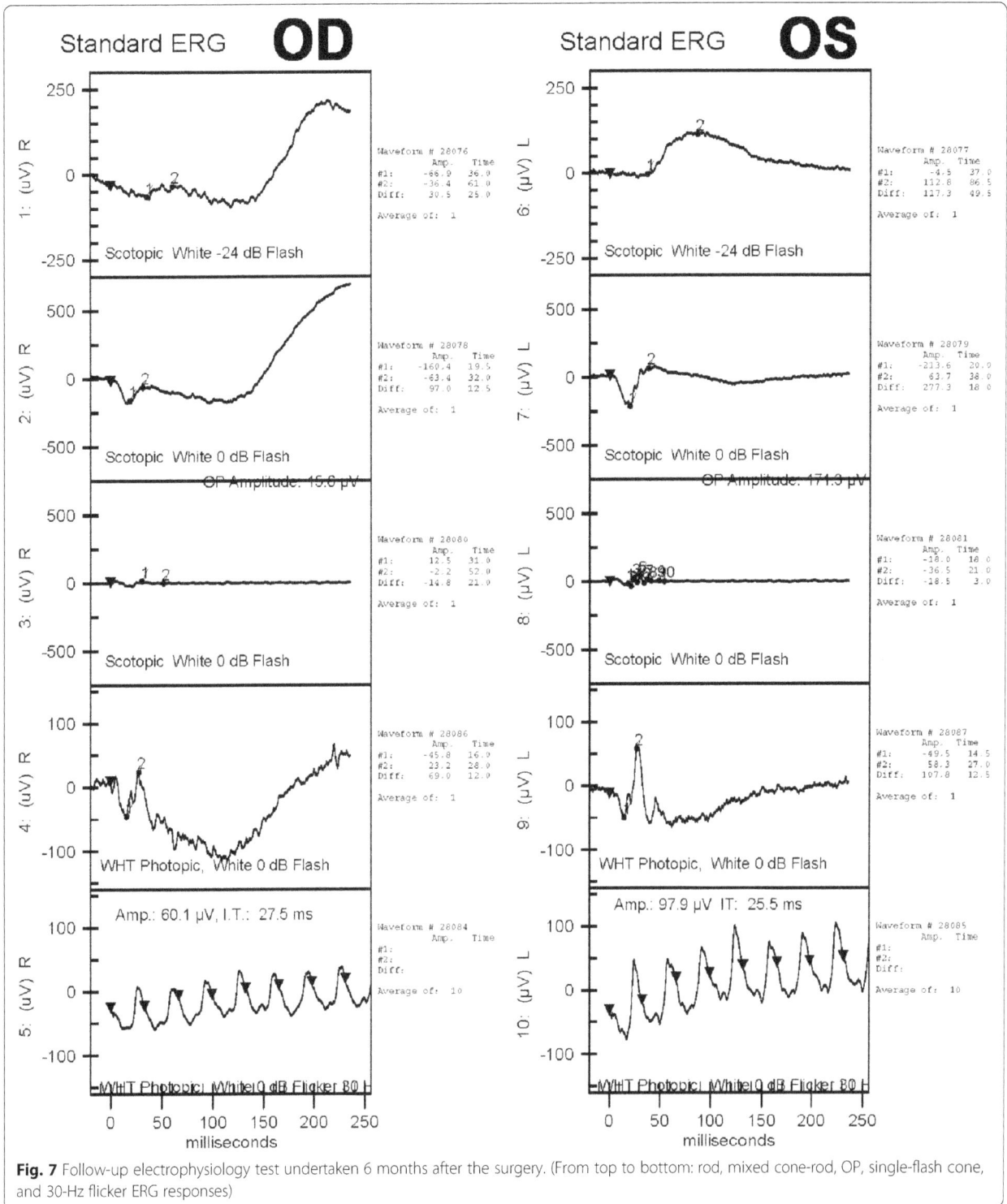

Fig. 7 Follow-up electrophysiology test undertaken 6 months after the surgery. (From top to bottom: rod, mixed cone-rod, OP, single-flash cone, and 30-Hz flicker ERG responses)

prognosis of ocular siderosis. According to previous studies, vision may be excellent in siderosis with ERG amplitudes of up to 50%, and complete reversal is possible following successful removal of the intraocular foreign body in the early stages of the condition and with amplitudes of up to 40% [8, 11]. Over this limit,

macrophage activity may be overwhelmed by the amount of iron load, leading to direct cellular toxicity [4].

With regard to the treatment of cataract associated with ocular siderosis, implantation of an IOL with a capsular tension ring has been recommended in some

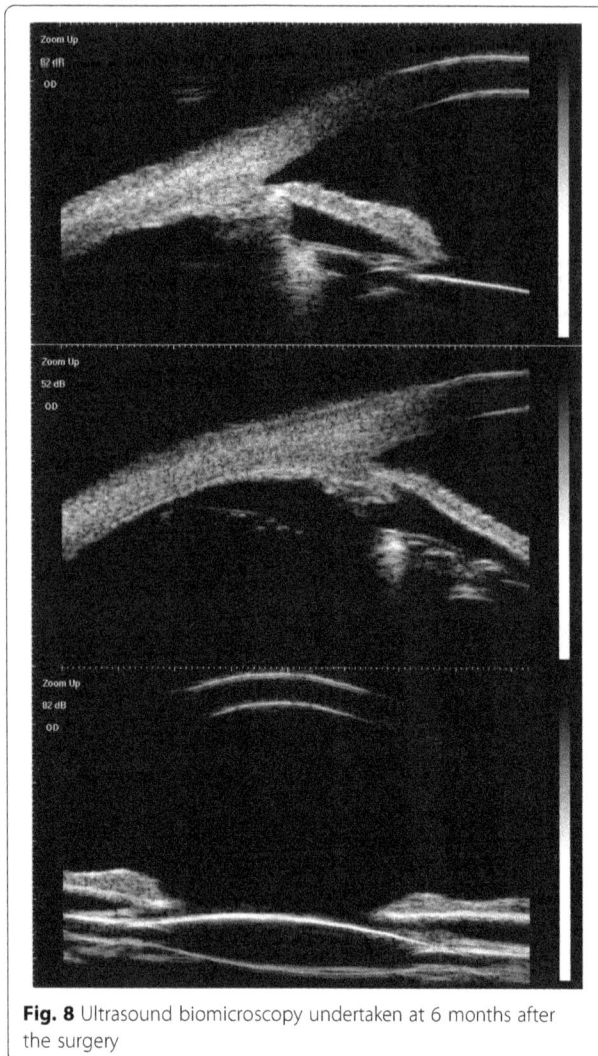

Fig. 8 Ultrasound biomicroscopy undertaken at 6 months after the surgery

previous studies. In patients who are strongly suspected to have a history of eye trauma, the lens ligament may be more fragile and too loose to maintain the stability of a posterior chamber IOL. A capsular tension ring is appropriate for patients with ocular siderosis.

Conclusions

This case report underscores the importance of close monitoring of patients with a history of trauma or previous penetrating injury to the eye, even if there is no intraocular foreign body, because they could develop ocular siderosis at a later stage. All primary care physicians and ophthalmologists should be aware of the possibility of a retained intraocular foreign body in a penetrating ocular injury, particularly when there is a history of high-velocity metallic injury [7]. In view of the sight-threatening complications of siderosis, prompt intervention is indicated to preserve visual acuity and

prevent progression of siderosis to involve the posterior segment [3].

Therefore, when decreased visual acuity and lens opacity with brownish pigment is noted in these patients following trauma, cataract surgery followed by histopathologic analysis is of substantial value for further diagnosis. ERG prior to cataract surgery and during follow-up remains important in the prognosis of ocular siderosis.

Additional file

> **Additional file 1: Figure S1.** Optical coherence tomography images of the right eye before and after surgery. Optical coherence tomography vaguely indicated no retinal detachment in the posterior pole region of the patient's right eye. (TIF 1859 kb)

Abbreviations
(ERG): Electroretinography; (IOL): Intraocular lens; (OD): Right eye; (OS): Left eye

Funding
This research was funded by research grants from the National Natural Science Foundation of China (Grant No. 81270989 and 81470613), the National Health and Family Planning Commission of People's Republic of China(Grant No. 201302015), and the Cutting-Edge Technology Combined PR Project of Shanghai Shen Kang Hospital Development Centre (Grant No. SHDC12012104).

Authors' contribution
Design of the study (XJZ); conduct of the study (KKZ); collection and management of the data (KKZ); analysis and interpretation of the data (KKZ and WWH); manuscript drafting (KKZ and WWH); review and approval of manuscript (XJZ and YL). All authors read and approved the final manuscript.

Competing interest
The authors declare that they have no competing interests.

Consent for publication
Informed consent was obtained from the patient for publication of this case report and any accompanying images.

Author details
[1]Eye Institute, Eye and Ear, Nose, and Throat Hospital, Fudan University, Shanghai 200031, China. [2]Department of Ophthalmology, Eye and Ear, Nose, and Throat Hospital, Fudan University, Shanghai 200031, China. [3]Key Laboratory of Myopia, Ministry of Health PR China, Shanghai 200031, China. [4]Shanghai Key Laboratory of Visual Impairment and Restoration, Fudan University, Shanghai 200031, China.

References

1. Siantar RG, Agrawal R, Heng LW, Ho BC. Histopathologically proven siderotic cataract with disintegrated intralenticular foreign body. Indian J Ophthalmol. 2013;61:30–2.
2. O'Duffy D, Salmon JF. Siderosis bulbi resulting from an intralenticular foreign body. Am J Ophthalmol. 1999;127:218–9.
3. Hope-Ross M, Mahon GJ, Johnston PB. Ocular siderosis. Eye (Lond). 1993;7: 419–25.
4. Faure C, Gocho K, Le Mer Y, Sahel JA, Paques M, Audo I. Functional and high resolution retinal imaging assessment in a case of ocular siderosis. Doc Ophthalmol. 2014;128:69–75.
5. Wu TT, Kung YH, Sheu SJ, Yang CA. Lens siderosis resulting from a tiny missed intralenticular foreign body. J Chin Med Assoc. 2009;72:42–4.
6. Lee W, Park SY, Park TK, Kim HK, Ohn YH. Mature cataract and lens induced glaucoma associated with an asymptomatic intralenticular foreign body. J Cataract Refract Surg. 2007;33:550–2.
7. Kannan NB, Adenuga OO, Rajan RP, Ramasamy K. Management of ocular siderosis: visual outcome and electroretinographic changes. J Ophthalmol. 2016;2016:7272465.
8. Imaizumi M, Matsumoto CS, Yamada K, Nanba Y, Takaki Y, Nakatsuka K. Electroretinographic assessment of early changes in ocular siderosis. Ophthalmologica. 2000;214:354–9.
9. Marra KV, Yonekawa Y, Papakostas TD, Arroyo JG. Indications and techniques of endoscope assisted vitrectomy. J Ophthalmic Vis Res. 2013; 8(3):282–90.
10. Yang X, Li QY, DU S, Ren H, Jia CY, Tang XH. Extraction of intraocular foreign body at or near the ciliary body under endoscopic vitrectomy. Zhonghua Yan Ke Za Zhi. 2013;49(8):691–5.
11. Weiss MJ, Hofeldt AJ, Behrens M, Fisher K. Ocular siderosis: diagnosis and management. Retina. 1997;17:105–8.

31

MiRNAs regulate oxidative stress related genes via binding to the 3' UTR and TATA-box regions: a new hypothesis for cataract pathogenesis

Changrui Wu[1], Zhao Liu[1], Le Ma[2], Cheng Pei[1], Li Qin[1], Ning Gao[1], Jun Li[3] and Yue Yin[3]*

Abstract

Background: Age-related cataracts are related to oxidative stress. However, the genome-wide screening of cataract related oxidative stress related genes are not thoroughly investigated. Our study aims to identify cataract regulated miRNA target genes that are related to oxidative stress and to propose a new possible mechanism for cataract formation.

Methods: Microarrays were used to determine the mRNA expression profiles of both transparent and cataractous lenses. The results were analyzed by significance analyses performed by the microarray software, and bioinformatics analysis was further conducted using Molecular Annotation System. The Eukaryotic Promoter Database (EPD) was used to retrieve promoter sequences and identify TATA-box motifs. Online resource miRWalk was exploited to screen for validated miRNAs targeting mRNAs related to oxidative stress. RNAhybrid online tool was applied to predict the binding between significantly regulated miRNAs in cataract lenses and target mRNAs.

Results: Oxidative stress pathway was significantly regulated in cataractous lens samples. Pro-oxidative genes were half up-regulated (11/20), with a small number of genes down-regulated (4/20) and the rest of them with no significant change (5/20). Anti-oxidative genes were partly up-regulated (17/69) and partly down-regulated (17/69). Four down-regulated miRNAs (has-miR-1207-5p, has-miR-124-3p, has-miR-204-3p, has-miR-204-5p) were found to target 3' UTR of pro-oxidative genes and could also bind to the TATA-box regions of anti-oxidative genes (with the exception of has-miR-204-3p), whilst two up-regulated miRNAs (has-miR-222-3p, has-miR-378a-3p) were found to target 3' UTR of anti-oxidative genes and could simultaneously bind to the TATA-box regions of pro-oxidative genes.

Conclusions: We propose for the first time a hypothesis that cataract regulated miRNAs could contribute to cataract formation not only by targeting 3' UTR but also by targeting TATA-box region of oxidative stress related genes. This results in the subsequent elevation of pro-oxidative genes and inhibition of anti-oxidative genes. This miRNA-TATA-box/3' UTR-gene-regulation network may contribute to cataract pathogenesis.

Keywords: Cataract, Oxidative stress, miRNAs

* Correspondence: lycwr@hotmail.com
[3]Basic Research Center, Affiliated Shaanxi Provincial Tumor Hospital, School of Medicine, Xi'an Jiaotong University, Xi'an, Shaanxi Province 710061, China
Full list of author information is available at the end of the article

Background

Age-related cataract is till now still the dominant cause of blindness worldwide. Although cataract surgery is a satisfying solution for cataract caused vision impairment, this procedure is not easily available in developing countries [1]. There have been studies on the mechanism of age-related cataract aiming to discover new targets for cataract treatment. However, the specific molecular pathway of this disease still merits further investigation. It has been suggested that oxidative stress plays an important role in cataract formation. Lens proteins undergo non-enzymatic, post-translational modification, accumulate fluorescent chromophores and are more susceptible to oxidation along with aging [2], therefore oxidative stress is partially responsible for cataract formation. It has also been reported that oxidation plays a key role in nuclear cataract, but its causal roles in cortical and posterior subcapsular cataracts are substantially less important [3]. Other groups have published gene profiling results from either cataract tissue samples or cell lines [4, 5]. There are also studies on the function of specific genes in cataract formation, particularly oxidative stress related genes, such as SOD1, TXNIP, etc. [6–8]. Thereupon oxidative stress related gene regulation is worth investigating.

MicroRNAs (miRNAs) are a group of small non-coding RNAs that modulate many pathways related to various diseases. Our previous work has shown that multiple miRNAs are regulated in human cataractous lenses [9]. However, the targets of these miRNAs still warrant further investigation. In this study, we used gene profiling to screen for differentially regulated mRNAs in human cataractous lenses compared with post mortem clear lenses. Then bioinformatics analysis was applied to examine the gene-pathway distribution and the regulation of oxidative stress related genes in cataract lenses. We compared our previously published cataract regulated miRNAs and these differentially regulated mRNAs, screening for miRNA 3′ UTR binding targets that could contribute to cataract pathogenesis. Our previous work indicated miRNAs could bind to the TATA-box region and promote gene transcription as well as 3′ UTR binding-mediated gene silencing [10, 11], so we also screened for TATA-box targets of the miRNAs reported in our previous publication [9]. Our study establishes a miRNA-TATA-box/3′ UTR-gene-regulation network that may contribute to cataract formation.

Methods

Human lens epithelium-capsule sample collection

Lens samples were obtained from Department of Ophthalmology, the First Affiliated Hospital of Medical School of Xi'an Jiaotong University. Epithelium-capsule samples were obtained after capsulorrhexis during surgery (15 age-related cataract patients, age ranges from 60 to 68, no other ocular diseases) or obtained from postmortem transparent lenses within 24 h after death (15 donors, age ranges from 58 to 65, no history of ocular diseases). The degrees of lenticular opacification of patients were determined by the Lens Opacities Classification System III (LOCSIII) [12, 13]. The lenticular opacification of postmortem lenses were grade 1 ~ 2 and cataract lenses were grade 4 ~ 6 (Additional file 1: Table S1). There was no significant difference between transparent and cataractous human lens samples respect to the age of donors in two groups (Additional file 1: Table S1, unpaired t test, $p > 0.05$).

Total RNA preparation

Five samples were randomly pooled into one lens sample to insure the quality and quantity of extracted total RNA. Total RNA of six pooled samples (three cataractous and three transparent samples) was extracted with Trizol reagent (Invitrogen, Shanghai, China) according to the manufacturer's instructions. The quality of RNA samples was confirmed by measuring OD260/280 ratio using NanoDrop spectrophotometer (Thermo Scientific, Shanghai, China) and the integrity of RNA samples was verified by agarose electrophoresis.

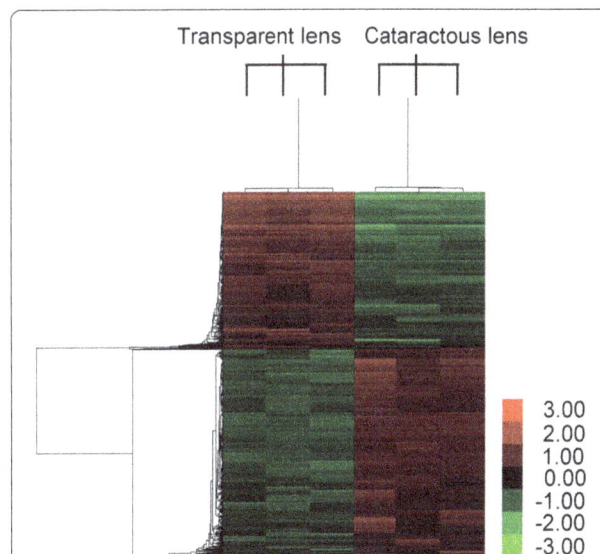

Fig. 1 Heatmap shows differentially expressed mRNAs in cataractous lens samples compared with transparent lens samples. Six separate microarray assays were performed to determine the genome-wide mRNA expression in the central epithelium of transparent and cataractous human lenses. Microarray data were processed by CapitalBio Corporation. Heatmap shows differentially expressed mRNAs in cataractous lens samples compared with transparent lens samples. Relative expression value from high to low was shown by gradient of red to green in the heatmap. Colors indicate relative mRNA expression. Red and green indicate higher or lower expression of mRNAs relative to those in transparent lens samples, respectively. FDR (false discovery rate) adjusted p-value <0.05

Microarray analysis

Gene expression profiling was performed for each pooled RNA sample using a Gene Chip-Human Genome Array (HG-U133 Plus 2.0, Affymetrix, Santa Clara, CA) at CapitalBio Corporation (Beijing, China). Gene Chip microarray service of CapitalBio Corporation is certificated by Affymetrix. Microarray processing was performed according to Gene Chip Expression Analysis Technical Manual provided by Affymetrix. In brief, 1 μg of total RNA was used to synthesize double-stranded cDNA. Biotin-tagged complementary RNA (cRNA) was produced using the MessageAmp II aRNA Amplification Kit (Ambion, Austin, TX). The resulting cRNA was fragmented and hybridized to the microarray. After hybridization the GeneChip arrays were washed, stained and then scanned on a GeneChip Scanner 3000 (Affymetrix).

Data processing and analysis

Microarray raw data were processed at CapitalBio Corporation. Briefly, the hybridization data were analyzed using GeneChip Operating software (GCOS 1.4, Affymetrix) and normalized using a DNA-chip analyzer. Significant Analysis of Microarray software (SAM) was used to identify mRNAs that exhibited significant differences in expression between transparent and cataractous samples (average fold change >2 or <0.5). Results were

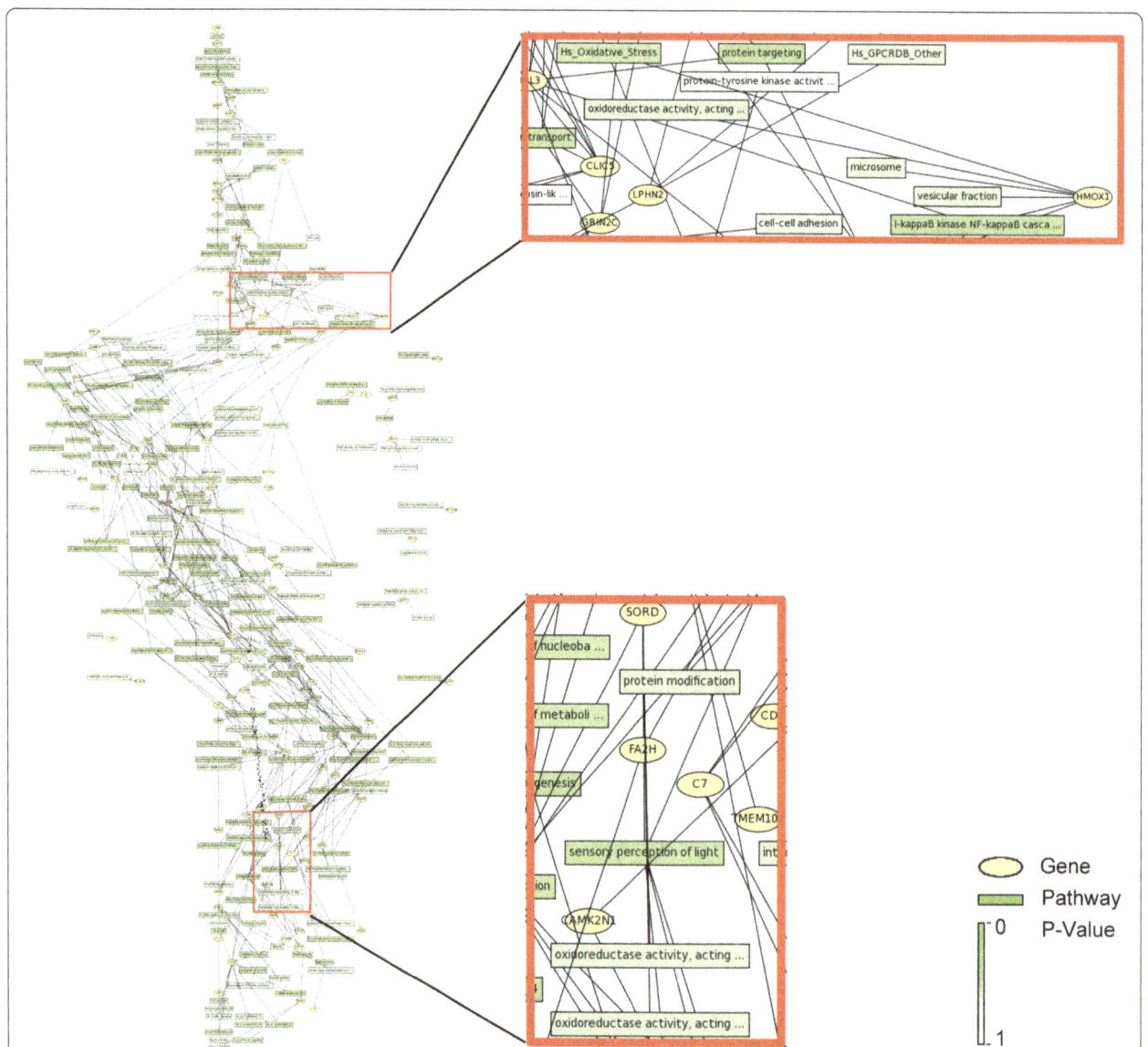

Fig. 2 Gene-pathway network graph shows oxidative stress related pathway in the regulated gene-pathway network. Gene symbols of 100 up-regulated genes and 100 down-regulated genes were uploaded to MAS 3.0 system. Then gene-pathway network graph was generated by MAS 3.0 sponsored by CapitalBio Corporation using GenMAPP database. Red-boxed areas show enlarged parts of the gene-pathway network graph related with oxidative stress pathway

screened for mRNAs with FDR (false discovery rate)-corrected p values < 0.05.

Bioinformatics analysis

Bioinformatics analysis was conducted via the online Molecular Annotation System (MAS 3.0) provided by CapitalBio Corporation. Gene symbols of mRNAs with average fold change >2 of <0.5 were uploaded in the MAS 3.0 system for Gene Ontology (GO) and gene-pathway network analysis. Heatmaps were either provided by Capi-talBio Corporation (Fig. 1) or generated by using Heatmap illustrator 1.0 according to the user's manual (Fig. 4) [14]. The Eukaryotic Promoter Database (EPD) [15, 16] was used to retrieve promoter sequences of selected oxidative stress related mRNAs and to identify TATA-box motifs as described in our previous publications [10, 11]. Online resource miRWalk [17, 18] was used to screen for validated miRNAs targeting mRNAs related to oxidative stress. RNAhybrid online tool [19] was applied to predict the binding between significantly regulated miRNAs in cataract lenses in our previous findings [9] and target mRNAs.

Statistical analysis

Differences between the two groups in microarray data were assessed using FDR (false discovery rate)-corrected p values ($p < 0.05$) provided by SAM. Age differences between the two groups were estimated using unpaired t test ($p < 0.05$ was considered statistically significant).

Results

Gene profiling in microarrays shows oxidative stress pathway is regulated in cataractous lenses

Gene profiling was determined by six separate micro-array assays, which identified 2223 up-regulated genes and 1829 down-regulated genes in cataractous lenses compared with transparent lenses (average fold change >2 or <0.5) (Fig. 1). Gene symbols of the top 100 up-regulated genes and top 100 down-regulated genes were uploaded to MAS 3.0 system to generate gene-pathway network graph using GenMAPP database, as it was too complex to generate graph by Graphviz if more than 200 gene symbols were included (Fig. 2). It is shown that oxidative stress related pathway was involved in cataract related gene regulation (Fig. 2). The overall distribution of cataract-regulated genes within different categories of the Gene Ontology (GO) classification system (the "biological process" and "pathway in Kegg database" categories) was examined (Fig. 3). Several classes of cataract-regulated genes in the biological process such as signal transduction, transcription, ion transport, etc. were consistent with previous work [4]. Interestingly, oxidation reduction was one of the top eight classes of GO enriched functional categories (Fig. 3a, Additional file 1: Table S2). We also found several pathways that were involved in cataract-mediated gene regulation, such as calcium signaling pathway, MAPK signaling pathway, TGF-beta signaling pathway, etc. (Fig. 3b).

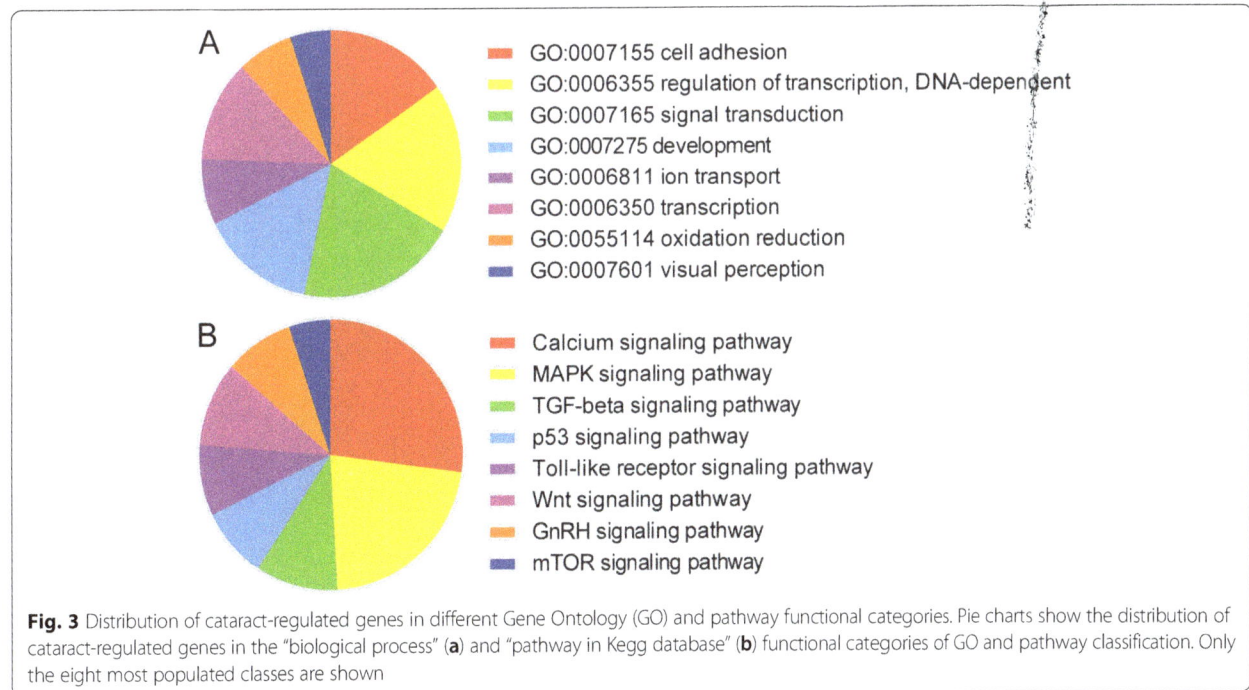

Fig. 3 Distribution of cataract-regulated genes in different Gene Ontology (GO) and pathway functional categories. Pie charts show the distribution of cataract-regulated genes in the "biological process" (**a**) and "pathway in Kegg database" (**b**) functional categories of GO and pathway classification. Only the eight most populated classes are shown

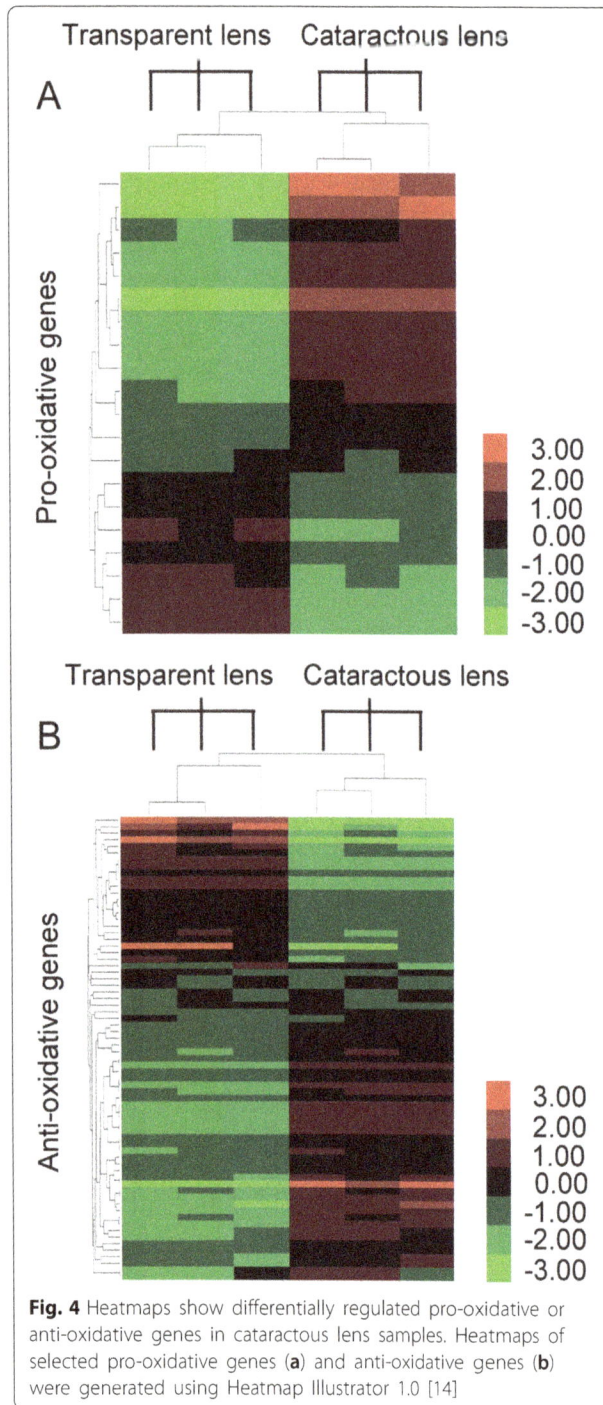

Fig. 4 Heatmaps show differentially regulated pro-oxidative or anti-oxidative genes in cataractous lens samples. Heatmaps of selected pro-oxidative genes (**a**) and anti-oxidative genes (**b**) were generated using Heatmap Illustrator 1.0 [14]

Table 1 Regulated miRNAs in Cataractous Samples and Target mRNA Gene Symbols

miRNA names	regulation	Average fold change[a]	3' UTR target	TATA-box target
has-miR-1207-5p	down	0.22	CYCS	FTL, MT1E, MT1G, MT1H, MT1M
has-miR-124-3p	down	0.36	CYB5A, CYP1B1	TXN
has-miR-204-3p	down	0.43	CYP1B1	None
has-miR-204-5p	down	0.43	TXNIP	ALDH1A3, TF
has-miR-222-3p	up	2.60	PRDX4, TXN	CYP1A2, CYP1B1
has-miR-378a-3p	up	2.80	SOD1	TXNIP

[a]Average fold change values were means of 3 separate array results (fold change = cataractous lens sample/transparent lens sample)

significantly regulated. So the oxidative stress related genes were generally up-regulated in cataractous samples. However, there were equal numbers of up-regulated and down-regulated anti-oxidative genes (17 of 69 for both) (Fig. 4b, Additional file 1: Table S3). The up-regulation of anti-oxidative genes was probably due to the response to elevated oxidative stress in cataractous lenses. The down-regulated anti-oxidative genes and up-regulated pro-oxidative genes could lead to the progression of oxidative stress, thus may contribute to cataract formation.

Table 2 Oxidative Stress Related Genes with miRNA Targets in Cataractous Samples

Gene Symbol	Pro-oxidant[a]	Anti-oxidant[a]	Regulation	Average fold change[b]
ALDH1A3	N	Y	down	0.50
FTL	N	Y	down	0.50
MT1E	N	Y	down	0.50
MT1G	N	Y	down	0.32
MT1H	N	Y	down	0.50
MT1M	N	Y	down	0.15
PRDX4	N	Y	down	0.50
SOD1	N	Y	down	0.50
TF	N	Y	down	0.17
TXN	N	Y	down	0.50
CYB5A	Y	N	up	2.00
CYCS	Y	N	up	2.73
CYP1A2	Y	N	up	2.00
CYP1B1	Y	N	up	7.11
TXNIP	Y	N	up	6.36

[a] "Y" = yes; "N" = no
[b] Average fold change values were means of 3 separate array results (fold change = cataractous lens sample/transparent lens sample)

Expression of oxidative stress pathway related genes in cataractous lenses

To further investigate the regulation of oxidative stress related genes in cataractous lenses, we generated heatmaps consisting only genes related to oxidative stress (Fig. 4). As it is shown there were more significantly up-regulated pro-oxidative genes (11 of 20) than down-regulated genes (4 of 20) in cataractous lenses (Fig. 4a, Additional file 1: Table S3). The rest 5 genes were not

MiRNAs bind to the TATA-box/3′ UTR of oxidative stress related genes

Since miRNA has been suggested to play a role in cataract formation by our previous work as well as publications of other colleagues [9, 20, 21], we used miRWalk database [17, 18] to screen for miRNA-target oxidative stress related genes. Four down-regulated miRNAs (has-miR-1207-5p, has-miR-124-3p, has-miR-204-3p, has-miR-204-5p) were found to target 3′ UTR of pro-oxidative genes whilst two up-regulated miRNAs (has-miR-222-3p, has-miR-378a-3p) were found to target 3′ UTR of anti-oxidative genes (Tables 1 and 2). To further investigate the part played by these miRNAs, we retrieved the promoter sequences of oxidative stress related genes and predicted the binding between the aforementioned miRNAs and the TATA-box regions of promoters. We found three out of four down-regulated miRNAs could specifically bind to the TATA-box regions of anti-oxidative genes, whilst the two up-regulated miRNAs could target the TATA-box regions of pro-oxidative genes (Table 1). For instance, miR-204-5p could specifically bind to the 3′ UTR of *TXNIP*, which is a regulator of the bioavailability of thioredoxin in the lens, and may promote oxidative stress-induced apoptosis [7]. MiR-204-5p could also bind to the TATA-box region of *ALDH1A3*, which is a member of gene family protecting the eye against cataract formation via detoxification function [8]. Since miR-204-5p was down-regulated in cataractous lenses, it is hypothesized miR-204-5p up-regulates *TXNIP* expression through the reduction of post-transcriptional gene silencing, while down-regulates *ALDH1A3* expression via reduced promoter activation-mediated transcription (Fig. 5a). On the other hand, miR-378a-3p could bind to the 3′ UTR of *SOD1*, a gene preventing hydrogen peroxide -induced oxidative damage to the lens [6]. MiR-378a-3p could also

specifically bind to the TATA-box region of *TXNIP*, a pro-oxidative gene [7]. Because miR-378a-3p was up-regulated in cataractous lenses, we propose that miR-378a-3p down-regulates *SOD1* expression via post-transcriptional gene silencing and up-regulates *TXNIP* expression through promoter activation-mediated transcription (Fig. 5b). Our results suggest up-regulated miRNAs down-regulate anti-oxidative genes via 3′ UTR binding, meanwhile up-regulate pro-oxidative genes via TATA-box binding-mediated transcription activation, and it is the opposite for down-regulated miRNAs. This results in the elevation of pro-oxidative genes and inhibition of anti-oxidative genes, which may lead to cataract (Fig. 6).

Discussion

Age-related cataract is believed to be the result of post-translational modification, the accumulation of fluorescent chromophores, increasing susceptibility to oxidation, etc. [2]. Oxidative stress plays an important role in nuclear cataract formation, therefore in this study we exploited genome microarray to determine the genes regulated in cataractous lenses, especially genes related with oxidative stress. Pro-oxidative genes were nearly half up-regulated (11/20), with a small number of genes down-regulated (4/20) and the rest of them with no significant change (5/20). Interestingly, anti-oxidative genes were partly up-regulated (17/69) and partly down-regulated (17/69). The possible explanation of this discrepancy is oxidative stress is not the only cause of nuclear cataract and other mechanism might contribute to this disease as well. Furthermore, there may be a compensation mechanism towards oxidative damage, and the up-regulation of some anti-oxidative genes and the down-regulation of some pro-oxidative genes may act as a response to

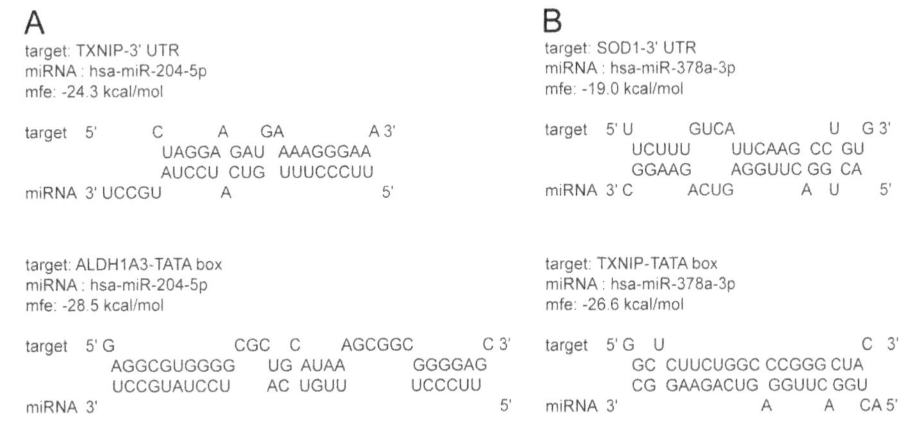

Fig. 5 Predicted binding between cataract-regulated miRNAs and the TATA-box region/3′ UTR of oxidative stress related genes. Online resource miRWalk [17, 18] and RNAhybrid [19] was used to predict binding between miR-204-5p/miR-378a-3p and the 3′ UTR of target mRNA *TXNIP/SOD1* (**a** and **b**, *upper part*). The Eukaryotic Promoter Database [15, 16] and RNAhybrid [19] were used to predict binding between miR-204-5p/miR-378a-3p and the TATA-box region of target mRNA *ALDH1A3/TXNIP* promoters (**a** and **b**, *lower part*). mfe: minimum free energy

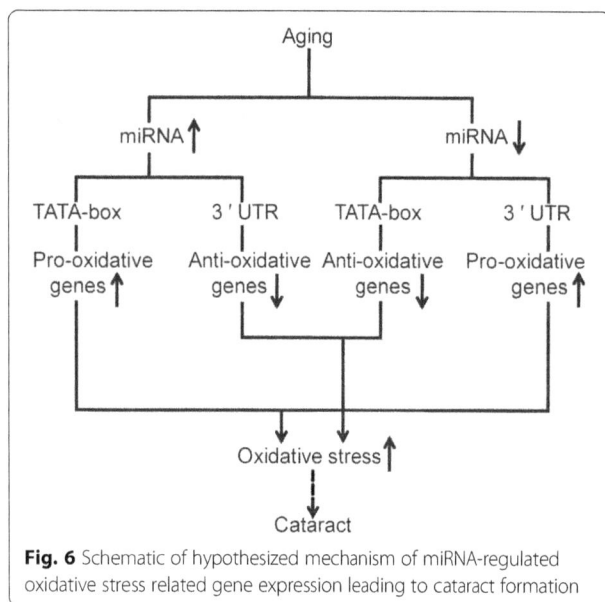

Fig. 6 Schematic of hypothesized mechanism of miRNA-regulated oxidative stress related gene expression leading to cataract formation

oxidative stress. Finally, there are limitations in our study such as the limited number of genes selected related to oxidative stress, lack of experimental validations, etc.

MiRNAs have been linked to cataract pathogenesis in studies from us and others as well [9, 20–25]. It would be worth exploring the relationship between these miRNAs and oxidative stress related genes. The classic pathway of miRNA regulated gene expression is via 3′ UTR binding-mediated post-transcription gene silencing. Our previous work indicated miRNAs could also bind to the TATA-box region and act as a gene transcription activator [10, 11]. Therefore, we took advantage of bioinformatics web tools and online resources to screen for targets of cataract regulated miRNAs. In this study, we found cataract regulated miRNAs could contribute to cataract formation not only by targeting 3′ UTR, but also by binding to the TATA-box region of oxidative stress related genes. This resulted in the subsequent elevation of pro-oxidative genes and inhibition of anti-oxidative genes. The elevated level of oxidative stress may lead to cataract formation.

Conclusions

In conclusion, we propose a hypothesis that this miRNA-TATA-box/3′ UTR-gene-regulation network may contribute to cataract pathogenesis. Our next step would be to validate these aforementioned miRNAs and mRNAs, to certify the target relationship between these miRNAs and their corresponding mRNAs, and to elucidate the specific mechanism of miRNA-TATA-box/3′ UTR-gene-regulation network during cataract formation.

Additional file

> **Additional file 1: Table S1.** Degrees of Lenticular Opacification Determined by Lens Opacities Classification System III (LOCSIII). **Table S2.** Top 8 Populated Gene Ontology Terms of the Biological Process Category. **Table S3.** Selected Oxidative Stress Related Genes (DOCX 23 kb)

Abbreviations
cRNA: Biotin-tagged complementary RNA; EPD: The Eukaryotic Promoter Database; FDR: False discovery rate; GO: Gene ontology; LOCSIII: Lens Opacities Classification System III; MAS 3.0: Molecular Annotation System; miRNAs: MicroRNAs; SAM: Significant Analysis of Microarray software

Acknowledgements
Not applicable.

Funding
The founding sponsors had no role in the design of the study; in the collection, analyses, or interpretation of data; in the writing of the manuscript, or in the decision to publish the results. This study was supported by the Fundamental Research Funds for the Basic Research Operating Expenses Program of Central College sponsored by Xi'an Jiaotong University (xjj2013067), Youth Foundation of the First Affiliated Hospital, Medical College, Xi'an Jiaotong University (2014YK7) and the National Natural Science Foundation of China (No. 81602698, No. 81470614).

Authors' contributions
YY and CW conceived and designed the experiments; CW performed the experiments; CW and YY analyzed the data; ZL, LM, CP, LQ, NG and JL performed capsulorrhexis during cataract surgery and provided clinical samples for this study; CW and YY wrote the paper. All authors read and approved the final manuscript.

Authors' information
Not applicable.

Consent for publication
Not applicable.

Competing interests
The authors declare they have no competing interests.

Author details
[1]Department of Ophthalmology, the First Affiliated Hospital of Medical School of Xi'an Jiaotong University, Xi'an, Shaanxi Province 710061, China. [2]School of Public Health, Xi'an Jiaotong University Health Science Center, Xi'an, Shaanxi Province 710061, China. [3]Basic Research Center, Affiliated Shaanxi Provincial Tumor Hospital, School of Medicine, Xi'an Jiaotong University, Xi'an, Shaanxi Province 710061, China.

References

1. Vrensen GF. Early cortical lens opacities: a short overview. Acta Ophthalmol. 2009;87(6):602–10.
2. Michael R, Bron AJ. The ageing lens and cataract: a model of normal and pathological ageing. Philos Trans R Soc Lond Ser B Biol Sci. 2011;366(1568): 1278–92.
3. Beebe DC, Holekamp NM, Shui YB. Oxidative damage and the prevention of age-related cataracts. Ophthalmic Res. 2010;44(3):155–65.
4. Ruotolo R, Grassi F, Percudani R, Rivetti C, Martorana D, Maraini G, Ottonello S. Gene expression profiling in human age-related nuclear cataract. Mol Vis. 2003;9:538–48.
5. Zhao W, Zhao J, Wang D, Li J. Screening of potential target genes for cataract by analyzing mRNA expression profile of mouse Hsf4-null lens. BMC Ophthalmol. 2015;15:76.
6. Lin D, Barnett M, Grauer L, Robben J, Jewell A, Takemoto L, Takemoto DJ. Expression of superoxide dismutase in whole lens prevents cataract formation. Mol Vis. 2005;11:853–8.
7. Liyanage NP, Fernando MR, Lou MF. Regulation of the bioavailability of thioredoxin in the lens by a specific thioredoxin-binding protein (TBP-2). Exp Eye Res. 2007;85(2):270–9.
8. Lassen N, Bateman JB, Estey T, Kuszak JR, Nees DW, Piatigorsky J, Duester G, Day BJ, Huang J, Hines LM, et al. Multiple and additive functions of ALDH3A1 and ALDH1A1: cataract phenotype and ocular oxidative damage in Aldh3a1(–/–)/Aldh1a1(–/–) knock-out mice. J Biol Chem. 2007;282(35): 25668–76.
9. Wu C, Lin H, Wang Q, Chen W, Luo H, Zhang H. Discrepant expression of microRNAs in transparent and cataractous human lenses. Invest Ophthalmol Vis Sci. 2012;53(7):3906–12.
10. Zhang Y, Yin Y, Zhang S, Luo H, Zhang H. HIV-1 infection-induced suppression of the let-7i/IL-2 Axis contributes to CD4(+) T cell death. Sci Rep. 2016;6:25341.
11. Zhang Y, Fan M, Zhang X, Huang F, Wu K, Zhang J, Liu J, Huang Z, Luo H, Tao L, et al. Cellular microRNAs up-regulate transcription via interaction with promoter TATA-box motifs. RNA. 2014;20(12):1878–89.
12. Chylack LT Jr, Wolfe JK, Singer DM, Leske MC, Bullimore MA, Bailey IL, Friend J, McCarthy D, Wu SY. The lens opacities classification system III. The longitudinal study of cataract study group. Arch Ophthalmol. 1993;111(6):831–6.
13. Grewal DS, Brar GS, Grewal SP. Correlation of nuclear cataract lens density using Scheimpflug images with lens opacities classification system III and visual function. Ophthalmology. 2009;116(8):1436–43.
14. Deng W, Wang Y, Liu Z, Cheng H, Xue Y. Heml: a toolkit for illustrating heatmaps. PLoS One. 2014;9(11):e111988.
15. Dreos R, Ambrosini G, Perier RC, Bucher P. The eukaryotic promoter database: expansion of EPDnew and new promoter analysis tools. Nucleic Acids Res. 2015;43(Database issue):D92–6.
16. Dreos R, Ambrosini G, Cavin Perier R, Bucher P. EPD and EPDnew, high-quality promoter resources in the next-generation sequencing era. Nucleic Acids Res. 2013;41(Database issue):D157–64.
17. Dweep H, Sticht C, Pandey P, Gretz N. miRWalk–database: prediction of possible miRNA binding sites by "walking" the genes of three genomes. J Biomed Inform. 2011;44(5):839–47.
18. Dweep H, Gretz N. miRWalk2.0: a comprehensive atlas of microRNA-target interactions. Nat Methods. 2015;12(8):697.
19. Rehmsmeier M, Steffen P, Hochsmann M, Giegerich R. Fast and effective prediction of microRNA/target duplexes. RNA. 2004;10(10):1507–17.
20. Qin Y, Zhao J, Min X, Wang M, Luo W, Wu D, Yan Q, Li J, Wu X, Zhang J. MicroRNA-125b inhibits lens epithelial cell apoptosis by targeting p53 in age-related cataract. Biochim Biophys Acta. 2014;1842(12 Pt A):2439–47.
21. Dong Y, Zheng Y, Xiao J, Zhu C, Zhao M. MicroRNA let-7b induces lens epithelial cell apoptosis by targeting leucine-rich repeat containing G protein-coupled receptor 4 (Lgr4) in age-related cataract. Exp Eye Res. 2016;147:98–104.
22. Li Y, Liu S, Zhang F, Jiang P, Wu X, Liang Y. Expression of the microRNAs hsa-miR-15a and hsa-miR-16-1 in lens epithelial cells of patients with age-related cataract. Int J Clin Exp Med. 2015;8(2):2405–10.
23. Dong N, Tang X, Xu B. miRNA-181a inhibits the proliferation, migration, and epithelial-mesenchymal transition of lens epithelial cells. Invest Ophthalmol Vis Sci. 2015;56(2):993–1001.
24. Dong N, Xu B, Benya SR, Tang X. MiRNA-26b inhibits the proliferation, migration, and epithelial-mesenchymal transition of lens epithelial cells. Mol Cell Biochem. 2014;396(1–2):229–38.
25. Wang Y, Li W, Zang X, Chen N, Liu T, Tsonis PA, Huang Y. MicroRNA-204-5p regulates epithelial-to-mesenchymal transition during human posterior capsule opacification by targeting SMAD4. Invest Ophthalmol Vis Sci. 2013;54(1):323–32.

32

Congenital aniridia with cataract

Jin Da Wang[1], Jing Shang Zhang[1], Ying Xiong[2], Jing Li[2], Xiao Xia Li[1], Xue Liu[1], Jing Zhao[1], Frank F. Tsai[3], Jhanji Vishal[4], Qi Sheng You[1], Yao Huang[2] and Xiu Hua Wan[1*]

Abstract

Background: This study evaluates patients with congenital aniridia and cataract who underwent phacoemulsification, capsular tension ring placement, and foldable intraocular lens implantation.

Methods: In this prospective case series, 10 patients (17 eyes) underwent cataract surgery via a 3.2 mm clear corneal incision. A continuous circular capsulorhexis with <6 mm diameter was employed. A capsular tension ring and HOYA yellow foldable posterior chamber intraocular lens was implanted. All patients wore color contact lenses postoperatively. Paired t test was used to compare visual acuity, intraocular pressure, and corneal endothelial changes before and after surgery.

Results: A single surgeon performed all surgeries. The best-corrected visual acuity improved from value 1.03 ± 0.27LogMAR preoperatively to value 0.78 ± 0.26LogMAR postoperatively ($p = 0.000$). The photophobic symptoms improved significantly after surgery. The mean corneal endothelial cell density before and after surgery was 3280 ± 473 cells/mm2 and 2669 ± 850 cells/mm2, respectively ($p = 0.006$). None of the patients developed corneal endothelial decompensation or secondary glaucoma after surgery.

Conclusions: Treatment of congenital aniridia and coexistent cataract by phacoemulsification, posterior chamber foldable lens implantation, capsular tension ring placement was safe and effective. Use of colored contact lenses in the postoperative period can reduce photophobic symptoms in this group of patients.

Trial registration: ChiCTR-OOC-17011638 (retrospectively registered at 12,June,2017)

Keywords: Congenital aniridia, Cataract removal surgery, Color artificial lens, Capsular tension ring

Background

Congenital aniridia is a rare genetic eye disease due to PAX6 mutation. It is associated with neuroectodermal and mesodermal dysplasia [1, 2]. Congenital aniridia is often associated with cataract that may require surgery [1–5]. These cataracts are characterized by an early age of onset, higher risk of complications, and limited post-operative visual improvement [6–10].

Implantation of prosthetic iris devices during cataract surgery has been described to alleviate the photophobia symptoms induced by aniridia, although serious complications such as secondary glaucoma and corneal endothelial decompensation may occur after surgery [6, 11].

In this study we describe the surgical and visual outcomes of cataract surgery in cases with congenital aniridia using phacoemulsification, posterior chamber foldable lens implantation, and capsular tension ring (CTR) placement.

Methods

Subjects

The study complied with the tenets of the Declaration of Helsinki and was approved by the Ethics Board of the Beijing Tongren Hospital. Written, informed consent was obtained from all patients before surgery. A total of 10 patients (17 eyes) with congenital aniridia and cataract were operated between January 2011 and December 2014. Patients with serious keratopathy (effect the

* Correspondence: xiuhuawan@126.com; xiuhauwan@163.com
[1]Beijing Institute of Ophthalmology, Beijing Tongren Eye Center, Beijing Tongren Hospital of Capital Medical University, Beijing Key Laboratory of Ophthalmology and Visual Sciences, Beijing 100005, China
Full list of author information is available at the end of the article

patients' visual acuity), glaucoma or lens dislocation were excluded.

Examinations

All patients underwent preoperative slit lamp examination of the anterior segment and intraocular pressure (IOP) measurement. Fundus photography and macular optical coherence tomography (OCT) were performed. Optometry examination was performed to determine the refraction and best-corrected visual acuity (BCVA). Corneal endothelium cell density was measured using endothelial microscopy. The corneal curvature was measured with computerized keratometry and axial length was measured with A scan ultrasound. The SRK-T formula was used to calculate intraocular lens (IOL) power. Postoperative follow-up was performed at 1 week, then at 1, 3, 6, 12, and 24 months.

Surgery

A single surgeon (WX) performed standard phacoemulsification and IOL implantation in all cases. All patients received tropicamide eye drops 1 h before the surgery. Topical anesthesia was applied 3 times within the conjunctival fornix 5–10 min before surgery. A 3.2-mm clear corneal wound was created with a keratome. Continuous circular capsulorhexis (CCC) was performed making sure that the largest diameter of the CCC was less than 6 mm. After phacoemulsification and irrigation-aspiration of the residual cortical matter, a capsular tension ring was implanted in the capsular bag through the 3.2 mm incision. Subsequently, a blue light absorptive yellow HOYA (manufacturer details needed, Japan) posterior chamber foldable IOL was implanted in the capsular bag. Postoperative treatment was started in the form of antibiotic eye drops (levofloxacin) and corticosteroid eye drops (prednisolone acetate) for 6 weeks. Patients were instructed to wear colored contact lenses 6–8 weeks after the surgery.

Statistical analysisStatistical analysis was performed using SPSS for Windows (version 22.0; IBM-SPSS, Chicago, IL, USA). Paired t-test was used to compare preoperative and postoperative BCVA, IOP, and corneal endothelial cell density. P-values represent results for 2-sided tests, with values less than 0.05 considered statistically significant.

Results

A total of 17 eyes of 10 patients (6 males and 4 females) with congenital aniridia and cataract were included in this study (Tables 1 and 2). The mean age of the patients was 25.4 ± 14.77 years (range: 4 to 50 years). The mean preoperative LogMAR BCVA was 1.03 ± 0.27 (range: from 0.7 to 1.3) and the mean IOP was 16.35 ± 3.9 mmHg (range: 8-24 mmHg). The mean corneal endothelial cell

Table 1 Demographic and clinical information

Characteristics	Results
Gender	
Male	6
Female	4
Age at surgery	
Range	4 to 50 years
Mean	25.4 ± 14.77 years
Family history	
Yes	8 patients
No	2 patients
Laterality	
Bilateral	17 eyes
Unilateral	0
Extent of aniridia	
Total eyes	16 eyes
Partial eyes	1 eyes
Follow-up period after surgery	
1 month	1 eye
6 months	9 eyes
18 months	6 eyes
Lost	1 eye

density was 3280 ± 473 cells/mm^2 (range: 1825 ~ 3829 cells/mm^2) and mean axial length was 22.83 ± 1.98 mm (range: 20.44~26.14 mm). Only 1 eye had a portion of iris present, while all of the other cases only had an iris root. All patients' lenses were fully exposed with visible lens zonules at the time of the surgery (Fig. 1). All patients suffered from severe photophobia symptoms and varying degrees of nystagmus. Although most fundus photos appeared fairly normal, OCT images showed an absent or abnormal foveal morphology.

All surgeries were performed successfully completed without any intraoperative complications. The power of implanted IOL ranged between 19.5 and 30.00D with an average of 24.44 ± 4.30 D.

All patients followed up for a mean period of 10.2 ± 6.4 months postoperatively. One patient (1 eye) was lost to follow-up. One eye was followed up for 1 month after the surgery, 9 eyes were followed up for 6 months after the surgery, and 6 eyes were followed up for 18 months after the surgery. The mean postoperative LogMAR BCVA was 0.78 ± 0.26 (range: 0.5 to 1.3), (p = 0.000). The photphobic symptoms improved subjectively after surgery that was more obvious after wearing cosmetic contact lenses. All corneas remained clear at last follow up. There were no complications from wearing the colored contact lenses. The capsule bags of

Table 2 Clinical manifestations

Clinical features	Results
Lens opacity type	
Nuclear	5 eyes
Posterior capsule	4 eyes
Cortex	8 eyes
Cornea	
Mild surounding opacity	3 eyes
Normal	14 eyes
Foveal hypoplasia	17 eyes
Glaucoma	0
Nystagmus	17 eyes
IOP	
Range	8 to 24 mmHg
Mean	16.35 ± 3.9 mmHg
Central corneal thickness	
Range	530 to 688 um
Mean	612 ± 37 um
Endothelial cell count	
Range	1825 to 3829 cells/mm2
Mean	3280 ± 473 cells/mm^2
Axial length	
Range	20.44 to 26.14 mm
Mean	22.83 ± 1.98 mm
IOL diopter	
Range	19.5 to 30 D
Mean	24.44 ± 4.3 D

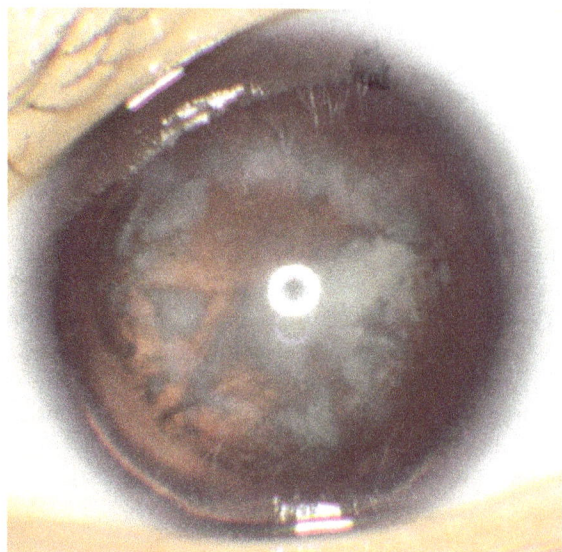

Fig. 1 The lens opacity of the congenital aniridia complicated with cataract patient before surgery

complications associated with cataract surgery in this group, careful preoperative planning should be done. Li et al. [13] performed cataract surgery in 12 patients (24 eyes) with congenital aniridia. Most patients had some improvement in visual acuity and quality.

In our study, no lens dislocation occurred. CTR implantation was performed to stabilize the zonules and prevent intraocular lens dislocation in the future. Postoperative visual acuity generally improved.

4 eyes appeared fibrosed 6 months after the surgery. YAG laser treatment was performed for posterior capsule opacification (PCO) in 2 adult patients (4 eyes) 6 months after surgery (Fig. 2). There were no cases of IOL dislocation due to zonular weakness. No secondary glaucoma was observed. The mean corneal endothelial cell density decreased from 3280 ± 473 cell/mm^2 *to* 2669 ± 850 cells/mm^2 ($p = 0.006$), but no case with secondary corneal endothelial decompensation was observed.

Discussion

The currently reported incidence of cataract in patients with congenital aniridia is approximately 50–85% [12]. Most researchers believe congenital aniridia complicated with cataract does not need to be treated when lens opacity and its effects on the visual acuity are mild. These patients can wear colored contact lens to relieve photophobia symptoms. However, the lens opacity may often progress and impact vision, which requires surgery. Due to the congenital structural anomalies and increased

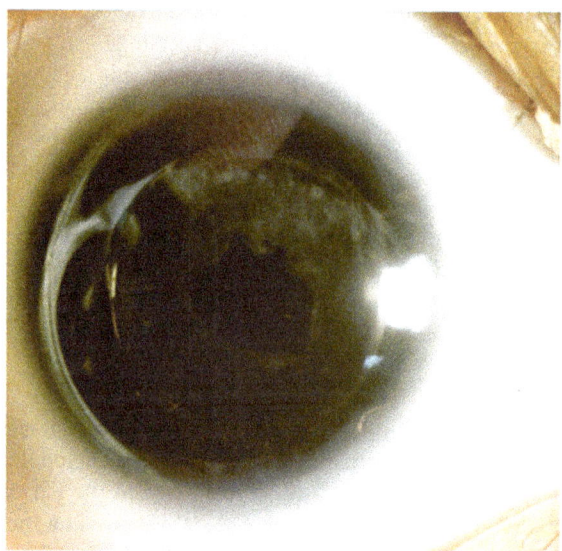

Fig. 2 The posterior capsule opacity were treated by YAG laser at 6 months after cataract surgery

In hopes of avoiding secondary glaucoma, corneal endothelial decompensation or other complications, as well as to alleviate the postoperative symptoms of photophobia, the CCC diameters in this group of patients were less than 6 mm. The anterior capsule may form an artificial pupil after fibrosis at 12 months after the PCO treated by YAG laser (Fig. 3). Moreover, the light absorbing yellow posterior chamber IOL may exert some light-shielding effects. Wearing cosmetic contact lenses postoperatively can also alleviate some of the photophobic symptoms. There were no instances of secondary glaucoma or corneal endothelial decompensation in our case series.

While iris prosthetic devices have been used to reduce the postoperative photophobic symptoms in patients with congenital aniridia and cataract, it was found to be associated with postoperative secondary glaucoma and corneal endothelial decompensation after long-term follow-up [6, 11, 14–17]. Reinhard et al. [11] reported outcomes of black diaphragm IOL implantation in 19 eyes with congenital aniridia. Deterioration in glaucoma occurred postoperatively in 4 out of 5 eyes with preoperative glaucoma whereas 4 out of 14 eyes without preoperative glaucoma developed postoperative chronic glaucoma. It was postulated that although glaucoma is a common endogenous complication of congenital aniridia [18], the blood–aqueous barrier (BAB) may be altered by the black diaphragm aniridia IOL thereby accelerating glaucoma progression.

There are some surgical tips for cataract surgery in patients with congenital aniridia. Firstly, the CCC must be treated with considerable care. Histological studies have demonstrated that the anterior capsules of patients with congenital aniridia are thin and fragile with degenerative changes in the epithelial cells [19, 20], which may predispose to the occurrence of capsular tears. It has been reported that the use of CTR can significantly reduce the probability of postoperative lens dislocation, PCO and anterior capsule fibrosis [21]. Moreover, patients with congenital aniridia are usually young, so the incidence of PCO is very high. However, many of these patients may have nystagmus that poses difficulty during YAG laser treatment. One possible option is to perform posterior CCC with anterior vitrectomy at the time of cataract surgery in these eyes.

In summary, the visual acuity and quality of vision in patients with congenital aniridia complicated with cataract can be improved through a carefully planned surgery. An appropriate individualized surgical method should be selected to minimize complications and give the best chance of postoperative success. Treatment of congenital aniridia and cataract with phacoemulsification, posterior chamber lens implantation, capsular tension ring placement, and post-operative colored contact lenses can improve the visual acuity and significantly reduce photophobic symptoms.

Conclusions

Treatment of congenital aniridia and cataract with phacoemulsification, posterior chamber lens implantation, capsular tension ring placement, and post-operative colored contact lenses are effective for some patirents.

Abbreviations

BAB: The blood–aqueous barrier; BCVA: Best-corrected visual acuity; CCC: Continuous circular capsulorhexis; CTR: Capsular tension ring; IOL: Intraocular len; IOP: Intraocular pressure; OCT: Optical coherence tomography; PCO: Posterior capsule opacification

Acknowledgements

We thank Prof JB Jonas and Prof PANG Chi Pui for giving help in the writing of the manuscript.

Funding

This work was financially supported by Beijing new star of science and technology (H020821380190, Z131102000413025), Fund of work committee for women and children of China State department (No.2014108), The national natural science fund projects of China (No.30471861).

Authors' contributions

WXH and WJD, design, conduction of the study, collection and analysis of clinical data, preparation, review and approval of this manuscript. LX and ZJ, conduction of the study, collection and analysis of clinical data, preparation, review and approval of this manuscript. XY and LJ, conduction of the study, review and approval of this manuscript. ZJS and LXX, clinical data collection and analysis, review and approval of this manuscript. YQS and HY design of the study, review and approval of this manuscript. FFT and JV, clinical data analysis, review and approval of this manuscript. All authors read and approved the final manuscript.

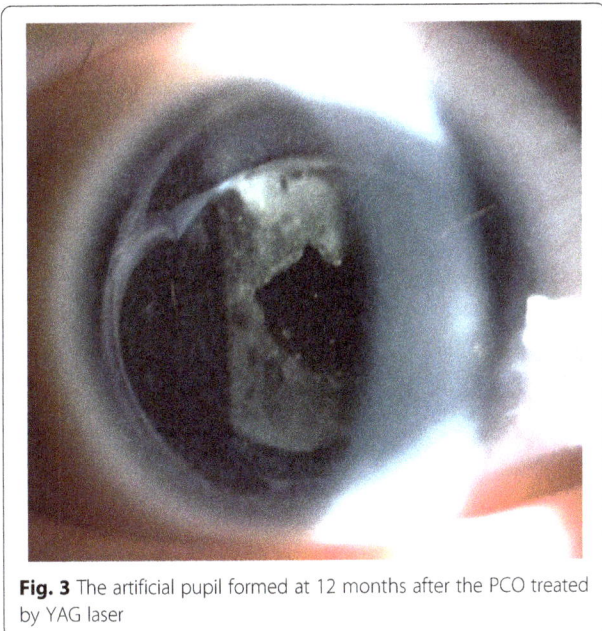

Fig. 3 The artificial pupil formed at 12 months after the PCO treated by YAG laser

Consent for publication

All patients voluntarily participate in this study and agreed to publish the personal data under the premise to protect the privacy. Written, informed consent was obtained from all patients before study.

Competing interests

No authors have a financial and proprietary interest in any material and method mentioned. The authors declare that they have no competing interests.

Author details

[1]Beijing Institute of Ophthalmology, Beijing Tongren Eye Center, Beijing Tongren Hospital of Capital Medical University, Beijing Key Laboratory of Ophthalmology and Visual Sciences, Beijing 100005, China. [2]Beijing Tongren Eye Center, Beijing Tongren Hospital of Capital Medical University, Beijing Key Laboratory of Ophthalmology and Visual Sciences, Beijing 100005, China. [3]Jacobs Retina Center, Shiley Eye Institute, and Department of Ophthalmology, University of California, La Jolla, San Diego, California, USA. [4]Department of Ophthalmology and Visual Sciences, the Chinese University of Hong Kong, Hong Kong, China.

References

1. Lee H, Khan R, O'Keefe M. Aniridia: current pathology and management. Acta Ophthalmol. 2008;86(7):708–15.
2. Singh B, Mohamed A, Chaurasia S, et al. Clinical manifestations of congenital aniridia. J Pediatr Ophthalmol Strabismus. 2014;51(1):59–62.
3. Netland PA, Scott ML, Boyle JW, Lauderdale JD. Ocular and systemic findings in a survey of aniridia subjects. J AAPOS. 2011;15(6):562–6.
4. Park SH, Park YG, Lee MY, Kim MS. Clinical features of Korean patients with congenital aniridia. Korean J Ophthalmol. 2010;24(5):291–6.
5. Edén U, Beijar C, Riise R, Tornqvist K. Aniridia among children and teenagers in Sweden and Norway. Acta Ophthalmol. 2008;86(7):730–4.
6. Neuhann IM, Neuhann TF. Cataract surgery and aniridia. Curr Opin Ophthalmol. 2010;21(1):60–4.
7. Edén U, Lagali N, Dellby A, et al. Cataract development in Norwegian patients with congenital aniridia. Acta Ophthalmol. 2014;92(2):e165–7.
8. Shiple D, Finklea B, Lauderdale JD, Netland PA. Keratopathy, cataract, and dry eye in a survey of aniridia subjects. Clin Ophthalmol. 2015;9:291–5.
9. Lee H, Meyers K, Lanigan B, O'Keefe M. Complications and visual prognosis in children with aniridia. J Pediatr Ophthalmol Strabismus. 2010;47(4):205–10. quiz 211-2
10. Tornqvist K. Aniridia: sight-threatening and hard to cure. Acta Ophthalmol. 2008;86(7):704–5.
11. Reinhard T, Engelhardt S, Sundmacher R. Black diaphragm aniridia intraocular lens for congenital aniridia: long-term follow-up. J Cataract Refract Surg. 2000;26(3):375–81.
12. Nelson LB, Spaeth GL, Nowinski TS, Margo CE, Jackson L. Aniridia. A review. Surv Ophthalmol. 1984;28(6):621–42.
13. Li H, Li JJ, Hu ZL, Wei CL. Treatment of congenital cataract accompanied by iridocoboma. Chinese Journal of Strabismus and Pediatric Ophthalmology. 2011;19(2):58–60.
14. Chang JW, Kim JH, Kim SJ, Yu YS. Congenital aniridia: long-term clinical course, visual outcome, and prognostic factors. Korean J Ophthalmol. 2014;28(6):479–85.
15. Gramer E, Reiter C, Gramer G. Glaucoma and frequency of ocular and general diseases in 30 patients with aniridia: a clinical study. Eur J Ophthalmol. 2012;22(1):104–10.
16. Sundmacher T, Reinhard T, Althaus C. Black diaphragm intraocular lens in congenital aniridia. Ger J Ophthalmol. 1994;3(4–5):197–201.
17. Sundmacher R, Reinhard T, Althaus C. Black-diaphragm intraocular lens for correction of aniridia. Ophthalmic Surg. 1994;25(3):180–5.
18. Brémond-Gignac D. Glaucoma in aniridia. J Fr Ophtalmol. 2007;30(2):196–9.
19. Hou ZQ, Hao YS, Wang W, Ma ZZ, Zhong YF, Song SJ. Clinical pathological study of the anterior lens capsule abnormalities in familial congenital aniridia with cataract. Beijing Da Xue Xue Bao. 2005;37(5):494–7.
20. Schneider S, Osher RH, Burk SE, Lutz TB, Montione R. Thinning of the anterior capsule associated with congenital aniridia. J Cataract Refract Surg. 2003;29(3):523–5.
21. Kim HJ, Yoon SH. The long-term effect of in the bag implantation of capsular tension ring on posterior capsular opacification in cataract surgery. ARVO 2015. 2015. Annual Meeting Abstracts, Program Number: 669.

Permissions

All chapters in this book were first published in OPHTHALMOLOGY, by BioMed Central; hereby published with permission under the Creative Commons Attribution License or equivalent. Every chapter published in this book has been scrutinized by our experts. Their significance has been extensively debated. The topics covered herein carry significant findings which will fuel the growth of the discipline. They may even be implemented as practical applications or may be referred to as a beginning point for another development.

The contributors of this book come from diverse backgrounds, making this book a truly international effort. This book will bring forth new frontiers with its revolutionizing research information and detailed analysis of the nascent developments around the world.

We would like to thank all the contributing authors for lending their expertise to make the book truly unique. They have played a crucial role in the development of this book. Without their invaluable contributions this book wouldn't have been possible. They have made vital efforts to compile up to date information on the varied aspects of this subject to make this book a valuable addition to the collection of many professionals and students.

This book was conceptualized with the vision of imparting up-to-date information and advanced data in this field. To ensure the same, a matchless editorial board was set up. Every individual on the board went through rigorous rounds of assessment to prove their worth. After which they invested a large part of their time researching and compiling the most relevant data for our readers.

The editorial board has been involved in producing this book since its inception. They have spent rigorous hours researching and exploring the diverse topics which have resulted in the successful publishing of this book. They have passed on their knowledge of decades through this book. To expedite this challenging task, the publisher supported the team at every step. A small team of assistant editors was also appointed to further simplify the editing procedure and attain best results for the readers.

Apart from the editorial board, the designing team has also invested a significant amount of their time in understanding the subject and creating the most relevant covers. They scrutinized every image to scout for the most suitable representation of the subject and create an appropriate cover for the book.

The publishing team has been an ardent support to the editorial, designing and production team. Their endless efforts to recruit the best for this project, has resulted in the accomplishment of this book. They are a veteran in the field of academics and their pool of knowledge is as vast as their experience in printing. Their expertise and guidance has proved useful at every step. Their uncompromising quality standards have made this book an exceptional effort. Their encouragement from time to time has been an inspiration for everyone.

The publisher and the editorial board hope that this book will prove to be a valuable piece of knowledge for researchers, students, practitioners and scholars across the globe.

List of Contributors

Kazuki Matsuura and Yuki Terasaka
Nojima Hospital, 2714-1, Sesaki-machi, Kurayoshi-city, Tottori 682-0863, Japan

Shiro Hatta
Maejima ganka, 226, Motomachi, Tottori-city, Tottori 680-0037, Japan

Yoshitsugu Inoue
Tottori University, 36-1, Nishi-cho, Yonago-city, Tottori 683-504, Japan

Young Choi, Youngsub Eom, Jong Suk Song and Hyo Myung Kim
Department of Ophthalmology, Korea University College of Medicine, Seoul, South Korea

Youngsub Eom
Department of Ophthalmology, Ansan Hospital, Korea University College of Medicine, 123, Jeokgeum-ro, Danwon-gu, Ansan-si, Gyeonggi-do 15355, South Korea

Ryosuke Ochi, Bumpei Sato, Seita Morishita and Yukihiro Imagawa
Department of Ophthalmology, Osaka Kaisei Hospital, Osaka-City, Osaka, Japan

Ryosuke Ochi, Bumpei Sato, Seita Morishita, Yukihiro Imagawa, Masashi Mimura, Masanori Fukumoto, Takaki Sato, Takatoshi Kobayashi, Teruyo Kida and Tsunehiko Ikeda
Department of Ophthalmology, Osaka Medical College, 2-7 Daigaku-machi, Takatsuki City, Osaka 569-8686, Japan

Chia-Yi Lee, Shih-Chun Chao and Hung-Yu Lin
Department of Ophthalmology, Show Chwan Memorial Hospital, No.2, Ln. 530, Sec. 1, Zhongshan Rd., Changhua City, Changhua 50093, Taiwan

Shih-Chun Chao
Department of Electrical and Computer Engineering, National Chiao Tung University, Hsinchu, Taiwan
Department of Optometry, Central Taiwan University of Science and Technology, Taichung, Taiwan

Chi-Chin Sun
Department of Medicine, Chang Gung University, College of Medicine, Taoyuan, Taiwan
Department of Ophthalmology, Chang Gung Memorial Hospital, Keelung, Taiwan
Department of Chinese Medicine, Chang Gung University, College of Medicine, Taoyuan, Taiwan

Hung-Yu Lin
Institute of Medicine, Chung Shan Medical University, Taichung, Taiwan
Department of Optometry, Chung Shan Medical University, Taichung, Taiwan
Department of Optometry, Yuanpei University of Medical Technology, Hsinchu, Taiwan

Chi-Chin Sun
222, Mai-Chin Road, Keelung, Taiwan

Konstantinos Andreanos, Petros Petrou, George Kymionis, Dimitrios Papaconstantinou and Ilias Georgalas
First Division of Ophthalmology, School of Medicine, National and Kapodistrian University of Athens, "G. Gennimatas" General Hospital of Athens, Athens, Greece

Konstantinos Andreanos
22str Digeni E.O.K.A, Nea Penteli, 15236 Athens, Greece

Tetsuhiro Kawata
Department Ophthalmology, Okayama University Medical School and Graduate School of Medicine, Dentistry, and Pharmaceutical Sciences, 2-5-1 Shikata-cho, Okayama City 700-8558, Japan

Tetsuhiro Kawata and Toshihiko Matsuo
Department of Ophthalmology, Fukuyama City Hospital, Fukuyama City, Japan

Kanmin Xue, Jasleen K. Jolly, Sonia P. Mall, Shreya Haldar, Paul H. Rosen and Robert E. MacLaren
Oxford Eye Hospital, Oxford Universities Hospitals NHS Foundation Trust, Oxford, UK

Kanmin Xue, Jasleen K. Jolly and Robert E. MacLaren
Nuffield Laboratory of Ophthalmology, Nuffield Department of Clinical Neurosciences, University of Oxford, Level 6 West Wing, John Radcliffe Hospital, Headley Way, Oxford OX3 9DU, UK

Hoon Dong Kim
Department of Ophthalmology, College of Medicine, Soonchunhyang University, Cheonan, Korea

Jae Min Kim and Jong Jin Jung
Myung-Gok Eye Research Institute, Department of Ophthalmology, Kim's Eye Hospital, Konyang University College of Medicine, 136, Yeongsin-ro, Yeongdeungpo-gu, Seoul 07301, Korea

Alfonso Vasquez-Perez, Andrew Simpson and Mayank A. Nanavaty
Sussex Eye Hospital, Brighton & Sussex University Hospitals NHS Trust, Eastern Road, Brighton BN2 5BF, UK

Mayank A. Nanavaty
Brighton & Sussex Medical School, University of Sussex, Falmer, Brighton BN1 9PX, UK

Danmin Cao and Yong Wang
Wuhan Aier Eye Hospital, Aier Eye Hospital Group, Wuhan, China

Danmin Cao, Shiming Wang and Yong Wang
Aierc School of Ophthalmology, Central South University, Changsha, China

Shiming Wang
Ningbo Aier Guangming Eye Hospital, Aier Eye Hospital Group, Ningbo, China

Yuko Hayashi, Shuko Fujita, Katsuo Tomoyose, Nobuyuki Ishikawa, Masahide Kokado, Takayoshi Sumioka, Yuka Okada and Shizuya Saika
Department of Ophthalmology, Wakayama Medical University, 811-1 Kimiidera, Wakayama 641-0012, Japan

Takeshi Miyamoto
Department of Ophthalmology, Wakayama Medical University Kihoku Hospital, 219 Myoji, Katsuragi-cho, Itogun, Wakayama 649-7113, Japan

Hong He, Xiaolian Chen, Hongshan Liu, Jiaochan Wu and Xingwu Zhong
Hainan Eye Hospital and Key Laboratory of Ophthalmology, Zhongshan Ophthalmic Center, Sun Yat-sen University, 19 Xiuhua Road, Haikou, China

Xingwu Zhong
Zhongshan Ophthalmic Center and State Key Laboratory of Ophthalmology, Sun Yat-sen University, Guangzhou, China

Peiqing Chen, Yanan Zhu and Ke Yao
Eye Center of the 2nd Affiliated Hospital, School of Medicine, Zhejiang University, #88 Jiefang Road, Hangzhou, Zhejiang 310009, China

Seung Pil Bang and Jong Hwa Jun
Department of Ophthalmology, Keimyung University School of Medicine, #56, Dalseong-ro, Jung-gu, Daegu 700-712, Korea

Gabriel de Almeida Ferreira, Luisa Fioravanti Schaal, Marcela Dadamos Ferro, Antonio Carlos Lottelli Rodrigues, Rajiv Khandekar and Silvana Artioli Schellini
Universidade Estadual Paulista Julio de Mesquita Filho Faculdade de Medicina Campus de Botucatu Botucatu, Sao Paulo, Brazil

Ji-guo Yu, Jie Zhong, Zhong-ming Mei, Fang Zhao, Na Tao and Yi Xiang
Department of Ophthalmology, the Central Hospital of Wuhan, Tongji Medical College, Huazhong University of Science and Technology, No, 26 Shengli Street, Wuhan, Hubei Province 430014, China

Chan Min Yang, Dong Hui Lim, Sungsoon Hwang and Tae-Young Chung
Department of Ophthalmology, Samsung Medical Center, Sungkyunkwan University School of Medicine, #81 Irwon-ro, Gangnam-gu, Seoul 06351, South Korea

Dong Hui Lim
Department of Preventive Medicine, Catholic University School Yang et al. BMC Ophthalmology of Medicine, Seoul, South Korea

Joo Hyun
Department of Ophthalmology, Saevit Eye Hospital, Goyang, South Korea

Karin Allard and Madeleine Zetterberg
Department of Ophthalmology, Sahlgrenska University Hospital, Mölndal, Sweden

Madeleine Zetterberg
Department of Clinical Neuroscience/ Ophthalmology, Institute of Neuroscience and Physiology, The Sahlgrenska Academy at University of Gothenburg, SE-431 80 Gothenburg, Sweden

Yi-Ju and Hung-Chi Chen
Department of Ophthalmology, Chang Gung Memorial Hospital, Linkou, Taiwan

Chi-Chin Sun
Department of Ophthalmology, Chang Gung Memorial Hospital, 6F, Mai-Jing Road, An-Leh District, Keelung, Taiwan, Republic of China
Department of Chinese Medicine, College of Medicine, Chang Gung University, Taoyuan, Taiwan

Aiwu Fang, Peijuan Wang, Rui He and Jia Qu
Wenzhou Medical University Eye Hospital, Wenzhou 325027, China

Alastair Porteous and Laura Crawley
Western Eye Hospital, London, UK

Keith Davey
Calderdale and Huddersfield NHS Foundation Trust, Huddersfield, UK

Bernard Chang
Leeds Teaching Hospitals NHS Trust, Leeds, UK

Christine Purslow
Thea Pharmaceuticals, Keele, UK

Emilie Clay and Anne-Lise Vataire
Creativ-Ceutical, Paris, France

Sho Ishikawa and Naoko Kato
Department of Ophthalmology, Saitama Medical University, 38 Morohongo, Moroyama, Saitama 350-0495, Japan

Sho Ishikawa, Naoko Kato and Masaru Takeuchi
Department of Ophthalmology, National Defense Medical College, 3-2 Namiki, Tokorozawa, Saitama 359-8216, Japan

Wei Wang, Shuang Ni, Xi Li, Xiang Chen, Yanan Zhu and Wen Xu
Eye Center of the 2nd Affiliated Hospital, School of Medicine, Zhejiang University, No.88 Jiefang Road, Hangzhou, China

Yana Fu and Qi Dai
The Eye Hospital of Wenzhou Medical University, 270 Xueyuan West Road, Wenzhou City 325027, Zhejiang Province, People's Republic of China

Liwei Zhu and Shuangqing Wu
Department of Ophthalmology, Hangzhou Red Cross Hospital, Hangzhou City 310003, Zhejiang Province, People's Republic of China

Young-Sool Hah
Biomedical Research Institute, Gyeongsang National University Hospital, Jinju, South Korea

Hye Jin Chung and Sneha B. Sontakke
College of Pharmacy and Research institute of Pharmaceutical Sciences, Gyeongsang National University, Jinju, South Korea

In-Young Chung, Seong-Wook Seo, Ji-Myong Yoo and Seong-Jae Kim
Department of Ophthalmology, Gyeongsang National University Hospital, Gyeongsang National University School of Medicine, Jinju, South Korea
Gyeongsang Institute of Health Science, Gyeongsang National University, Jinju, South Korea

Sunmi Ju
Division of Pulmonology and Allergy, Department of Internal Medicine, Gyeongsang National University Hospital, Jinju, South Korea

Wojciech Rokicki, Dorota Pojda-Wilczek, Serap Ogultekin and Ewa Mrukwa-Kominek
Department and Clinic of Ophthalmology, School of Medicine in Katowice, Medical University of Silesia, Ceglana 35, 40-514 Katowice, Poland

Jolanta Zalejska-Fiolka and Alicja Hampel
Department of Biochemistry, School of Medicine with the Division of Dentistry in Zabrze, Medical University of Silesia, Katowice, Poland

Wojciech Majewski
Radiotherapy Department, Maria Sklodowska-Curie Memorial Cancer Center and Institute of Oncology, Gliwice Branch, Poland

Guan-hong Zhang and Xin-guo Jia
Department of Ophthalmology, Shengli Oilfield Central Hospital, Shandong Province, Dongying 257000, China

Xiang Zhang and Tian Tian
Department of Ophthalmology, Xin Hua Hospital Affiliate of Shanghai Jiao Tong University School of Medicine, Shanghai 200092, China

Jia-song Yang and Rui Zeng
Vitreous & Retinal Department, Apex Eye Hospital, Xincai 463500, Henan Province, China

Chun-li Chen
Department of Ophthalmology, Tianjin Medical University Eye Hospital, Tianjin 30000, China

Zhennan Zhao, Qi Fan, HongFei Ye, Lei Cai and Yi Lu
Department of Ophthalmology, Eye and ENT Hospital of Fudan University, 83 Fenyang Road, Shanghai 200031, People's Republic of China

Peng Zhou
Department of Ophthalmology, Parkway Health Hong Qiao Medical Center, Shanghai 200336, People's Republic of China

Ke-Ke Zhang, Wen-Wen He, Yi Lu and Xiang-Jia Zhu
Eye Institute, Eye and Ear, Nose, and Throat Hospital, Fudan University, Shanghai 200031, China
Department of Ophthalmology, Eye and Ear, Nose, and Throat Hospital, Fudan University, Shanghai 200031, China
Key Laboratory of Myopia, Ministry of Health PR China, Shanghai 200031, China
Shanghai Key Laboratory of Visual Impairment and Restoration, Fudan University, Shanghai 200031, China

Changrui Wu, Zhao Liu, Cheng Pei, Li Qin and Ning Gao
Department of Ophthalmology, the First Affiliated Hospital of Medical School of Xi'an Jiaotong University, Xi'an, Shaanxi Province 710061, China

Le Ma
School of Public Health, Xi'an Jiaotong University Health Science Center, Xi'an, Shaanxi Province 710061, China

Jun Li and Yue Yin
Basic Research Center, Affiliated Shaanxi Provincial Tumor Hospital, School of Medicine, Xi'an Jiaotong University, Xi'an, Shaanxi Province 710061, China

Jin Da Wang, Jing Shang Zhang, Xiao Xia Li, Xue Liu, Jing Zhao, Qi Sheng You and Xiu Hua Wan
Beijing Institute of Ophthalmology, Beijing Tongren Eye Center, Beijing Tongren Hospital of Capital Medical University, Beijing Key Laboratory of Ophthalmology and Visual Sciences, Beijing 100005, China

Ying Xiong, Jing Li and Yao Huang
Beijing Tongren Eye Center, Beijing Tongren Hospital of Capital Medical University, Beijing Key Laboratory of Ophthalmology and Visual Sciences, Beijing 100005, China

Frank F. Tsai
Jacobs Retina Center, Shiley Eye Institute, and Department of Ophthalmology, University of California, La Jolla, San Diego, California, USA

Jhanji Vishal
Department of Ophthalmology and Visual Sciences, the Chinese University of Hong Kong, Hong Kong, China

Index

www.ingramcontent.com/pod-product-compliance
Lightning Source LLC
Chambersburg PA
CBHW082017190326
41458CB00010B/3212